The Complete Guide to
Alzheimer's-Proofing Your Home

The Complete Guide to Alzheimer's-Proofing Your Home

Revised and Updated Edition

Mark L. Warner

PURDUE E, INDIANA

04 03 02   5 4 3 2

The paper used in this book meets the minimum requirements of American National
Standard for Information Sciences—Permanence of Paper for Printed Library Materials,
ANSI Z39.48-1992.

⊖ Printed in the United States of America

Interior design by inari

Cover design by Lisa Hasbargen

Ageless Design® is a registered trademark of Ageless Design, Inc.

Library of Congress Cataloging-in-Publication Data

Warner, Mark L., 1948–
     The complete guide to Alzheimer's proofing your home / Mark L. Warner.
        p.   cm.
     Includes bibliographical references and index.
     ISBN 1-55753-220-6 (cloth : alk. paper) —ISBN 1-55753-202-8 (pbk. : alk. paper)
     1. Alzheimer's disease—Patients—Home care. 2. Home accidents—Prevention.   I. Title.
  RC523.W36   2000
  362.1′96831—dc21   99-462016
                                                               CIP

Contents

Chapter 2: Thinking-Related Issues 83

In recognition of our modern-day heroes—the caregivers, special people who make daily sacrifices to take care of loved ones, or even strangers, and dedicate with unselfish devotion and kindness their lives, knowledge, and energies to making others more comfortable.

To our parents and grandparents, who taught us to care, to love, and to want to give back.

But most of all, to my dear wife, Ellen. Without her help, guidance, and support, this book could never have been possible.

Preface

The illnesses we associate with aging are many, and the treatments diverse. As a practicing architect and gerontologist, I have long been struck by the lack of information available on living alternatives for those with chronic illnesses associated with aging. A wealth of ready information exists on institutions such as nursing homes, assisted-living facilities, and hospices, which are appropriate when the requirements for care are too demanding. But until now, no one has stepped up to provide information about one of the best places for long-term health care: the home.

Many loving caregivers already provide compassionate and effective treatment for their spouses, elderly parents, and relatives in their homes, allowing their family members a quality of life and feeling of contentment that are themselves a form of therapy.

Others would like to care for their relatives at home, but feel it's not properly equipped and don't know how to prepare it. Most often they are burdened by homes that make care more difficult, and they lack the answers to key questions: How can I set up my home to provide an efficient, safe, and thoughtful living environment that is sensitive to the needs of my loved one? How can I satisfy my own needs for peace and privacy and well-being?

Most people with chronic diseases prefer to remain at home. Few prefer to seek out nursing homes, skilled care, or assisted-living facilities. So there is a vital need for frank discussion of the challenges involved in making homes accessible, safe, and comfortable for people with debilitating diseases like Alzheimer's, Parkinson's, and diabetes.

Homes That Care

With this book, we at Ageless Design, Inc., are introducing the Homes That Care® series to provide information necessary for modifying or building a home that addresses the needs of those enduring long-term illnesses and the needs of their caregivers. Many of the principles and some of the adaptations herein are well understood in institutional settings, where architectural gerontology has long been practiced. Few have been applied in the one setting most people prefer over an institution: their own homes.

A great deal of research has gone into this first book in the series. Alzheimer's is a particularly difficult disease to deal with because of its many phases and the hardships it imposes upon the person with AD and the caregiver. However, there are a great many things you can do or plan for to make life better for all concerned.

Many difficult problems can be solved by simple home modifications. Your doctor can prescribe medications, and a therapist can rehabilitate, but they lack the knowledge and training to help you address the role your home can play. This book shows you how to create a home that can help you cope with the many difficulties of Alzheimer's disease. It identifies useful products, old and new, and tells you where to get them. We sincerely hope that the suggestions, advice, and ideas presented here will make it safer and more possible for you to care for someone at home, to anticipate and avoid many problems, and to create a calm and less threatening environment. If your goal is to avoid a nursing home for your loved one, we hope this book will help you do so for as long as is reasonably possible.

"Ageless Design®"

Up until now, architects, interior designers, residential designers, builders, and other design professionals have had only two standards to guide them in designing for people with age-related or other disabilities: accessible design and universal design.

Accessible design, a major leap forward, demonstrates how buildings can be designed to help people with special needs, particularly those who are deaf or blind or have mobility impairments. Universal design goes one step further, showing how homes can address the needs of all generations, from the smallest child to the oldest adult.

While both of these concepts have been revolutionary, neither directly addresses the many age-related conditions, dysfunctions, and diseases that affect so many of us and our loved ones and that make it so hard to live independently in our own homes.

Ageless Design concepts recognize the specific burdens of such debilitating age-related conditions as Alzheimer's, Parkinson's disease, arthritis, stroke, visual and hearing impairments, heart condition, diabetes, and osteoporosis—and offers solutions that make it possible for people living with these conditions to remain at home much longer than was ever before possible.

To do this we have to take a hard look at how aging and age-related diseases really affect people and how caregivers care for them. Where should you put grab bars to help someone getting into a bathtub, sitting down, standing back up, and getting out? How long should a ramp be for an elderly woman pushing her husband in a wheelchair? How does an older person with a visual impairment really see? How can one's home help to minimize the injury that might occur from falls? How might a home contribute to hallucinations, paranoia, and the delusions associated with dementia, and what can be done to avoid this? These kinds of questions are critical in responding to the needs of older people, especially those with debilitating diseases. Only a hard look and resulting answers lead to the concepts created by Ageless Design®.

About This Book

This book is many things: a home guide, a reference, a catalog, and (I hope) a companion. But it is not a caregiving book for those dealing with Alzheimer's. There are many fine books available today for caregivers and medical professionals. In addition, organizations such as the Alzheimer's Association and your local Area Agency on Aging offer valuable information and support.

One part of this book provides room-by-room detail on how a home should be set up to facilitate care. You can judge the strengths and weaknesses of your own home against the information that appears in this part of the book and gain some understanding of what preparations you may need to make. This book also focuses upon behavioral and cognitive issues and specific kinds of impairment. Those coping with difficult problems, such as wandering or incontinence, can go directly to the appropriate section and find candid discussion of these subjects and specific suggestions for how the home can be adapted to help cope with them. Throughout the book we also refer to products available to help make changes in your home that can make a difference. Highlight the products and ideas you like, refer to the directory of products and manufacturers, and call for information or a catalog.

Please take the time to review the book in its entirety. Not all of the suggestions and techniques and products it presents will apply to your situation, but those that do can help you identify and address many difficulties. For those terms that you are not familiar with or would appreciate a little clarification, refer to the glossary in the back of the book.

If this book helps you understand the options available to you and provides you with a sense that what you are trying to do is not just worthwhile and good, but actually achievable in your home, then you will take away from it the most valuable thing of all: hope.

Acknowledgments

Our deepest heartfelt thanks go out to the experts on our review committee. These truly genuine artists, professionals, and masters added so much to the book that words cannot describe:

Benjamin Barnea, M.D.

Margaret Calkins, Ph.D.

Deborah Marks Carlson, MSN, RNC, CS

Geri Richards Hall, Ph.D.(c), ARNP, CNS

Brian Kirkland, D.O.

Susan Klein, BSW, MA

Sue Maxwell, MSW

Beverly Bigtree Murphy, MS, CRC

Beth Witrogen McLeod

Our special thanks go also to the following people and organizations for their help, support, and contributions to making this book possible: Tricia Andryszewski, Thomas Bacher, Mary M. Barnes, Michael Barry, Alan Beck, Barbara Cusano, Jack Green, Judy Heath, Margaret Hunt, Beth Lewis, Juliet Mason, Carl Myrus, Phyllis Perlick, Beth and Ben Schatman, Rose Schreiber, Adele Shapiro, Michele and Harris Sokoloff, Edward Steinfeld, Greg and Louise Warner, E. Leland Watkins, Battalion Chief Thomas Murphy and Palm Beach County Fire Rescue (Station 23, "C" Shift), the Syracuse University Gerontology Center, all of the manufacturers who donated photos, products, and information, and the many caregivers who so generously shared their stories with us.

The Complete Guide to Alzheimer's-Proofing Your Home is the result of years of research and talking with dedicated professionals in various fields. I would also like to recognize these wonderful people for their unselfish willingness to share their knowledge, wisdom, and unique insights into this disease. Many of the ideas in this book have been developed from knowledge gained by personal communications. My most grateful appreciation goes out to these people, who in so many ways have contributed to making this book possible:

> Elizabeth Brawley
> Margaret Calkins
> Geri Richards Hall
> Mitchell L. Hewson
> David Hoglund
> Diana McGowin
> Eunice Noell
> Richard Olsen

Introduction
About Alzheimer's
Disease

Take a good look at your own set of keys. Do you know what
lock each key opens? If you have forgotten what some of
those keys do, you're pretty normal. But if you were a victim
of Alzheimer's disease, you might see just a jangling mass of
metal and wonder what those odd shapes were.

Alzheimer's was "discovered" as a disease in 1907 by Dr.
Alois Alzheimer. Until recently, little was known about it or
about effective treatment. In the past decade, though, Alzheimer's has become the focus of much research. We are learning more about it every day.

Alzheimer's disease (AD) and memory loss are not a normal
part of aging, as once was suspected. It is a disease, one that
progressively affects the brain and limits its ability to transmit
and process information. Initially appearing as simple forgetfulness, it progresses to an inability to execute basic tasks and,
eventually, an inability to interpret and comprehend sensory
data. Ultimately, the body is no longer able to control its own
functions, and in time the person dies.

People with Alzheimer's slowly but surely forget what has
happened to them over the past 10, 20, or 30 years. Memory is
erased and recognition fails. Your loved one may no longer know
his own spouse, his home, or even his own room. A toaster may
become strange and unusable, a bathtub forbidding. Activities

we take for granted, like dressing or shaving, become difficult and require assistance.

To those of us who know someone with Alzheimer's disease, she or he seems to be living in a world where nothing makes sense and rules no longer apply. A person with Alzheimer's may get lost in a hallway, or be unable to find her kitchen or bathroom in the house she's lived in for 20 years. But that doesn't mean the environment is extraneous. Because the individual has such difficulty coping with her world, her home, her room, the characteristics of those spaces become crucial.

More than four million people in the United States now have Alzheimer's, and projections by the federal government indicate that some 20 to 35 million people in our aging population will have it by the year 2050. Because it afflicts the elderly, the disease also burdens the young, who are called on to provide increasingly demanding care for their parents and grandparents. Nonetheless, as new medical treatments are emerging to alleviate some of the suffering, care in the home is clearly an option that many caregivers and care receivers prefer.

Not long ago, I attended an Alzheimer's meeting that brought together experts and caregivers to share experiences. I was one of maybe a thousand attendees who were listening and seeking advice from a distinguished panel of experts. When the panel called for questions from the audience, I stepped to the microphone and asked, "How can I modify my home to help me care for a person with Alzheimer's disease?"

There was an uncomfortable silence as members of the panel looked at each other. Finally one of the panelists suggested, "One thing that you should do is remove the knobs from the stove."

That exchange was the incentive for this book. As an architect and gerontologist, I had been interested in the problems of home health care for several years. I knew very well there are many more things you can and should do when you are living with someone with Alzheimer's disease.

We must be realistic. Alzheimer's is a disease of the mind, not of the home. The environment is not a treatment, and it offers no cure. But many problems related to the disease can be lessened for the person with AD and especially for the caregiver by making changes in the home environment. The modifications, products, and services described in this book can go a long way to help you cope with the frustrations of this disease. The stories caregivers have shared with us, and the unexpected challenges they have faced, are the heart of this book. What has worked for them can work for you!

Two principles regarding this disease play important roles when considering the home environment. One is that the disease gradually destroys the neurological or informational paths in the brain. Though your loved one may know what she wants, the message just doesn't get to the right place. Thoughts may become like an airport with no air traffic control, flying around with nowhere to land or be understood. When the brain isn't able to complete the task with what it has, it makes substitutions, such as "Please pass me the *sugar*," when in fact it is the *spoon* that is being sought. In modifying the home, it is thus important to recognize that individual cues, landmarks, and signals may not work. Multiple cues may be necessary, increasing the likelihood that one of them will find a path intact and successfully complete the neurological trip from concept to action.

The second principle is that the mind erases memories on the basis of "last in, first out." The most recent memories (short-term memory) go first, followed by long-term memory, and finally even the most basic bodily functions seem to be forgotten, as though retracing the knowledge, abilities, and skills of one's entire life, from present to infancy. This concept will help you understand many of the principles suggested in this book.

The Stages of Alzheimer's Disease

What is most noteworthy about this disease in its early stages is that people hardly notice it. People with Alzheimer's disease rarely look ill and may be in excellent physical condition. The decline they suffer may be so gradual as to take years of observation to detect. And some individuals who sense their loss of memory may out of shame or fear disguise their declining abilities quite cleverly.

What makes Alzheimer's disease so difficult to recognize is the different rates at which the mind and body decline. The afflicted may appear perfectly normal, yet they may be completely unable to make rational decisions or judgments. They may be strong and handsome, yet unable to recognize a loved one, balance their checkbooks, or follow simple instructions. We may find its ravages hard to believe or accept. What we see with our eyes is not what we know in our hearts.

One day may be much better or worse than another. Your loved one can improve or regress mysteriously, appearing to skip a stage or to recover long-lost faculties for a moment. He or she may settle into routines making life more or less comfortable, then all of a sudden engage in irrational behavior. There may be rare but wonderful "windows" when your family member miraculously emerges from his or her confusion for a brief period and then just as strangely returns, as if nothing ever happened. The signs of this disease are all too inconsistent, making acceptance and understanding difficult.

That said, Alzheimer's does have a progressive quality that is often described as stages. No matter how you describe the disease, it can take anywhere from two to thirty years to complete. By considering researchers' descriptions of Alzheimer's stages, we gain a better grasp of the way this disease progresses through time.

In the early stages memory is slightly impaired. Items become lost; names, events, and people forgotten. As some forgetfulness is typical of the aging process, these symptoms may be dismissed or disregarded. The first person to notice something wrong is often the afflicted person himself. He may admit it, hide it, or attempt to compensate.

As the disease progresses, life becomes a struggle for mental survival where forgetting simple things causes complex reactions of embarrassment, anger, denial, fixation, or overcompensation. For example, a doctor's appointment, though met and completed, may not be remembered. The fear of missing it causes anxiety: notes on the refrigerator or calendar, phone calls, and dressing over and over for the appointment . . . now long past.

Though irritating and embarrassing, enough memory remains that some of the routines of daily living may not change. The person is still comfortable and secure at home. But as time goes by, less is remembered and more is forgotten. Life becomes frantic and bizarre, for both the person with AD and caregiver.

As the middle stages approach, life becomes a series of short stories, at best, connected only by the thinnest threads of memory or logic. Instructions become useless, quickly forgotten. But while what happened moments before may not be remembered, the person may dwell upon events or people from decades ago, in remarkably vivid detail.

Though the person may act as though he or she understands, explanations are quickly forgotten. An activity like raiding the refrigerator may be out of the question. Opening the refrigerator can lead to eating a piece of raw chicken or drinking from a bottle of seasoning. At this point, a caregiver must enter the picture; constant supervision and assistance with activities of daily living are now necessary.

Things that once made sense no longer do. Your loved one may be unable to recognize you or other people close to him, and indeed, may not know who the person staring back in the mirror really is. And decision making becomes equally frustrating. Choosing between different brands of cereal may be impossible, with fear and embarrassment over making the "wrong" choice.

Activities may be performed over and over. Simple activities may be the only ones your family member can accomplish. The analogy of "returning to childhood" is often used. If, as a child, your loved one helped her parents clean and put away the dishes, this may again become a pleasurable and satisfying responsibility.

In the final stages of the disease, even these simple, pleasurable activities are no longer possible. The body, in response to the mind's continuing decline, is unable to respond to stimulation. Your loved one may be bed- or wheelchair-bound, unable to care for herself. She may not be able to hold her head upright or sit straight up in her chair. Communication declines, until it is rare to see even a smile. (For a more precise description of the stages of Alzheimer's disease refer to the appendix in this book.)

A Special Plea to the Caregiver

Remember, if anything happens to you, both of you will be in hot water!

The biggest and most important factor in providing safe and loving care in the home is consideration for the caregiver. The success of home care depends upon your ability to balance caregiving with the needs of everyday living—a job, caring for children, privacy.

You may be used to taking care of yourself, a spouse, and children—but your dependent with Alzheimer's is much more demanding, of up to 100 percent of your attention and 100 percent of your time. You may feel you have no time to yourself or to perform such necessary everyday tasks as paying bills or even to go to the bathroom. Alzheimer's sufferers may be active both day and night, and that can cause severe stress and sleep deprivation for you. Many caregivers say their lives are in turmoil.

The parent becomes the child, and the child becomes the parent in the twilight zone inhabited by people with Alzheimer's disease. For much of your life, your father or mother may have taken care of you, looking out for your well-being and protecting you from danger. Now, because of this disease, you find that you must do these things for him or her, explaining what is safe and what isn't, even taking charge of dressing and feeding.

Since the caregiver's job is so stressful, time for healing is critical. Temporary care and respite services can look after your loved one and provide you with much-needed relief. You'll need the time to attend to personal matters or just to catch up on sleep.

Adult day care can also provide valuable respite and quality care specific to the needs of those with Alzheimer's disease. Explore the resources in your community, so that you'll know what is available to help you in the crises ahead.

Support groups can refer you to local resources, furnish answers to difficult questions, and provide opportunities to discuss your problems with others who are going through the same things you are experiencing. Contact your local Alzheimer's Association chapter for information about support groups and other resources in your area.

For those of you with computers, two rich sources are on-line chat groups and list servers. List servers are bulletin boards where people ask questions and others respond. There is no charge, and you can post your questions or read responses at your convenience. Be warned, however: if you subscribe, you will get a lot of mail and information.

For more information and a list of chat groups and list servers, visit our web site at: http://www.agelessdesign.com.

Finally, one must come to grips with the possibility that the home may not be the best place for your loved one. Notwithstanding your best and devoted efforts and the one-to-one care that you can give, specialized care facilities do have specially trained personnel and offer the added benefit of socialization. This is a personal decision for which you must take a lot of factors into consideration, the most important being what is best for your loved one and your family.

One thing that you must remember is that moving your loved one to an institution is not a failure; it may very well be the only way both of you can survive and achieve the best quality of life for everyone. Keeping your family member at home for as long as reasonably possible is an accomplishment itself, one in which you can take tremendous pride.

1

Preparing Your Home

Caring for someone with Alzheimer's disease (AD) need not be an overwhelming burden. The more planning, thinking, and constructive action you take early in caregiving, the easier it will be for the entire family to cope. Preparing your home and family for living with Alzheimer's is not so difficult, when you know what to do. The difficulties you encounter are not unique. They have been faced by many other families coping with this disease. Because caregivers have been so willing to share their stories with us, we have practical advice to offer that will help get you started and keep you going as you confront new behaviors and seemingly impossible situations.

The one consistent piece of advice we have heard from families is that you definitely need to arrange your home to care for a person with Alzheimer's. You may assume that you'll need to make changes to create a home that will serve you best in these difficult times. You should start with a plan.

Developing a Plan

This is a step-by-step process, one that you'll need to think about, write out, or draw. You can start by reading through this book to decide what steps you should take now and those that can wait. It's far better to plan and do the job right, rather than react to a crisis, pay premium prices, or do the job only half right. As you read through this book, make a to-do list. This will give you a better idea of what steps you will need to take and when you should take them.

Let's consider the steps.

Start as Soon as Possible

Alzheimer's disease is progressive and incurable. Although some medical treatments may slow its progression, none have been shown to reverse it. As time goes on, more and more problems are likely to arise, compounding the difficulties you face. For example, you may need to have work done (installing grab bars, railings, or locks, for example) that require workers to be in your home for several days. These strangers may upset your loved one, make noise, or destroy walls during construction. A person with Alzheimer's may feel threatened, accuse workers of stealing her things, or take tools and hide them. Getting work done as early as possible means the stress created can be better managed, during a time when your loved one needs less supervision and your family can better adjust to the changes.

Stay at Least One Step Ahead

Constant change is one of the more frustrating aspects of this illness. As soon as you get a grip on certain behaviors or problems—the rules change! You can't expect to win if you and your home remain stagnant while the disease continues to progress.

Though your loved one may appear to be functioning normally most of the time, you'll want to stay one step ahead. Learn all that you can about Alzheimer's disease. Plan for each stage of the illness, both mentally and physically. Constantly and coolly be on the lookout for new behavioral patterns, and for appropriate or better ways to deal with them. Your loved one may insist on using dangerous tools or objects (even nail clippers can be dangerous if used improperly!), or want to go into rooms with hazardous appliances. Avoid the crises to come by taking preventive action now.

A simple lock can prevent injury, even save a life. At least, it might prevent aggravation and worry. Create storage space for dangerous items and a safe home for your loved one. Look for available wall space in less frequently used rooms where you can add lockable cabinets. Identify the doors leading to dangerous rooms or outside of the house (if wandering away from home is a concern) and add locks or alarms. (See chapter 6 for more ideas.)

Make the Big Changes Early, Then Modify Gradually

By planning early, you can ease your way through the later stages of the disease. You may need to create secure storage space for dangerous items, or rethink the layout of your home to accommodate someone who may one day be unable to get up and down the stairs, who may be in a wheelchair or bed-bound. In the future you may need to position medical equipment near the bed. Are there enough outlets available? Are they in the right places? You may need to add lights, move a TV, or install new electrical outlets. Have an electrician do the electrical work early, rather than create a more serious problem with extension cords or an overloaded circuit breaker.

Now is the time to start looking for a dependable handyman. You can be sure there will be many occasions when you will need his or her help. Look for someone you can trust, who lives nearby, and who doesn't have a workload that will require weeks to get to you. If someone in your family fits this description, you are very lucky!

Visualize Your Home as You Want It to Be

A home should be many things: familiar, comfortable, safe, and easy to live in. It should accommodate the needs of caregivers and the person with Alzheimer's. If your loved one is moving into your home, talk together about the things he or she may need. Who knows better the difficulties he or she is having, or what modifications might be helpful? For example, if your loved one has trouble finding her way to the bathroom, or gets lost, ask what might help: maybe a small sign on the wall with an arrow pointing toward the bathroom, and another pointing back to the bedroom. Or a pathway laid out with tape on the floor showing the correct route. Such cues are nothing to be embarrassed about, especially if they help your loved one avoid episodes of getting lost or requiring help. Asking what might help often leads to surprisingly simple and effective solutions!

You don't have to make all of the decisions and do all of the planning yourself. Besides talking with your loved one, talk with your family about their needs and feelings. Seek the wisdom to be found in your local Alzheimer's support group. These are people who have already been through many of the situations confronting you. Their insights can be valuable in helping you prepare for the future.

Safety-Proof Your Home

This is probably the number one concern as you prepare to care for someone with Alzheimer's disease. All homes need to be safe, but now your home must help you avoid accidents, minimize injuries in the event of an accident, and remove triggers or causes of agitation or catastrophic reactions.

Your home should protect everyone from dangers, real and perceived. This is a confusing time for your loved one. A soft, familiar, and comfortable environment is reassuring and safe. Provide her with her own room and special places, where she can feel safe and protected, allowing her to keep a comfortable distance from strangers and sources of agitation.

You will need to survey your home thoroughly before making changes. And not just once, but in an ongoing effort to improve it, as often as appropriate. New situations will arise and new dangers will be found in the most ordinary objects or utensils. It's easier to overlook dangers than it is to see them. For example, certain common house and garden plants are toxic. If your family member begins to play with them, or put them in his mouth, it's important to remove them now.

Remove items that are clearly dangerous to your loved one or are valuable to you: medicines, kitchen utensils, jewelry. (See chapter 9.) Objects, utensils, and appliances that might cause problems should be moved to another part of the house that is less accessible, especially to someone who may wander. Make safe objects in accessible rooms easy to reach and see.

Eliminate unnecessary furniture, especially low, decorative items that are easy to trip over and can be hard to see in the dark. Use path or accent lighting in dark places, especially along normal paths of travel or wandering paths.

Relocate pieces of furniture that block your view of your loved one and his view of you. This lets you keep an eye on him and encourages conversation and interaction. This can also minimize fears of isolation, exclusion, or abandonment.

Child-Proof Your Home

Look at your home in much the way you would for a small, inquisitive child. Your loved one may no longer be able to distinguish good from bad, harmful from safe, or appropriate from inappropriate. Like a child, she may want to touch things she shouldn't, out of curiosity or desire for attention. For example, wall outlets may seem to be strange little holes for paper clips, dirt in a planter may be tempting to eat, or coats hanging in a dark closet may appear to be someone hiding.

Strategies for Change

Simplify, Simplify, Simplify

The wisdom that Thoreau gained from his little cabin at Walden Pond equally applies in your home. A simpler, easier-to-understand home benefits your loved one in many ways. As Alzheimer's disease progresses, it becomes more difficult to process environmental information. The familiar can become increasingly strange, entrances and exits to rooms may become harder to recognize. The simpler things are, the fewer environmental inputs there are to interpret.

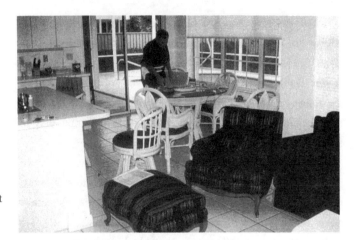

Extra furniture can block and complicate room exits, making it difficult for those with AD to recognize the way out of a room. Photo courtesy Ben and Beth Schatman.

Simplify pathways, make trips from point A to point B as straight and direct as possible, with no hazards or distractions along the way. Make them clear and easy to follow. Use your furniture to define them.

Reduce clutter. Many older people move from large homes to smaller apartments. Often they bring with them far more than will fit in their new home. As a result, excess furniture and decoration crowd rooms and hallways. These become hazards when a path four feet wide is reduced to two feet.

People with AD often spend hours hiding things and rummaging. The simpler the environment, the easier it will be for you to detect changes. It's easier to discover where items may have been hidden or which ones are now missing when the room is kept neat and orderly. Imagine trying to discover

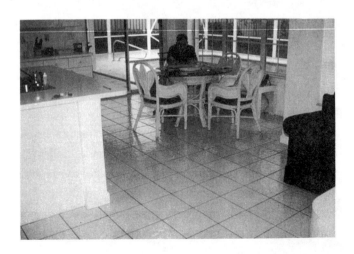

By removing unnecessary furniture, entrances and exits are a lot easier to recognize. Photo courtesy Ben and Beth Schatman.

changes in a bedroom where clothes are strewn around, with lots of clutter on shelves and in corners. Items out of place or missing may also confuse or upset your loved one. Make it easier on everyone by reducing clutter and simplifying the room to reveal things hidden, favorite rummaging sites, or hard-to-find items suspected of being "stolen."

Finally, limit your changes to only those that are necessary. Some modifications to your home environment may also confuse your family member so that he doesn't recognize otherwise familiar features. New furniture arrangements, for example, may be difficult to understand, especially if done all at once. Whatever modifications that you do make need to take this into consideration. Some may add to the confusion rather than avoid it. Once again, trial and error may be your best test.

Think Therapeutically

A therapeutic environment is one that helps and contributes, rather than hinders and creates barriers. Glaring light can reflect on floors, making them look slippery and dangerous. Reducing the glare with adjustable blinds would create a more therapeutic environment. An additional outlet located for a night light would help illuminate the path, guide your loved one, and make nighttime visits to the bathroom safer and easier. Grab bars in showers and tubs offer safety and calming security when bathing. A therapeutic environment can benefit everyone in the house, not just the person with Alzheimer's disease.

Put yourself in their place. Imagine that one night you wake up in a strange bed in an unfamiliar house. You have no idea how you got there, or whose house this might be. At that moment, you need to go to the bathroom. You turn on a light, get out of bed, and look for the bathroom. You enter a hallway, but the doors are all closed, and they all look alike: *problem number one*. Finally you find the right door and go in. When you come out and look for your room, once again all the doors look alike: *problem number two*.

Seek modifications that guide and attract your loved one when guidance is needed. If the door to the bathroom is more prominent than the door to a closet, then it is more likely that the bathroom door will be opened.

Create a home that encourages correct decisions and avoids wrong ones. To make the bathroom easier to find, you could install a nightlight with a photocell that always goes on when it gets dark; and to help your loved one find his own bedroom, you could paint the door trim his favorite color (and not paint the trim on other doors). To help him find where the plates are in the kitchen, you could paste a picture of a plate on the correct cabinet. (See chapter 5 for more ideas.) To camouflage the intent of such alterations, make this a fun event by including the grandchildren. Have them cut out the pictures and paste them to doors. Turn the signs into items of pride rather than prosthetic tools.

Encourage successful decisions and completion of tasks. Quite often the person with Alzheimer's disease is aware of the difficulties she is having. This may lead to denial, fear, or a disproportionate concern over the burden of caring for her. Things that are reminders of her condition may inhibit tasks, create new concerns, or even lead to emotional outbreaks or crises. It is in everyone's best interest to avoid reminders of the forgetfulness caused by the disease or the inability to complete more difficult tasks.

Encourage independence. Create opportunities for activities your loved one enjoys and can perform safely. If your mother has always loved to cook, provide ingredients for her to prepare simple meals, such as cereal and milk, rather than brisket or Stroganoff. Group and locate items logically—bowl, spoon, and sugar together so there is no need for searching. Label drawers and cabinets, and arrange boxes for maximum visibility. The failure to complete a task should not be caused by something as simple and unnecessary as not being able to find where the bowl or spoons are kept.

"Aunt Peggy just can't make up her mind. Even choosing her cereal in the morning seems too difficult for her."

A therapeutic home offers choices rather than avoids them. Choosing from two boxes of cereal may be easier than choosing from four. More is not better when dealing with someone with AD, so get rid of the extra boxes. This concept also applies

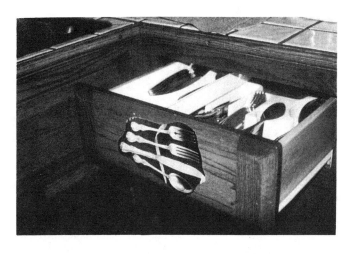

To help your family member locate things, attach pictures illustrating a drawer's contents to the face of the drawer. Make it a family affair.

to the bedroom closet and drawers, where decisions have to be made on what to wear today.

If you make the backyard safe and impossible to wander out of, your family member will be able to go outside if she chooses. We all need to make decisions and act on them, no matter how simple they may be. This reinforces feelings of autonomy, independence, and freedom, which your family member may perceive to have been taken away. (See chapter 5 for special precautions on making the backyard safe.)

Provide opportunities for conversation and interaction. Picture albums and family photos provide excellent conversation starters. Locate comfortable chairs in front of a sliding glass door, or put benches on a porch or in the backyard, where there are views of activity or a landscaped area designed to attract birds or other wildlife. An area with a sandbox for the grandchildren or with people walking by are also opportunities for conversation. Create such an area where a mess or accident can do no harm, where your loved one can be safe and secure, and where he can easily be supervised.

Consider Family and Friends

Like many other diseases, Alzheimer's is said to have numerous victims, not just the person afflicted. Though your primary focus has to be on her needs, don't overlook the needs of other family members, visitors, grandchildren, or yourself.

This is a difficult time for everybody. It requires understanding and patience. Making caregiving as easy as possible for everyone involved will reduce the trauma and increase the pleasure and sense of well-being derived from caring for a loved one at home.

Identifying the Zones of Your Home

A good way to approach many of the issues we've been considering is to examine your home in terms of zones that are appropriate for a family living with Alzheimer's disease. Rooms and areas (cabinets, drawers, and doors) can be categorized as one of three types: Danger Zone, Respite Zone, or Safe Zone.

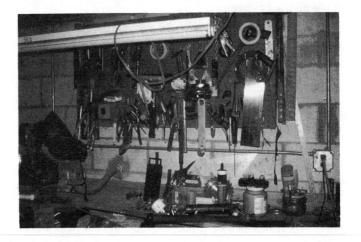

A hobby workshop contains many dangerous tools and/or chemicals and needs to be off-limits.

The Danger Zones

The first type of area that will be off-limits to your loved one we refer to as Danger Zones. They include places with objects or features that may be dangerous. These rooms can be used to store valuable, breakable, or unsafe items, such as tools and chemicals. Doors leading into Danger Zones (or outside the home) should be kept locked and alarmed, or controlled with wander-prevention devices. Such areas may include:

Garage	Computer room
Hobby rooms	Kitchen
Workshops	Playroom

Offices	Cellar
Laundry room	Pool area
Sewing room	Attic
Storage closets	Staircases
Basement	

The Respite Zone

The other portion of the home that is off-limits to your loved one is that area reserved for the caregiver. This is a sanctuary, an undisturbed, private place where you can relax, be by yourself, and conduct your affairs. It may be your bedroom and bathroom, a renovated room in the attic, or your office at home. Even something as simple as a bench in the backyard garden will do. Since burnout is a big problem for caregivers, you will need a place to get away and have time alone while your loved one rests or is cared for by someone else. Burnout is a primary cause for caregiver stress and prematurely admitting Alzheimer's patients to nursing homes.

The Safe Zone

The rest of your home needs to be safe and accessible. The person you are caring for has had the run of the entire house all her life. As much of the house as is safe and reasonable should remain available to her now, to wander, hide things, and rummage in, free from potentially agitating or harmful situations. (Refer to chapter 9 for more suggestions and discussion on safety.)

You may want to create special places in your home for certain activities to satisfy the needs and habits of your loved one. These places should be set up to enable the safe and successful completion of tasks, even simple crafts. For example, a place might be created in the den for reading "mail" or in the kitchen to make sure you make the pie "just right." A table in a well-lighted area can serve for playing cards or doing puzzles. Locate it where you can see what's going on so you'll be able to monitor activities and carry on with your daily routines at the same time.

Mary cares for her 76-year-old mother-in-law with Alzheimer's. She has set aside a spare room upstairs as her "sanctuary." She decorated it with pillows and covered the bed in her favorite fabric. She moved a comfortable lounge chair in from the patio, and purchased a lovely new cushion. She also found an old tape player in the attic and placed a few of her favorite cassettes on shelves next to some good books, magazines, and family photos. Mary has been working on several knitting projects, which she finds relaxing. So she has moved them into her sanctuary as well. Once a day, or more, Mary schedules a visit to her special room. Upon leaving, she is refreshed and ready to care for her mother-in-law.

Take advantage of all the senses. Maintain a clean, neat, warm household that smells good. Flowers and the aroma of fresh-baked cookies are all reminders of comfort and pleasant memories.

Remember, each stage of the disease is different. In addition, behavior, degree of difficulty, and safety are all affected by environmental factors, often in ways that are hard to imagine. Locks and accessible drawers for safe objects limit hiding and rummaging, grab bars help with bathing and toileting, and child-proofing reduces accidents.

Create a Comfortable Environment

Try to discover your loved one's comfort zone. It's probably not the same as yours. Consider the home's temperature, lighting, and sounds (just to name a few). Be extra-sensitive in doing so—even the motion or draft from a ceiling fan can be annoying. Your loved one may not know what is wrong, only feel uncomfortable. Her only means of expression may be agitation or desperate efforts to escape the discomfort.

Avoid foreign, institutional-looking equipment and furnishings whenever possible. No one makes a home homier by bringing in a hospital bed or scary lifting equipment.

Encourage Memories

One of the more noteworthy and confusing characteristics of Alzheimer's disease is the gradual loss of short-term memory, often accompanied by incredibly accurate and detailed recollections of events that occurred decades ago.

"Mom doesn't know what she had for lunch an hour ago, but she can tell me the dress she wore and the change she received buying a flower thirty years ago when she met Dad."

Many people with AD progressively retreat to earlier times and places in their lives. Perhaps as recent memories become erased, all that remain are those from further and further in the past. They may include an old home or neighborhood where your loved one grew up or a time when she was younger, protected and provided for by her parents.

So when you think "familiar," think "old-fashioned." Take advantage of resurfacing memories. As memories of past times and places surface, encourage and embellish them. What your mother grew up with may be what helps her remember and feel comfortable. Surround your loved one with pictures of people from years ago, of old neighborhoods, scenes from his past, and photos representing personal interests or achievements. In fact, it may be easier for your loved one to recognize pictures of himself when he was younger than himself in more recent photographs.

Observe their behavior, and look for clues. More than just memories, routines from the past may be the best way your loved one can function today. Maybe ceramic handles on the faucets are more familiar than single-handled levers. Perhaps a clothes line in the backyard would offer an opportunity for your loved one to help with the laundry in a way that she can understand and enjoy.

Of course, this window of familiarity is different for each generation. What seems familiar to someone seventy or eighty years old could date back to 1920. What may be familiar to Baby Boomers might be 8-track tapes or black-and-white televisions.

For friends and visitors not familiar with the disease, it is all too easy to see your family member as a patient, rather than a colorful interesting person. Photos and memorabilia will remind them and create opportunities to stimulate interest and conversation. Look for things that make your family member smile, even if it is the same thing, over and over. (See chapter 2.)

When you create a home that allows your loved one to enjoy the best quality of life possible, he probably will. Adapt your home to him, in positive and encouraging ways. The result will promote better health and better quality of life. If your home and lifestyle modifications are simply to extend life, with little regard to human needs, that will be noticed. Don't forget that inside, despite your loved one's confusion, there remains a loving, and perhaps frightened human being.

"Uncle Al used to work on the railroad. We found books on trains at the flea market, cut out pictures, framed them, and lined the walls in his special area with them. Here he spends hours working on train puzzles and looking through his books, telling story after story (half of which we think he makes up). We even found an old train light which he swears came off one of the trains he used to ride."

Lighting

One of the most important components to creating a truly safe home is sufficient lighting. When you brighten a room, you make it easier to see obstacles and distinguish changes in direction or elevation. Older people need as much as three times the amount of light than they did when they were younger.

Proper lighting plays many important roles in the home. Lighting:

- improves safety;
- helps family members see where they are going and recognize pathways;
- can improve one's appearance, self-image, and self-esteem;
- allows us to distinguish colors (important when distinguishing pills or foods from one another and avoiding obstacles);
- contributes to the successful completion of tasks; and
- can even minimize depression. (Brighter homes are more cheerful and less gloomy.)

By reducing shadows and dark areas in your home, you also help your loved one understand his world, and you eliminate sights that might be misinterpreted or trigger hallucinations.

Maximize Storage

We often joke about not having enough storage space. Families living with Alzheimer's never have too much! You will now need areas for safekeeping valuable and dangerous items, as well as space for medical, caregiving, and cleaning supplies. "Safekeeping" storage needs to be out-of-the-way and locked. Space for important supplies should be convenient and close to where the items will be needed.

Take a long look around your home for lockable rooms and storage areas (consider the attic and basement), out-of-the-way cabinets, and unused wall space for new cabinetry. Is there room in the garage or in an outside toolshed?

Other ways to maximize storage include:

- getting rid of things you've stored for years to make room for others,
- reserving prime and reachable locations for the most important items,
- not wasting space with four bottles of something

when you only need one. Check supplies often and replenish them when they become low.

Use the same strategies in all storage locations (kitchen, bathroom, etc.). Install sliding shelves or lazy Susans in cabinets or attach shelves to the inside of the cabinet doors to make items easier to reach.

Lazy Susans and sliding shelving:

Rev-A-Shelf, home improvement centers.

Every home has rooms that are used less than others, that we use rarely or only for specific purposes. If you observe where your loved one goes, you can convert less-frequented rooms into lockable storage areas. After all, you cannot make the entire house off-limits. Using less-frequented rooms for storing off-limits items and reserve supplies will minimize agitation and reactions to locked doors.

Bathroom Storage

Once your family member requires more attention and supervision, you won't want to leave her alone in the bathroom. Leaving her alone for only a few seconds might be not only unsafe, but could result in panic or fear of being abandoned.

Have a plan. Maximize bathroom storage, even for "luxury" items that you might not need immediately. For example, storing a blanket in the bathroom to keep your family member warm when sitting on the toilet or grooming could be comforting and calming. Such a luxury might be appreciated by those who constantly complain that they are cold.

Take advantage of space that may have been overlooked in the bathroom. A shelf unit that hangs over the door can provide valuable storage on the back side of the door. How about installing shelves or a cabinet on the wall over the toilet? Some companies even make free-standing shelf units that go over the toilet, providing storage space that you might not even realize you had it.

Free-standing shelves for over and behind the toilet:

Get Organized, Hold Everything, Renovator's.

If room allows, consider adding a bathroom pantry or linen closet. Look for unused areas in your bathroom. Or, if you have a closet next to the bathroom, consider using part of it by creating an opening from the bathroom. It might be worthwhile to call

Susan used to stock her father's bathroom every Sunday morning. Her checklist included:

   toilet paper (two rolls)

   tissues (one extra box)

   paper towels (one extra roll to clean up accidents and spills)

   clean towels and wash cloths (at least three of each)

Because she planned, Susan never left her father alone or un-attended. It was safer for him, and made less tension and worry for her.

a contractor for an estimate and expert advice, and to see if he can come up with other ideas for maximizing storage.

Provide and store items to help the caregiver. Design and adapt your home for everyone, including visiting caregivers. Make sure that supplies are well stocked and located conveniently, visibly and logically. This will allow the caregiver to focus attention on your loved one, rather than on searching for a roll of toilet paper or having to leave momentarily for a needed supply.

Some items belong on open shelving, visible and easy to find, while others need to be put away for caregiver access only. You'll also want to make space for more frequently needed items. This space will need to be convenient and creative. Is there space over your toilet where more shelves could be added?

Planning Major Projects

Adding a Bathroom

A home with only one bathroom can be a problem, especially if the bathroom is upstairs, or a long walk from your loved one's room or favorite chair. It can even be a silent cause for incontinence—if you can't get to or find the bathroom, you can't use it!

Having only an upstairs bathroom limits your loved one. And the sense of urgency that using the bathroom entails can cause hurried reactions that lead to slips and falls. It also places demands on the caregiver, who will probably be doing most of the traveling up and down those stairs. The greater the distance, the greater the problems.

Adding a bathroom may not mean a full bathroom. A first-floor closet may be just big enough for a sink and toilet (or just a portable commode). A local contractor or architect can examine your home and offer suggestions. Another benefit of adding a bathroom, according to the National Association of Realtors, is that it's the single most cost-effective addition you can make to most homes. All or most of its cost can be recouped when you sell your home!

Converting a Room

Consider converting a first-floor room to a bedroom. Relocating your loved one's room downstairs can have many advantages. Having him close by during the day makes it easier to keep an eye on him, and it allows him to be closer to you and easier to participate in family activities. Neither one of you wants to spend time going up and down stairs that can make a difficult situation truly a hardship!

If possible, choose a room with a sliding glass door, or install one. It will offer an increased viewing area and can provide someone who is bed-bound with hours of visual pleasure every day. Furthermore, in an emergency it's likely to be the safest and most direct exit out of the house.

Taking advantage of a guest house or "granny flat" is another solution that may work, at least for a while. When closer supervision is needed, it may be wiser to have Mom or Dad move into the main house, and then convert the guesthouse or flat into a caregiver's apartment.

Preparing a Caregiver's Room

You may eventually need a professional caregiver. If so, he or she may come on an hourly, a daily, or a live-in, 24-hours-a-day basis. Where will she stay? When thinking about a caregiver's room, take into consideration both privacy and proximity to the care-receiver. That may mean relocating your loved one's room.

Adding a Washer/Dryer

These useful appliances are not always located conveniently. They may be downstairs in a basement, on the side of the house away from the bedrooms, or otherwise accessible only with difficulty. I've seen laundry rooms next to workshops and furnaces, when they should be close to where most of the laundry is generated (the bedroom and bathroom). Adding a washer/dryer is a good idea. You may need it close to an outside wall for venting the dryer exhaust, and close to plumbing lines for the washer. Often a kitchen or bathroom can meet these requirements. Talk to a contractor for help, and see chapter 7 for more ideas and products.

Your Home's Interior Spaces

Now let's look at your home room by room, taking into consideration the special concerns that Alzheimer's disease imposes. (Refer also to the discussions later in the book on specific behaviors and challenges.)

The Bathroom

Comfort

For people with Alzheimer's disease, recognizing or communicating even basic concerns may eventually become difficult. Your loved one may not realize that the bathroom is too cold, only that she is uncomfortable. She may not associate the room temperature with her discomfort or have the ability to communicate it to you. The result is often frustration, vented anger or desperate attempts to escape the discomfort.

Though your loved one may not appear to think rationally, the desire for privacy and dignity remains an active and important concern. Often privacy needs to be sacrificed for safety, yet certain compromises should be made to preserve both. For example, the bathroom may need to be accessible in the event of an emergency, or to ensure that your loved one cannot lock himself inside. At the same time, the bathroom is a private place. Replacing privacy locks with passage locks or the bathroom door with a heavy shower curtain may provide both sufficient privacy and the necessary access.

"Grandma Esther is a survivor of the Holocaust. Whenever we try to give her a shower she begins to scream and do everything she can to escape."

Bathrooms should be warm and comfortable. Forcing someone who is already confused to take a shower in a cold, ceramic tile room (with horrible experiences in her long-term memory) might logically result in a catastrophic reaction. Paintings on the wall, carpeting on the floor, cheerful wallpaper, curtains on the window, and warm colorful towels are characteristic of a home, not an institution.

What makes a bathroom warm and comfortable?

- Soft materials—carpeting and warm, colored towels.
- Temperature—not too cold or too warm, and no drafts. Heat lamps installed in the ceiling provide warmth and comfort and cannot be knocked over, dropped into a tub of water, or touched by wet hands. They are out of reach and safe. Use a timer switch so your loved one can never forget to turn off the heat lamp.
- Familiar features—residential-style sink, tub, shower, and toilet.
- Sunlight brightening the room, coming through a window decorated with pretty curtains.
- Interior design—calming colors and patterns for tile, paint, and wallpaper.
- Odors—the bathroom usually has its own smell, whether fresh and clean, or otherwise. Good household cleaning habits can go a long way in creating a more inviting (rather than offensive) environment.
- Safety—a shower or bathtub seat, grab bars to hold, non-slip floor surfaces. (See chapter 9.)
- Little extras—paintings, curtains on the windows, a place to hang a bathrobe or a blanket to keep warm when sitting on the toilet.
- Sounds—don't overlook certain sounds in the bathroom that may be confusing or irritating: rushing water, the toilet flushing, the exhaust fan whirring, and noises from outside the window (traffic or neighbors arguing).

Little touches like these go a long way in creating a comfortable room for bathing that will not remind Grandma Esther of terrible events in her past.

Bathroom acoustics may be great for singing in the shower, but not for those who are irritated or upset by noise bouncing around in hard, ceramic tile environments. Soften the bathroom as much as possible to absorb confusing and overwhelming sounds. Use soft towels, shower curtains, and carpeting.

One simple way to make a bathroom more comfortable is

to invest in a good quality shower curtain. A heavy, pretty cloth curtain helps to create a safer, more inviting and comfortable bathroom. Choose a calming color and pattern for the curtain. Look for a strong shower curtain that won't come down if grasped for extra support. Subtle touches, like these, are appreciated by everyone.

Minimize bathroom clutter. Simplicity is key to creating an environment that is easier to understand and less threatening.

Consider locating a washer/dryer somewhere near the bathroom. Warm-from-the-dryer towels for after the bath or for sitting on the toilet are a nice touch. In addition, if incontinence becomes a problem, a washer/dryer upstairs (near the bed and bedroom) will minimize the distance for carrying heavy, wet sheets and towels (several times a day).

If you're planning to build or renovate a bathroom, keep in mind that the larger the bathroom, the easier it will be to care for someone there. Most bathrooms, bathtubs, toilets, and showers are designed to be used by one person, not by someone caring for another. Extra space will be especially appreciated if a wheelchair becomes necessary. In addition, those who suffer from contractures or rigidity have limited arm movement and mobility. To ease moving about, they need more space and fewer obstructions.

One way to make a bathroom larger is to remove extra items that make it smaller! Find a better location for decorative items and floor pieces that get in the way—that magazine rack, wastepaper basket, hamper, etc.

If room allows, provide a comfortable chair to sit on while drying off. Your family member may have difficulty standing or balancing and feel more comfortable sitting down. Certainly there's the toilet to sit on (with a soft, comfortable cover), but a chair, if there is room, is more comfortable and dignified.

Safety

The bathroom may be the smallest, but it is often regarded as the most dangerous room in your home. It poses dangers in all six categories of common home injuries: slips and falls, burns, poisoning, cuts, electrocution, and drowning. In the bathroom

Combination washer/dryer that requires no venting:

Bendix, Equator Corp.

Stacking washer/dryers:

Maytag, Westinghouse. Also check with your local appliance dealer for compact units that fit in apartment closets.

are wet, slippery floors conducive to slips and falls. The bathroom is frequently visited during the night when family members may be alone and half asleep, when lighting is poor. In addition, medicines, cleaning supplies, and other toxic agents are commonly stored there. Aspirin and other medications are not the only items in the bathroom that can be dangerous if swallowed. Don't overlook products like:

Shampoos	Shoe polish
Colognes	Nail polish remover
Hair cleaning products	Toilet cleaners
Antiseptics	Air fresheners
Nail polish	Drain openers
Alcohol	Perfumes
Petroleum jelly	Liquid soaps & cleansers

Many of these products are brightly colored and scented to smell like fruit, making them tempting to someone who may not know better than to taste them. Items meant to go in the mouth may not be meant to be swallowed. Be aware that even seemingly harmless products if ingested or taken in excess can cause serious illness:

"I found Granny in the bathroom last night eating the toothpaste."

Mouthwash	Sleeping pills
Laxatives	Cough syrup
Toothpaste	Other medicines

Examine your bathroom for dangerous accessories that could cause injury if your loved one falls against them. You may want to safety-proof, remove or relocate:

Bathtub spouts	Counter and cabinet edges
Wall hooks	Tub walls
Towel bars	Heaters & radiators
Soap dishes	Glass shower doors
Glass shelves	Decorative fixtures
Doorknobs	Shower door handles

Also look for hooks and other projections located on walls at head or eye level where they might be hit in a fall.

In general:

Bathtub faucet cushions:

Kids Club, Perfectly Safe, Safety 1st.

- Remove or relocate items that are in dangerous locations.
- Replace others with safer models.
- Cushion or soften those that cannot be removed or relocated, such as bathtub faucets.

Remove glass and fragile items from the bathroom. This includes the drinking glass used for brushing teeth, bottles of soap, ceramic vases, and glass shelving. Replace clear cups with colored, sturdy, plastic cups that are easier to see and hold. Clear plastic cups may be harder to see than ones that are colored. Glass shelving can be replaced with wood shelving with rounded, safer edges.

Unplug and/or remove small electric appliances that could be touched by wet hands or dropped in the sink, tub, shower, or toilet while still plugged into the outlet. Here are a few common household electrical appliances often found near water:

Hot lather dispensers	Irons
Electric razors	Hand-held vacuums
Electric toothbrush stands	Electric rollers
Lighted portable mirrors	Hair dryers
Curling irons	Radios or small TVs
Space heaters	Jewelry cleaners
Contact lens cleaners	Denture cleaners

Appliances do not have to be on to be dangerous, just plugged in! Make sure the outlets in your bathroom and kitchen are ground fault interrupted (GFI). GFI outlets and circuit breakers help protect you and your loved one from accidental shocks. However, even GFI outlets can fail to operate, and they should not be relied on 100 percent. But they are inexpensive and much better than no protection at all.

GFI protection can be accomplished in one of two ways: Either you have a GFI outlet, or the circuit breaker in your electrical panel is a GFI breaker. The advantage of having a GFI circuit breaker is that it protects all the outlets on that circuit. The way to identify GFI outlets or breakers is to look for a test or reset button either on the outlet itself or on the circuit breaker in your electrical panel. When the test button is pressed (or when a short circuit occurs) the mechanism should pop and turn off the electrical outlet. (You can also use this as a secret switch to turn off the outlet.) (See chapter 9 for more discussion on GFI outlets and breakers.)

If your electrical system is not protected or your GFI outlets are not working properly (or if you don't know how to check), ask your local electrician to help you. You could also take a lesson from parents of young children and install child-proof plug covers in outlets to prevent foreign objects from being inserted or electrical appliances from being plugged in and used dangerously. And finally, for added safety always unplug your electrical appliances when they are not in use.

Portable heaters and lamps also can be dangerous. Ceiling-mounted fixtures and heat lamps cannot be reached, tipped over, touched by wet hands, or dropped into a tub of water. They are much safer than portable heaters that sit on the floor. Consider talking to your local handyman or contractor about having a heater or heat lamp put in your bathroom ceiling.

Don't limit your safety-proofing to your loved one's bathroom only. *Your* bathroom is dangerous, too! You might want to install a child-proof lock on your medicine cabinet or a lock on your bathroom door. Trouble lurks almost everywhere, and you are dealing not with the cleverness of a small child, but rather with that of someone who can reach into more places and has enough life experience to realize that pills go into the mouth and are swallowed. Lock 'em up!

"Arlene went into our bathroom last night and ate a whole box of laxatives."

Grab Bars

Install grab bars in the bathroom. This is one of the most important safety investments that you can make—not only for your loved one, but for everyone in the household. At the very least, you'll need grab bars in the shower, in the bathtub, and on both sides of the toilet. They are also good next to the tub or shower to hold while standing or getting in and out, and to provide the caregiver with support when helping or lifting.

People sometimes fall off the toilet and hit their heads on the edge of the counter or wall of the bathtub. Some of these accidents are fatal.

"We can't leave Dad alone for a minute. If we take him into the bathroom and put him on the john, he falls over. Last night he hit his head on the edge of the counter."

Fold-down grab bars:

American Health Care Supply, ASI, Barclay, Basco, Bobrick, Carex, DSI, Elcoma, ETAC USA, Frohock-Stewart, Häfele America, HEWI, Invacare Continuing Care, Lumex, McKesson, Otto Bock, Sammons Preston, Tubular Specialties Mfg., or home improvement centers.

Install grab bars on both sides of the toilet. These will help confine and prevent falling. Where one side is open, next to the tub or too far away to install a side-wall-mounted bar, install a fold-down bar mounted on the rear wall or one that mounts to the floor and rear wall. (See chapter 9 for the different types of grab bars, their uses, and advantages.)

Install a grab bar on the front of the sink counter to provide your loved one with something to hold while standing at the sink. Grab bars, unlike the edge of the counter, are round, making them easier to hold and offering something familiar to grasp.

Replace towel bars with grab bars. Towel bars are not grab bars. They are not designed to hold a person's weight. But grab bars can be used as towel bars. Some grab bars on the market now come in decorator colors and are hardly recognizable as grab bars, but serve both purposes well. In emergencies, when you desperately need something to grab on to, you don't have time to make the distinction between a grab bar and a towel bar. This is especially true for someone with AD who may not know the difference or, because of instability or judgment difficulties, may need the extra support of a grab bar.

Install a small grab bar anywhere you or your loved one may need support. This includes next to the scale, next to the sink, where he gets dressed, or on the wall where he dries himself or gets dried off.

Slips and Falls

Slip-resistant flooring strips:

American Health Care Supply or home improvement centers.

Slip-resistant backing for rugs:

Alsto's Handy Helpers, Harriet Carter, Home Trends, Improvements, Joan Cook, Miles Kimball, Optimum Technologies, or home improvement centers.

Install nonslip or slip-resistant mats, strips, or appliques to the bathtub and shower floor.

Install nonslip flooring materials also on slippery floors *outside* of the shower or tub. These can be slip-resistant mats or inexpensive adhesive strips available at most home improvement centers.

Remove throw rugs or, at the very least, attach slip-resistant backing. An alternative to slip-resistant backing is double-faced carpet tape, available at most carpet, flooring, and hardware stores, and home improvement centers. Use this tape to attach the rug to your floor. Periodically check to make sure that the tape hasn't worn off, lost its sticky coating or allowed corners to curl and become "trippers."

Consider carpeting your bathroom floor. Carpeting is slip-resistant, warm, homey, soft to the touch, and more forgiving if there's a fall. One problem with carpeting is odor retention in the event of incontinence, but that too can be addressed. (See chapter 7.)

Often falls occur during times of agitation or catastrophic reactions, when your loved one is angry and not careful. Fits of rage include flailing or attempts to strike the caregiver. Balance can be lost and slips can occur, especially in spaces as confined and slippery as the bathroom.

To help you listen for accidents, consider purchasing a monitoring device or intercom for your family member's bathroom and, if she sleeps alone, for her bedroom. This would help you hear any nighttime calls for assistance as well as any falls.

Bathtubs

To help protect your loved one from injury caused by falling in the bathroom, cushion the tub wall or replace your bathtub with one that has soft, cushioned walls.

To help getting in and out of the tub install a bathtub transfer seat or a shower seat in your shower. A bathtub transfer seat allows a person to sit down outside of the tub and transfer to the tub without stepping over the tub wall. (See chapter 8 for the names of manufacturers.)

Bathtub transfer seats and shower seats offer several other advantages. Your loved one can bathe sitting down, minimizing movement and the potential of slipping and falling. Alternatively, some people use transfer seats just to enter the tub safely, then shower normally, standing up. A bathtub transfer seat allows the family member a little more dignity and independence, since she does not require as much help. It makes getting in and out easier and safer. Finally, it assists the caregiver, making the transition that much easier.

Consider replacing the tub with a roll-in shower. Although any shower stall will be helpful to both the caregiver and your loved one, down the line when a wheelchair enters the picture

"My husband got angry last night when I tried to give him a bath. He started swinging at me and fell down."

"Aunt Sue fell in the bathroom last night. We found her on the floor this morning."

Baby monitoring devices:

Gerber, Fisher-Price, Kids Club, The Right Start, The Safety Zone, Safety 1st, or baby supply stores.

Bathtub wall cushions:

KidKusions

Soft, cushion-walled bathtubs:

International Cushioned Products.

Soft, cushioned bathtub insert trays:

Diversified Fiberglass Products.

a roll-in, accessible shower will be a lifesaver. There are kits to replace tubs with accessible showers. (See chapters 4 and 8.)

Showers

Install a hand-held showerhead. Look for the ones that have an on-off or pause button on the hand-held part for better control of the water flow. This not only helps those with fears of water or bathing, but also helps prevent wetting hair, bandaged areas, or other body parts that need to be kept dry. (See chapter 4 for more suggestions.)

Install a fold-down shower seat so that the shower can be used safely by your family member and conventionally by others in the household who may not want to sit down while showering.

Make sure your shower doors and sliding glass doors are tempered glass, not plate glass. Plate glass is dangerous. When it breaks, the result is sharp pieces of glass versus the thousands of safer tiny glass pellets that result from breaking tempered glass. Prior to 1977 the installation of dangerous plate glass shower doors was permitted. If there is any doubt, have a glass contractor inspect your glass or replace your shower door (see page 66).

You can easily replace your shower door with one made from tempered (safety) glass or, better, a shower curtain. Shower curtains make access easier and safer. Removing shower doors will allow you more open space to bathe your loved one and assist him in getting in and out of the shower.

Sinks and Counters

Cushion the edge of the sink countertop to protect your loved one from injury caused by striking it, especially if it is sharp-edged, rather than smooth and round. Many stores catering to baby needs offer cushioned edge protectors for tables and other sharp furniture edges. Basically they are soft, padded cushion strips with adhesive on the back. Check your local baby store.

To provide a protective edge and save some money, go to your local home improvement center and buy inexpensive hot

---

Hand-held showerhead assemblies:

Access with Ease, Alsons, American Health Care Supply, Care Catalogue, Carex, Guardian Products, Jaclo, Lumex, M.O.M.S., McKesson, North Coast Medical Inc., Sammons Preston, Sears Home HealthCare Catalogue, Shamrock Medical Equipment.

Fold-down shower seats:

American Health Care Supply, ASI, Bradley, ETAC USA, Graham Field, Häfele America, Invacare Continuing Care, Lumex.

"Andrea hates to be bathed and struggles to avoid it tooth and nail. This evening she tried to fight off the nurse and wound up hitting her arm on the edge of the sink counter."

water pipe insulation. This is a soft, pliable foam cylinder that is split along its full length. It comes in various sizes, intended to fit around different sizes of pipe. You can easily install it on the projecting edge of your countertops. A couple of strips of adhesive-backed Velcro (also available at your local home improvement center) are all that is needed for a good installation.

Adhesive-backed Velcro:

Consumer Care Products, Sammons Preston, Smith & Nephew.

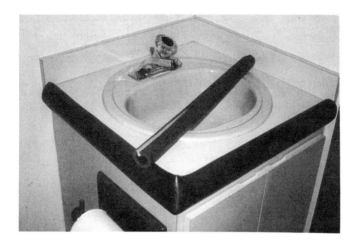

Foam pipe insulation provides an inexpensive cushion for sharp edges on countertops and tables.

Avoiding Burns

Whenever you are using both the hot and cold water (for example, when taking a shower) and the supply of cold water is diminished, the result can be a temporary surge of hot, perhaps scalding water. This temporary "stealing" of cold water can be caused by someone flushing a toilet, turning on another faucet (in the kitchen sink, another bathroom, or an outdoor hose), or the washing machine or dishwasher changing cycles. The results can be painful. Since people with Alzheimer's disease may be unable to express their discomfort appropriately, the result might be agitation, hostility, or some other act of desperation, and justifiably so.

A good safety precaution in anyone's bathroom is to install anti-scalding devices: in sinks, bathtubs, and showers. Showers and bathtubs should be equipped with a pressure-sensitive and/or temperature-limiting (anti-scalding) balancing valve. This device senses and compares the pressure in the hot and cold water lines. When there is a sudden change in pressure,

Pressure-sensitive, temperature-limiting anti-scalding bath and shower valves:

Delta, Kohler, Moen, Price Pfister, or a plumbing dealer.

Anti-scalding devices:

Accent on Living, AdaptAbility, Joan Cook, Independent Living Aids, Keeney, Memry Corporation, or home improvement centers.

Anti-scalding showerheads:

Accent on Living, AdaptAbility, Brookstone, Independent Living Aids, Keeney, Lighthouse Enterprises.

Anti-scalding devices for bathtub faucets:

Keeney.

Toilet bidet devices:

Access with Ease, AdaptAbility, American Health Care Supply, Enrichments, Hygiene Specialties, J. C. Manufacturing, Lubidet, Maddak, McKesson, MNO Sales, North Coast Medical, Sammons Preston, Self Care, Toto Kiki.

Inexpensive, hand-held toilet bidet/sitzbaths:

North Coast Medical, Sammons Preston.

Child-proof toilet seat locks:

Kids Club, Safety 1st or baby supply stores.

the valve compensates so that you don't get caught in a stream of too-hot water. You can pre-set the temperature-limiting valve not to let the water exceed a certain temperature.

Bathtub and sink faucets can be sources of scalding water too. Insert anti-scalding devices in all faucets that have both hot and cold water (including the laundry room, guest bathrooms, etc.). These devices fit into or onto your existing faucet pipe or showerhead. If the water gets too hot, they expand and shut off the water flow. They are inexpensive and easy to install.

There are also special anti-scalding showerheads. These can replace your existing wall showerhead.

The Toilet

Add a bidet to your toilet to help with toileting. These accessories attach to your john and provide a gentle spray of water to aid in cleansing one's private parts. Bidet devices range from simple to fancy. Some feature air dryers and adjustable water temperature settings. There are also inexpensive bidet devices with hoses that attach to your sink faucet and others that are held by hand.

One cause for incontinence is the inability to see the toilet well enough to use it. This is especially a problem for men. Imagine how difficult it might be to urinate into a white toilet in a bathroom with a white floor and white walls if you have difficulty with your eyes. Lighting plays an important role here, but there are other things you can do that might help also. Install colored electrical tape on the inside rim of the toilet bowl, or replace the toilet seat with one of a different, more contrasting color. This concept can also be applied to making the sink, sink counter, bathtub, and shower curb easier to see.

Another problem with toilets: They can be used for hiding or disposing of things that shouldn't go in the toilet bowl. Child-proof toilet locks are available—but they can also make the toilet harder to use. Special care and supervision will be necessary to assist family members when they really need to use the toilet, instead of using it improperly.

Finally, consider elevating the toilet to make getting up and down easier. Arthritic knees may make sitting and getting up from low toilets painful. Raising the height of the toilet seat reduces the vertical travel distance. For men it also puts the "target" closer when they're standing to urinate. A higher toilet seat with grab bars on both sides will make using the toilet much easier and less troublesome for both your loved one and the caregiver. (See chapters 4 and 8.)

The Bathroom Door

Replace the door with a shower curtain or change the door lock. You don't want your loved one locking herself in the bathroom. A passage lock is one that opens freely from both sides and cannot be locked from either. Your lockable door knob can easily be replaced with a much safer and more convenient passage lock. Or you can hide an emergency key close by, perhaps on the door frame overhead (if you can reach it) or in an unobtrusive location.

"Becky thinks people are coming to get her. She locks herself in the bathroom and stays for hours."

You may eventually need to widen the bathroom door for wheelchair access. (See chapter 8 for more discussion and ways of widening doors.)

Emergency paramedics receive countless calls informing them that someone has collapsed in the bathroom and no one can get to him because he is lying on the floor right behind the door. Changing an in-swinging door to one that opens outward, a pocket door, a bi-fold door, or even a curtain prevents this problem.

"Last week Grandpa collapsed in the bathroom. He fell right behind the door. We couldn't open the door to help him."

One warning, however: A door swinging into a hallway or other path of traffic, if opened when someone is walking by, may hit him. Give careful thought before changing the swing of the door.

Lighting

Lighting is important in the bathroom, not only for the person with AD but also for the caregiver. Often people identify and recognize their pills by their color, size, or shape. Without sufficient lighting, mistakes can easily happen.

"My husband got deathly sick last night. We had to rush him to the hospital. I thought I was giving him his little round, pink pills, but I gave him the violet ones instead!"

In addition, lighting affects how you see yourself and how you feel. Poor lighting creates a gloomy atmosphere. It can contribute to depression.

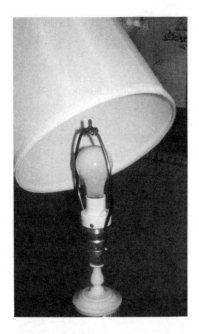

With a photocell adapter, ordinary light fixtures can be modified to turn on automatically at night.

Poor lighting also makes finding things that dropped to the floor, such as a small pill, much more difficult. It can therefore contribute to the unsuccessful completion of a task and upset your loved one, who may silently blame the difficulty on AD rather than poor lighting.

Older eyes need more light than younger eyes to perform the same tasks. If your bathroom is dark, install additional lights over the sink, in the shower ceiling, or wherever else you might need them. (Lights in the shower have to be GFI protected and vapor-proof. Discuss this with an electrician.)

Install lights or light adapters that turn lights on automatically when it gets dark. Hallway lights and lights in bathrooms located off common hallways can be controlled by photocells that automatically turn on at night and help your loved one quickly and easily find the bathroom. Photocell adapters that fit between the light bulb and the socket are available at your local home improvement center. Make sure the lampshade or cover will still fit once the adapter is installed.

If your loved one gets up in the middle of the night looking for the bathroom, walks out into the hallway, and sees a light in one doorway, she will naturally be drawn toward it. The light in the bathroom will help guide her to her destination.

Some night lights come with photocells. These too are available at your local hardware store or home improvement center.

Miscellaneous Suggestions

Sometimes confused people don't recognize their own reflections in the mirror. They may think their reflection is a departed spouse, brother or sister, stranger to be feared or fed, or friend to talk to. Except for the last category, you may want to discourage any concern over the "person in the mirror." (In the latter case, caregivers have told us stories about many pleasurable hours spent talking to the "person in the mirror.")

If the mirror becomes a problem, you can:

- remove the mirror
- turn it around
- cover the mirror

- paint the mirror with water-based paint
- paste decorative wallpaper or contact paper on the mirror.

Remove wastebaskets, hampers and other items resembling toilets (pots, planters, etc.) if they are being used as such. (See chapter 2 for more discussion on both of these problems.)

The Kitchen

Although most people don't consider the kitchen a dangerous place for adults, the kitchen is second on our list of the most dangerous rooms in your home. The unusual behavior that accompanies Alzheimer's makes trying to anticipate sources of trouble in the kitchen a monumental task. You will need to observe your loved one carefully in the kitchen. Often how she behaves during the day will provide hints of how she might behave when the caregiver is not there to supervise.

Many caregivers are very concerned about nightly visits to the kitchen. Even the thought of their loved one in the kitchen at night, unsupervised and confused, stirs up terrible images and possibilities. Modify the kitchen with two ideas in mind: safety and organization.

Safety

The kitchen is a place that you would rather make safe for as long as possible, rather than out of bounds. Potential problem areas include the sink drain, disposal, the trash can or compactor, electrical appliances, as well as the refrigerator. (See also chapter 9.)

In the kitchen, your loved one has perhaps prepared many meals, made cakes to the delight of the whole family, and demonstrated her love every day. It may be where you spend a great deal of time, and your loved one is naturally going to want to be around you and where the family action and conversations are happening. Denying her these pleasures and opportunities to contribute would be both cruel and difficult for her to understand.

The kitchen should be safety-proofed and simplified. Fewer items on shelves will simplify decisions and make items easier to find. Remove any products, appliances, or other items that may be dangerous and accessible. You may need to disconnect the disposal and remove knobs from the stove and inside the refrigerator. (See also chapters 5 and 9.)

Diminished ability to smell and taste sometimes affects people with Alzheimer's disease. This may contribute to your loved one's inability to realize that he is eating spoiled food or something inappropriate.

- Toxic products not designed or intended to be eaten, but colored, scented, and packaged attractively for marketing may be tempting. Colors, fragrances, and pictures of fruit or smiling faces on containers give wrong impressions that are easily misinterpreted by confused minds and may lead them to believe the product is tasty and harmless.
- Products intended to be eaten only sparingly can be consumed in larger, inappropriate amounts: spices, vinegar, pickle juice, vitamins, sweeteners, etc.
- Sometimes food is inadvertently left too long in the refrigerator and spoils. The person with AD may not have the ability to realize, for example, that all that fuzzy green stuff on moldy cheese is bad. Instead of throwing it out, he may eat it. Caregivers need to check the refrigerator on a regular basis.
- Some kinds of medication, such as antibiotics, require refrigeration and may be stored in the refrigerator. You may need to install a lock on the refrigerator, especially if it is used to store and keep medications cool. (See chapter 6 for more discussion and ideas on this subject.)

Don't overlook pet food and pet supplies, which are often stored in the kitchen or pantry. Some older people who grew up in the Depression when money was scarce may have been forced to eat pet food or products nearly spoiled. If those long-term memories are recalled, this behavior may not seem as unacceptable to them as it is to us. Remove pet supplies and store them in a safe place.

Remove (or hide) the temperature control knob in the refrigerator. You certainly wouldn't want the temperature to be turned up to the warmest level or turned off by your family member. You may also want to install an alarm to alert you to inappropriate temperatures in the freezer. (See chapter 6 for more information.)

Freezer alarm that alerts you if the temperature goes above 15 degrees:

Improvements, Independent Living Aids.

Burns can occur so easily in the kitchen. Night visits to the kitchen for a bite to eat can result in catching a sleeve on fire at the stove, or cooking something on the burner, then going back to sleep and forgetting to turn it off.

Some caregivers have told us that their loved ones have removed the burners from the stove and hidden things in the spaces beneath. When the burners were turned on later, the items caught on fire or melted.

Many older people use the oven for storage. After all, when you're not using it to cook why not take advantage of this extra storage space? Not a good idea! The oven can be turned on by mistake, and whatever is stored inside can catch on fire or become hot enough to burn someone.

Consider installing a child-proof lock on the oven, available at most baby supply stores and some home improvement centers. Look for other ways to maximize storage so you don't have to resort to using the oven. (See chapter 6.)

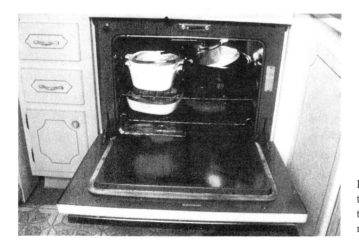

Items stored in an oven may be forgotten, catch fire, or become too hot to touch if the oven is turned on by mistake.

Appliances with automatic shut-offs:

Black & Decker or appliance dealers.

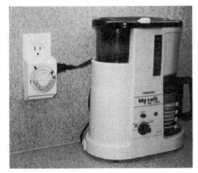

A common timer limits when a small appliance can be turned on, contributing to a safer kitchen at night.

Stove timers:

Grainger Electrical Supply, Logan Powell, or your local electrician.

Hand-held fire extinguishers:

BRK, The Fire Extinguisher Company, The Safety Zone, fire equipment supply companies or home improvement centers.

Fire extinguishers in a spray can:

The Safety Zone.

Don't overlook the microwave oven.

- "Explosive" items can be placed in the microwave— any sealed container cooked in the microwave can explode. Eggs, too!
- Inappropriate items can be cooked and ruined, including the TV remote control.
- Your loved one may put something metallic in the microwave, such as a jar with a metal cap or plate with a fork. This can damage the oven, set off sparks, start a fire, or heat up the metallic object, resulting in a serious burn.
- The microwave can heat food up to temperatures so hot that your loved one could be seriously burned trying to remove or eat it.

Disconnect the microwave, install a remote switch or timer, unplug it when not in use, or install a child-proof lock on the door. (See also chapter 6.)

When shopping for other appliances that heat (coffee makers, irons, etc.), look for those that automatically turn off after a certain period of time.

Timers can be installed in the kitchen to control electrical outlets for stoves and other appliances. They can be set to allow the outlet to be used only during certain hours, or to allow the outlet to be active only for preset limits of time: 10 minutes, 30 minutes, one hour, etc. Setting a timer so that the stove is inoperable after, say, 7:00 P.M. would guarantee a night's sleep safe from mischief involving the stove. You might also discuss with an electrician installing a pool pump or water heater timer at your electrical breaker box to serve the same purpose. Also ask him about common household timers that, if installed correctly, can limit the times when smaller electrical appliances are operable.

Install small, hand-held ABC fire extinguishers in key locations in the kitchen. ABC fire extinguishers will put out most types of fire. There should be at least one on each floor of your home. Do not locate the extinguishers right where a fire is likely to occur, but close by. In other words, do not store the extinguisher immediately next to the stove or fireplace, where fire may make the extinguishers inaccessible. (See also chapter 9.)

The RangeQueen automatic fire-extinguishing system is a unique product. Resembling a can of cat food, it comes with a magnet that attaches to the metal exhaust vent found over most stoves. Once it's in place, you just forget it. When it senses a fire, the contents inside expand, releasing a fire-supressing chemical onto the burners below. The manufacturer recommends one unit per two burners. It's no guarantee, but for those who are concerned about their loved one's starting a fire in the kitchen, this might be a great first line of defense. (Of course, once it's been used, you'll need to replace it.)

Certain utensils in the kitchen require more understanding for safe use than others. For example, a boiling tea kettle spews out raw steam that can cause serious injury. Do not store tea kettles on the stove. Put them in a safe cabinet to prevent any accidents.

And, if you own one, disconnect or unplug the instant hot water dispenser.

The kitchen is full of small objects and appliances that require skill and coordination to operate safely. Consider, for example, the sharp edge of a lid removed by most can openers. Other hazards are posed by blenders, food processors, and the garbage disposal (a popular spot for hiding and rummaging).

This might be a good time to switch to paper or heavy-duty plastic mugs and plates for everyday use. Remember, items dropped and broken are not only dangerous and require cleaning up, but they are also potential reminders to your loved one of the disease and burden he may feel he is imposing. Make sure also that you select colored plastic cups or mugs, rather than clear ones that may be difficult to see.

Remove or lock up dangerous knives, long forks, and other sharp-edged or pointed cooking implements that could be mishandled or used as weapons (if applicable). Install locks on the cabinets and drawers where they are stored.

RangeQueen fire-suppressing system:

Pyro Control.

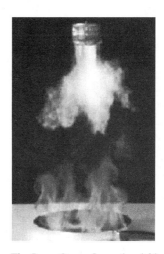

The RangeQueen fire-extinguishing system is automatic, inexpensive, and easy to install. Photo courtesy Pyro Control.

Unplug or disconnect the garbage disposal. This is not only for safety, but also to eliminate the possibility of it getting broken by a small item dropped down it, and to protect valuable items such as rings that may get hidden down there. (See chapter 6 for more ideas.)

Any portable electric appliance is dangerous, especially if it is close to a source of water. In the kitchen there may be several small, portable electrical appliances that can be touched by wet hands or dropped in the sink while still plugged in. Unplug and/or remove from the sink area appliances such as:

Can openers	Hot plates
Coffee makers	Electric teapots
Radios	Toasters
Televisions	Toaster ovens
Blenders	Waffle makers
Food processors	Bread makers

Once again, appliances do not have to be turned on to be dangerous. They only need to be plugged into an electrical socket. (Refer to the discussion on GFI outlets in the previous section on the bathroom, and in chapter 9.) Make a habit of unplugging your appliances and installing child-proof plug caps in the outlets to prevent them from being used when you're not there to supervise.

Survey your kitchen and look for appliances that are old or worn or that might not be in good repair. Maybe that hot plate that you have had for years has a cord that's a bit frayed or a bad switch. Any appliances that are not in a good state of repair should be either fixed or thrown out.

The kitchen is a popular spot for rummaging, hiding, and for removing food to be taken back to the bedroom (for the "friend" in the mirror or in case "supplies run out later"). Other potential sources of trouble in the kitchen include trash cans and trash compactors: Keys, remote controls, and other small valuables can be hidden there and ultimately crushed or thrown out.

Check your sink and drain. Make sure the trap underneath is accessible, just in case something of value happens to get dropped down the drain. Have a plumber look at your sink. If some plumbing modifications need to be made to provide an accessible trap, it is better to do it now than to lose something of value later.

Do not leave or keep bowls of small items in the kitchen or around the house. Even food such as chocolates or other candies can be dangerous if mishandled. For example, hard candy, popcorn, or nuts can cause someone to choke if they are not properly chewed and swallowed. People with Alzheimer's may eventually forget how to chew and swallow their food.

Remove stepladders that invite injury for someone who may not acknowledge his failing balance and coordination skills or recognize the side effects of his medications.

Organization

Organization is the other major consideration for the kitchen. The kitchen represents good feelings, sounds, and smells. It is also a family activity center and place of congregation. Encourage everyone in your family to continue enjoying these good feelings and invite your loved one to continue to be a part of them.

Create an environment that continues to foster the good feelings that come with raising a family or taking care of someone else. Minimize confusion by removing items that are now too difficult to understand or require skills that are no longer present. Simplify choices. Remove excess food products, utensils, and appliances. A drawer, counter, or cabinet with only a few items will be less intimidating than one full of every kitchen tool known to man. Use up or throw out extra boxes of cereal, for example, leaving only two or three to choose from.

Where possible, create a special place in the kitchen for your loved one, where she can sit, watch, and contribute to family activities safely. Frustrations may result from activities that are no longer wise for your loved one to perform, such as cooking. You may not be able to make it safe for your mother to use a blender, but you can create a special place in the kitchen for her to sit and share in other activities with you.

Stirring ingredients, setting the table, kneading dough,

folding napkins, cleaning up, and drying dishes are just a few of the things she might still enjoy. Continue to encourage as many meaningful activities for your loved one as possible. Providing her with her own space includes her in important family functions, protects her self-esteem, and prevents feelings of isolation or abandonment.

Create a simpler, easy-to-understand environment. Locate supplies close to where they will be needed. Minimize counter clutter. Store safe, commonly used items in the open or on shelving where they can be seen easily. Remove temptations and reminders of things that your loved one is no longer able to do, such as cake mixes.

Place pictures or labels on drawers and cabinets illustrating their contents. You may want to add large, readable labels to containers of frequently used drinks and foods to avoid possible confusion. (See chapter 2.)

In some cases, making the kitchen off-limits may be the only safe answer. (See chapters 5 and 6.)

The Bedroom

The bedroom is number three on our list of the most dangerous rooms for a person with Alzheimer's disease. The chief problem here is falls resulting from traveling to the bathroom, dressing, transferring (to wheelchairs), lifting and getting in and out of bed.

Simplify the bedroom as much as possible to reduce obstructions. The simpler the room, the easier it will be to get around and understand. In addition, minimize places to hide food and "stolen" articles.

Recognize, though, that for most people (and especially for those being cared for) the bedroom is a refuge and a personal space. Anyone tampering with their bedroom may be violating their privacy. Be careful when modifying your loved one's personal space, as this can contribute to agitation, delusions, or loss of trust. As much as possible, involve him in the discussion and changes you're making in his room, though understandably he may not remember later.

Empower your loved one by letting him feel the change helps you, not him. For example, move the bed against the wall to make it easier for YOU to clean the floor or put a railing on the wall because it will prevent YOU from hurting your back when helping him. This will often be more acceptable than changes made to help him!

Trips to the Bathroom

Simplify and clear the path to the bathroom. Make it as safe and direct as possible. Remove items that are difficult to see and might cause your family member to trip. Consider installing a handrail on the wall leading to the bathroom to help guide and support him along the way. Make sure the railing is strong, easy to grasp, and easy to see. One family's solution was to tie a rope leading from the bed to the bathroom, much like a railing.

Night lights along the way can help illuminate the railing and the floor. Few homes are designed with enough outlets, let alone outlets well located for night lights. Installing additional outlets may be another modification that you may want to make early. Talk to an electrician.

Paint or decorate the door to your family member's room to make it as unique and recognizable as possible. Making it different, attracting attention to it, making it stand out will go a long way to helping someone find his way back when the caregiver isn't available. (See chapters 2, 5, and 8.)

Install an intercom system or monitoring device to help the caregiver hear cries for help, nocturnal activity, or accidents.

The Bed

Sometimes spouses, who have slept in the same bed with their loved ones for years, now find that this is no longer an option, due to incontinence or nocturnal restlessness. The room may now have to be slightly rearranged, and twin beds may replace queen or king-sized.

Lower the bed. Remove the frame and the box spring. This way, if your loved one does fall out of bed, he won't have far to go. Though lowering the bed will minimize injury and reduce falls from bed, keep in mind that it will also make it more difficult to get up from bed. (See chapter 8 for more ideas on this topic.)

Wireless intercom:

Radio Shack, The Safety Zone, Solutions, or home improvement centers.

Baby Monitoring devices:

Fisher-Price, Gerber, Kids Club, The Right Start, Safety 1st, The Safety Zone, and most stores that sell products for babies.

"My husband keeps falling out of bed at night both when he is sleeping and just sitting on the edge. Last week he hit the floor and sprained his wrist."

Bed bars and handles:

AdaptAbility, Aids for Arthritis, Ali-Med, American Health Care Supply, Assist Equip., Bed Handles, Brown Engineering, Easy Street, Graham Field, J. C. Penney Special Needs Catalogue, Larkotex, LCM Distributing, Mobility Transfer Systems, North Coast Medical, Sammons Preston.

Bed railings:

AliMed, American Health Care Supply, Carex, Graham Field, Larkotex, Lumex, McKesson, Medreco, PCP-Champion, St. Louis Medical Supply.

Bed handles assist the caregiver and the person with AD when sitting on the edge or getting in and out of bed is difficult. Photo courtesy Bed Handles, Inc.

If you move the bed against the wall it will at least provide a barrier against falling out of one side. It will also help prevent the bed from moving when your loved one gets in and out.

Another solution might be bed railings or bed handles. Bed handles are small handles that attach to the side of a bed for you to hold onto and assist your loved one getting in and out of bed. Bed railings, on the other hand, are longer rails that keep your family member from falling out of bed.

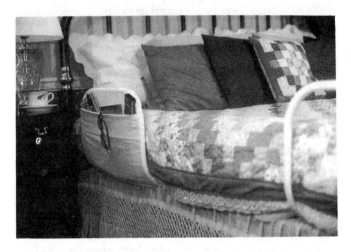

Finally, there are fall-prevention alarms that warn you of attempts to get out of bed. Some are also designed to work with chairs. (See chapters 5 and 8.)

Take a look at the electrical outlets near your loved one's bed. Are there enough or will you need more? Eventually, you may need extra outlets for normal bedside electrical appliances (a night table light, cordless telephone, radio, and clock), an electric hospital bed, and important medical equipment. Now is the time to add them, not later. Is there a possibility that you may transfer your loved one to a downstairs room eventually? Take a look at that room also.

Lighting

For a person with Alzheimer's, the world is complicated and confusing. Dimly lit rooms can add to confusion, frustration, and disorientation, making paths seem unfamiliar and rooms unrecognizable—especially to older eyes, which need as much as three times more light.

Can your loved one's bedside light be turned on from the door of his room so he doesn't have to enter a dark room? Some people forget where the bed is once the light is out. Make sure there is a light switch next to the door. If your home was designed without a light switch at the door, you can add one inexpensively. Install a wireless, remote light switch. These adhere to the wall, headboard, your night stand, or wherever you would like to place them, and look like a stan-

Remote wireless electrical switch:

Improvements or home improvement centers.

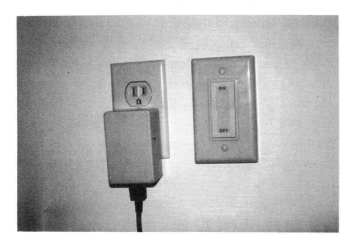

The adhesive-backed wireless wall switch (right) controls the plug-in adapter (left). Plug your lamp into the adapter, and you have a switch that controls your lamp from anywhere in the room.

dard light switch. They work like a TV remote control (the receiver fits between the lamp plug and the wall outlet), allowing you to easily control the light from anywhere.

You may want to discuss with an electrician installing (three-way) switches that will control the light from *both* the bed and the doorway.

If turning on the bedside light becomes difficult, a wireless remote switch located on the night stand might help—or consider installing a touch switch. These small devices also fit between the plug and the outlet and make it possible to turn a light on or off by simply touching any metallic part of the lamp or the cord. Some touch switches have a remote pad that you can place on the night table that allows the slightest touch on the pad to turn on the light. No more reaching, searching, or twisting little knobs or buttons!

Be aware that touch switches sometimes turn lights on due to a power surge or power shortage. Lights can mysteriously go on in the middle of the night, frightening or startling your

Touch switches and remote touch switches:

AdaptAbility, Home Trends, Sammons Preston, Westek, hardware stores or home improvement centers.

loved one. However, because touch switches also convert single-level lamps to three-level lamps, the lights usually go on dimly, making it easier for the eyes to adjust and less startling if they go on accidentally.

Sudden light is a strain on older eyes. It commonly results in temporary blindness, which in turn is a common cause for accidents. Compact fluorescent light bulbs can help. A compact fluorescent bulb replaces your regular light bulb. However, some go on at only about 25 percent of their full brightness then slowly, over about a minute, increase to full brightness. Though hardly noticeable, this allows older eyes a little more time to adjust to the change in light levels.

A dimmer switch also allows a gradual change in brightness. Dimmer switches can replace your flip switch and will allow you to turn on your incandescent light to any level that is comfortable. Dimmer switches are available at most hardware stores or home improvement centers. Any good electrician or handyman can install one for you.

Miscellaneous Suggestions

As Alzheimer's disease progresses, more time will be spent in the bedroom. Eventually your loved one will become bedbound. Early planning should take this into account. (See chapter 8.)

If reflections in mirrors frighten or agitate your loved one, remove mirrors in the bedroom. Since her image of herself may be based on how she looked years ago, she may not recognize herself now. Often reflections are misinterpreted as strangers, departed spouses, friends, or relatives.

Remove wastebaskets, potted plants, and other open containers that may be used to hide food, or as a toilet.

If rummaging and hiding are creating problems (especially with hoarding food in the bedroom until it spoils), consider installing an inexpensive surveillance camera to help discover hiding places before they become problems. Disguise or hide the cameras well. (If your loved one suffers from delusions, a visible camera may validate his concern!) One idea might be to blend and combine it with the television on a wall-mounted

---

Compact fluorescent screw-in light bulbs:

Philips Light Company, home improvement centers, hardware stores, and some grocery stores.

Surveillance cameras:

surveillance or security stores, Alsto's Handy Helpers, Canwood Products, Crest, J. C. Penney Special Needs Catalogue, Kids Club, Radio Shack, The Right Start, The Safety Zone, Vivitar, or home improvement centers.

TV shelf; or some companies make cameras already disguised as Teddy Bears, clock radios, etc. (See chapter 5 for more discussion on this topic.)

Den, Family Room, and Living Room

The den, family room, and living room, like the kitchen and dining room, are places where family activities and discussions take place. Your loved one will not want to be left out of these activities, regardless of his state of dementia or confusion. Even if he doesn't participate, listening can still be enjoyable.

To minimize potential confusion, try not to change familiar furniture layouts too much. Certain changes may be warranted, however. If pathways need to be widened or cleared, do so. Make the primary destinations easy to see and reach. Straighten pathways and simplify arrangements to create open spaces with only large, geometrical shapes and colors that are easy to see and navigate. Neither you nor your loved one should ever have to walk around obstacles to get to a destination.

Eliminate furniture that blocks routes to windows, doors, displays, or interesting table decorations. Make paths wide enough for a wheelchair or two people walking side-by-side, one assisting the other (minimum 4'-0"). (See chapter 8.)

Create a special place for your loved one to sit and enjoy views, family activities, and conversations with family and friends. Surround her with displays that represent her life and accomplishments: photographs of favorite subjects, events involving her, and items that she has made. Go through hobby magazines and find related pictures to frame. Place the items where they can be viewed by your loved one and visitors.

Be careful. If pictures of departed friends or loved ones upset your family member, causing her to mourn their loss over and over, don't use those pictures.

Locate your loved one's special place so that it allows a safe distance from "intruders." Often the main door of the home opens right into the family or living room, exposing and making your loved one feel vulnerable to strangers. If territorial issues or fear of strangers become a problem, lo-

Clock radio with hidden surveillance camera:

American Technology Network, The Edge Company, Independent Needs Centre.

cate your family member's special place in an area that has
perceptible boundaries and is out of the main paths of travel,
yet is within view of everything going on. Provide a comfortable chair for your loved one that is easy to get in and out of
and that won't be a problem if incontinence enters the picture. (See chapters 7 and 8.)

Don't forget to set aside space to store a walker or wheelchair. You'll want to have them close to your loved one's special place for both convenience and the security of knowing
they are nearby if needed.

Remove reminders of travel that might trigger desires of
wandering away from home or going to the office. These include everyday items such as hooks for keys, hat racks, suitcases, briefcases, garage door remote controls, shoes by the
door, etc.

Be extra-sensitive to what is comfortable for your loved
one. This may not be what you find comfortable. Drafty ceiling fans, scary TV programs, loud music that makes it hard to
hear, or your neighbors arguing may make him uneasy or
uncomfortable.

Background noise may make understanding and communicating more difficult. Softening the environment (adding carpeting, soft upholstery, curtains, and carpeted wall hangings)
can help absorb noise.

You may observe your loved one in the midst of a fall grasping for a wall that is ten feet away, or misjudging where the
floor ends and the wall begins. This often happens when the
floor and wall are similar colors, making it difficult for those
with visual impairments to tell where the wall begins. Consider
painting the wall or baseboard a contrasting color to make it
easier to see and to help with depth perception difficulties.

Furniture

Provide strong, sturdy furniture that will support your family
member, rather than furniture that might slide or fall over under
his weight. Avoid chairs that swivel, rock or roll, requiring skills
that your loved one may no longer have. Furniture may be
leaned upon in times of crisis or just used to steady oneself

when moving within the room. Remove chairs and tables on wheels that will move unexpectedly when leaned against.

Provide safe, "forgiving" furniture. Soft, cushioned furniture without sharp edges or corners will result in fewer and less severe injuries in cases of falls.

To make pieces of furniture easier to see, modify their colors to improve their contrast against the floor and the wall behind. This can be done by re-upholstering your furniture or simply by placing new cushions or a colored towel over the back to change its color. You could also define their edges with colored electrical tape. (Electrical tape in various colors is available at any hardware store or home improvement center.) This will make it easier for someone to see and grab the edges of furniture in the event of a fall, or just to guide himself along.

Too much patterned upholstery in a room can be overwhelming for your loved one, offering too much environmental information to be digested and understood. Solid colors for carpeting, furniture, walls, and curtains are better.

The Dining Room

The dining room is the one place in most homes where the whole family gathers together to eat and discuss the day's activities and concerns. As mentioned earlier, you'll want to include your loved one in these important activities. (See also chapter 4.)

Emphasize the features of the dining room to help your family member find and recognize it. Your dining room may have its own unique features: wallpaper, table, chairs, etc. In addition, set the table with colorful place mats and table cover to be seen, recognized, and further identify the room.

Decorate the dining room with pictures and paintings that reinforce the purpose of the room. Hang pictures of food or people eating and entertaining. Try to avoid excessive background noises—such as the dishwasher, water running in the sink faucet, or even phone conversations—to create a calm atmosphere conducive to hearing and understanding discussions.

Define tables and chairs in the dining room. Clearly outlining the edge of the table and chair simplifies the area and makes the table and chair easier to see. If the outlines are not clear, you can simply and inexpensively highlight the edges with colored electrical tape available at your local hardware store or home improvement center.

Make sure lighting in the dining room is sufficient, but not overpowering or glaring. Your family member's senses of taste and smell may not be as good as they once were. Give him every opportunity to see and recognize his food and appreciate its color and texture. The better the lighting, the easier it will be for your family member to see colors, textures and shapes; and the more appetizing the meal will appear. Lighter wall coverings and finishes will also help to reflect the light.

Do you have a chandelier over the table with multiple bulbs, each allowing a clear and irritating view of the bright filament? Replace the bulbs with frosted bulbs. They will be easier on the eyes, provide just as much light, and be less of an annoyance and distraction.

As is true for any room, too much going on in the dining room can be overwhelming to your loved one. The results may be confusion, agitation, or attempts to leave the room. Typical culprits include wallpaper or fabrics that are too busy—too many items on the dinner table, and multiple conversations and table arguments, all going on at the same time.

Professional Scotchgard carpet treatment:

3M Company or your local carpet treatment company.

Small, portable carpet cleaner:

Alsto's Handy Helpers, American Health Care Supply, Bissell, Eureka, Home Trends, Hoover Company, Improvements.

Spray cans of Scotchgard for furniture upholstery:

hardware stores, grocery stores, and home improvement centers.

Tables with perimeter lips:

Sunrise Medical.

Noise can also be a problem. Like so many restaurants, dining rooms are often designed with hard, reverberating materials. Reduce noise by softening the room with curtains and soft furniture. Also reduce background noise coming from the kitchen or other areas of your home (the dishwasher, radio, fan, etc.).

Anticipate and be prepared for accidents, spills, and messes. Protect the carpeting with Scotchgard and/or a mat that is flat and not conducive to tripping or sliding. Consider investing in a compact carpet cleaner that will clean up liquid messes as well as dry ones. Protect upholstered chairs and carpeting with plastic covers and Scotchgard.

A plastic table cloth and floor mat will protect the table and floor from spills. Some manufacturers offer special tables with perimeter lips to contain spills and prevent them from landing in your family member's lap. This is especially important when what's spilled is hot.

Offices, Workshops, Hobby Rooms

Your personal office should be a refuge, one of the rooms to be included in the Respite Zone. You store not only important papers here but also important equipment (computers, answering machines) that if tampered with could cause significant damage and loss. You need for your office space to be kept off-limits.

On the other hand, an "office" might play an important role for your family member. One of our favorite stories is about a man who gets up in the middle of the night, dresses himself, and attempts to "go to the office." To solve the problem, his caregiver creatively set up an "office" in their home (complete with typewriter, adding machine, and desk). We are told that he now spends hours "banging away at the calculator" and reading his mail. You could create a small office within your family member's own room with just a desk and a typewriter.

In the same vein, hobbies can be hard to give up. They may represent a life's worth of pleasure and accomplishment. However, some may now be dangerous and best avoided; for example, sewing may be dangerous for someone whose judgment skills are no longer what they used to be. If your loved one can no longer safely engage in her hobbies, you might surround her with products of them, such as pillows that she embroidered, awards or photos of related events.

Workshops, like offices, may be places where hours were spent in fixing broken appliances or constructing projects. Recollections rooted in long-term memory may lead your loved one to feel he still has the skills needed to use his tools, though that may now be dangerous. For example, men who enjoyed building model planes or constructing model railroads or carpentry projects might hurt themselves working with sharp tools, glue, or electricity.

The alternative may be to display the fruits of their labor and accomplishments. Create safe but spectacular displays and collections of their work. Locate them where they can be viewed by your loved one and visitors and be a source of pride and endless conversation. I'm sure each one has its own story.

If at all possible, modify the hobby room so your loved one may be able to continue and enjoy some past pleasures. For

"Dad used to be a photographer. His work was published in several well-known newspapers and magazines. We contacted a local developing company and asked them to set aside some of their photos instead of throwing them out. My brother picks them up once a week and we give them to Dad to put in his scrap book."

example, you wouldn't want your family member to develop photographs, but you could allow him to create collages of favorite photos (whether he took them or not).

If you have a hobby or workshop room accessible to your loved one, the same basic rules apply as in the rest of your home. Reduce clutter, provide room for maneuvering, and follow safety precautions. Remove dangerous chemicals, tools, and equipment. This includes paints and paint removers, photographic developers, tools that are sharp or require coordination and skill, etc. (See also chapter 9.)

In its place you could create a special area where limited activities could be performed. One with plenty of light and close to supervision, in case help is needed.

Your loved one may not be as strong or coordinated as he once was. Remove items that exceed his present abilities such as lawn and gardening tools, hammers, and saws. Failed attempts to use such tools often result in disappointment and agitation. Surround your family member with tasks and projects that he can complete. If you give him a puzzle to work on, it would be wiser to give one made up of only a few pieces rather than a few hundred.

The Laundry Room

"Momma always did our laundry and took tremendous pride in ironing everything to perfection. She won't give it up now, though we worry about her burning herself or starting a fire. So we disabled the outlet. Now she spends hours safely enjoying her ironing."

We have heard from caregivers that laundry and related activities (ironing, folding, and putting linens away) are greatly missed by those who have spent their lives taking care of their family. Unfortunately, along with the "joys" of laundry come the dangers. These include touching a hot iron, leaving the iron on or dropping it on one's foot, misusing detergents and bleaches, and the proximity of portable electrical appliances to the laundry sink.

Often laundry rooms are in remote locations where, if there were a fire or accident, it could go unnoticed for a long time. This further increases the need to safety-proof or lock your laundry room.

Relocate dangerous laundry tasks to a new location where your loved one can be supervised more easily; for example, move the ironing board to the kitchen, den, or craft area. This way dangerous irons can be put away when not in use, accidents will be easier to discover and prevent, and you can provide loving supervision.

With any dangerous electrical appliance that your loved one insists on using:

- remove the appliance and lock it up,
- place child-proof caps in all the outlets,
- disable certain outlets (see chapter 9),
- purchase and have available only lightweight appliances that turn themselves off automatically.

Faucets for your sinks and laundry tubs should be equipped with anti-scalding devices. These devices fit into or onto your existing faucet pipe. If the water gets too hot they expand and shut off the water flow. They are inexpensive and easy to install.

Provide lockable cabinets for bleach, dyes, detergents, fabric softeners, the iron, etc. Install locks on cabinets and drawers in the laundry room. This is not a complicated job; any competent handyman with a drill and a screwdriver can install them for you. (See chapter 6.)

Make sure the outlets in the laundry room are GFI (ground fault interrupted). (See chapter 9 and the discussion on how they can also be used to disable an outlet.) Install child-proof caps in the outlets. The laundry room is another room with access to both small, portable electrical appliances and water (the sink and washing machine).

Don't overlook the washer, dryer, and sink drain as potential hiding places. Any drain, including the laundry sink and floor drain, may be an attractive place to hide small items that fit through the holes. Make sure your sinks have accessible drain traps. If they don't, discuss this with a plumber.

Provide a comfortable chair in the laundry room to allow your loved one to assist and be with you as you do the wash. A small folding table would allow her to help fold or separate clothes while you either assist or continue with the laundry.

In so many homes the washer and dryer are in remote locations, sometimes down in the basement. Heavy loads may have to be carried down rickety stairs. The result is often an

Anti-scalding devices:

Accent on Living, AdaptAbility, Joan Cook, Independent Living Aids, Keeney, Memry Corporation, or home improvement centers.

Child-proof door and drawer locks:

Perfectly Safe, Rev-A-Shelf, The Safety Zone, The Woodworker's Store, and baby supply stores.

accident. If your washer/dryer is in your basement some prudent precautions might be:

- provide sufficient lighting on the stairs,
- make sure there is a light switch at both the top and bottom of the stairs,
- repair any broken steps or railings,
- provide clear indicators to alert you to the top and bottom step (see chapter 9),
- install railings if you don't have them—on *both* sides of the stairs, and
- install a telephone and a jack at the bottom of the stairs to use in case of an accident or just to catch a phone call.

Adding a small washer/dryer near the bedroom will reduce the number of trips to the "ol'" laundry room, as well as the amount of time you will have to spend there. This will be especially valued if you have to deal with incontinence, which could mean carrying heavy, damp sheets, towels, and clothing to the laundry room several times a day. Look for a small closet near the bathroom where access to water and drainage is available. Some of today's washer/dryers do not need exhaust vents to the outside of the home.

Consider your laundry room's other uses. Could they be dangerous? Many people who have cats, for example, keep the litter box in the laundry room. It is out of the way, unobtrusive, and easily forgotten. But if your loved one were to discover it, might he do something inappropriate, such as handle the contents?

The laundry room is also a candidate for flooding if someone puts too much detergent in the washer or leaves the water running. Consider installing a flood alarm that will alert you to water on the floor before it begins working its way to other rooms or apartments below.

Eventually the laundry room will probably become off-limits to your loved one and a good place to install more lockable cabinets to safely store valuable or dangerous items. Until then, you may want to restrict the laundry room so that it is used

Wireless remote telephone jacks:

Brookstone, Comtrad Industries, Hear More, Phonex, Radio Shack.

Combination washer/dryer that requires no venting:

Bendix, Equator Corp.

Stacking washer/dryer:

Maytag, Westinghouse. Also check with your local appliance dealer for compact units that fit in apartment closets.

Flooding alarm:

Home Trends, Improvements, The Safety Zone, or home improvement centers.

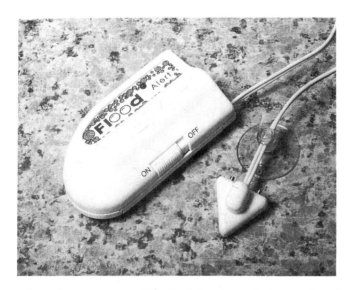

A flood alarm alerts you to water that may overflow from a sink, perhaps caused by a faucet accidentally left on. Photo courtesy Improvements.

only under your supervision. Install a strong lock or series of locks on the door. (See chapter 6 for some good ideas.)

Attics, Basements, and Cellars

Attics, basements, and cellars are rooms that fit in the category of dangerous areas that should be off-limits for someone who is confused, if for no other reason than that they are located at the top or bottom of potentially dangerous staircases. They should be protected with locks, alarms, and gates. (See chapters 5 and 6.)

Check the outside of your home for dangerous window wells. If you have windows wells that your loved one could fall into while wandering outside, it is best to install strong covers that will support a person's weight.

Hallways and Corridors

Hallways and corridors need to be kept clear. These are not good locations for furniture or decorations that can be walked into or tripped over. Remove furniture that restricts paths of travel. Pathways should be unobstructed and wide enough for two people (one assisting the other), a minimum of four feet wide. (See chapter 8.)

Be aware of items both on the ground and above—for example, shelves or lights that project from the walls at head

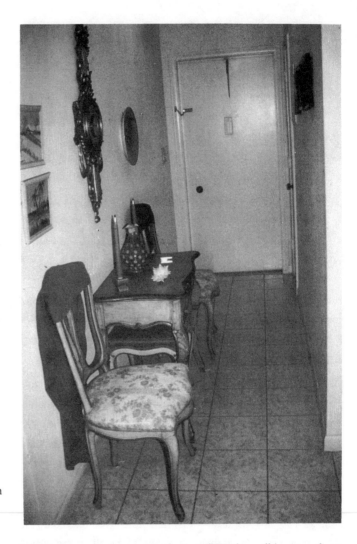

A crowded hallway is a hazard for both the person with AD and the caregiver trying to offer assistance.

height. Remember, a person having difficulty walking may focus only on what is on the floor and what her feet may trip over, completely forgetting about other obstacles. People with Alzheimer's sometimes develop a type of tunnel vision—they tend to see the world through a narrow "window," like a horse wearing blinders. Items outside the limits of that "window" may be overlooked.

Corridors and hallways are rarely properly lit. They are often shadowy, with dark carpeting and light only at either end or, at best, intermittently. Yet these are major arteries of travel within your home, used every day, over and over. Lighting should be generous and continuous, so no one has to travel through areas of light, then dark, then light. Contact an electrician and add lights if your hallways are too dark.

Place signs or labels in hallways to help direct your loved one:

DOROTHY'S ROOM

DINING ROOM $\rightarrow$

BATHROOM

Make up any excuse to put up signs that will help preserve her dignity: "Billy and Susie made them for you." (See chapters 2 and 8 for more suggestions on signage.)

Stairs, Steps, and Railings

At some point, to avoid stairs, you may feel it's in everyone's best interest to relocate your loved one to a downstairs bedroom. Though this may add to his confusion (moving out of a room that may have been his bedroom for years and into a strange, new one), it will offer several advantages:

- He no longer will have to go up or down the stairs, nor will the caregiver.
- He will now be closer to you during the day, allowing you and others to spend more time with him and making caring for him easier.
- His room may now be closer to the laundry room, so you won't have to carry heavy, moist sheets as far.
- If he is bed-bound, you'll be better able to hear him call you during the day than when he was upstairs.

Stairs and Single Steps

Meanwhile, inspect your steps and stairs to ensure that they are in good repair. Look for loose, worn or broken planks and nails that may be sticking up, and make sure all railings are secure and do not wobble. Pay particular attention to any worn or loose carpeting that could cause a fall.

Install highly visible, colored, slip-resistant strips and treads on stairs and steps. Locate slip-resistant strips at the front edge

Slip-resistant, visible treads:

American Health Care Supply, Consolidated Plastics, Mercer, Musson, R.C.A. Rubber Co., Reese.

of each step to identify it clearly, making each easier to see and understand. Cues to alert you that you've reached the first and last step are also helpful. (See chapter 9.)

To prevent unauthorized or accidental journeys up or down stairs, install secure gates at the top AND the bottom of staircases. If you only install one at the top, your loved one may go up the stairs and not know how to get back down, and may fall.

Install lockable gates at the top and bottom of outdoor stairs, too. Your family member, wandering outside, may go up the stairs leading to the second floor or downstairs to the basement. You can install a weather-resistant wrought iron gate, or have a handyman build a gate out of pressure-treated lumber. Regardless, don't overlook these dangerous steps.

Remove distractions along stairs. Anything that might distract your loved one's attention from a single step can be dangerous: She might pay more attention to the curious little boy in the painting on the wall than to where her foot needs to be placed on the stair tread. Distractions can include wallpaper with interesting figures, paintings, photographs or floor decorations. Remove distractions such as potted plants along outside steps as well.

Open stairs are distracting and difficult to understand. Open stairs have no risers (the vertical parts of each step; treads are the horizontal plates you step on) and thus allow you to see right through them while going up. This can be dangerous for people with AD for several reasons. They trigger fears of height and offer opportunities for distracting views through the steps. Open wooden stairs may be closed by adding plates to the back of each step. Those that cannot be modified might be best avoided, gated, or used with extra care.

Closed stairs are often one color: risers *and* treads. Monotone stairs can be hard to decipher, especially for people with visual impairments or difficulty with depth perception. Risers of one color and treads of another—the more the two colors contrast, the better—will make steps easier to see when going up. At the forward edge of each step place a slip-resistant, colored strip (also in a contrasting color). This makes them easier to distinguish both coming down. (The colors of treads should

Non-slip colored strips for stairs: home improvement centers.

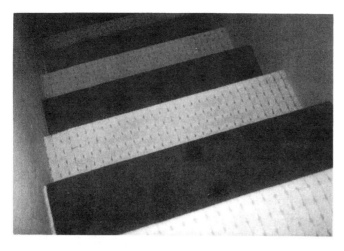

Alternating stair tread colors is an-other way to make each step easier to see.

also contrast with the normal colors of peoples' shoes—brown, black, and white).

Single steps in homes are also difficult to see. Sunken living rooms, the step from the garage to the house, and the one at the front door are often overlooked as causes of falls. Call attention to single steps by:

- installing a slip-resistant strip in a contrasting color to the front edge of the step.
- providing a convenient handrail or grab bar;
- placing a "Watch Your Step" sign nearby;
- making the step a bright color so it will be apparent to anyone about to use it; and
- adding extra light to make it easier to see.

Outdoors, you can install landscape lighting; indoors, you can have an electrician install lights in walls where they are needed. Color and railings are also successful tools for calling attention to steps.

Three-way light switches at both the top and bottom of your stairs will allow you to operate the light independently from either location, so that no one will ever have to go up or down a dark set of stairs. An electrician will be very familiar with this type of switch.

Do not place landmarks too close to single steps or other hazards along a pathway. You wouldn't want your loved one to trip and fall because she was looking at the landmark rather than at the dangerous step. Landmarks can be any items of interest, including bird feeders, benches (which she may be eager to get to), statues, etc. (See chapter 8 for more information on landmarks.)

To make it easier to negotiate difficult steps and to allow access by a wheelchair, add either a permanent or a portable ramp. (See chapter 8 for more ideas and sources for ramps.)

Railings

Railings for stairs (including stairs outside) should be easy for older hands to grasp strongly. Make sure that your railings allow your family member's hand to wrap fully around them. Older people in general need to be able to get their hands *all the way around* the railing to ensure the best grip to help pull themselves up stairways and to help prevent a fall in case they lose their balance or are having a little difficulty.

Residential railings:

IPC, Tepromark International, or have your local contractor provide and install them for you.

Install strong, secure railings on *both* sides of hallways and stairs. Often a person is more dependent or stronger on one side of his body than the other, especially if he has had a stroke. Providing railings on both sides makes the railings accessible to the user going in either direction, ascending or descending. If railings are installed on only one side, the railings and stairs may be usable by your loved one in only one direction—unless he backs down the stairs on the return trip!

Stair railing also need to extend at least 12" beyond the top and bottom steps. This allows your family member opportunity to prepare and adjust before taking the first step and after the last one.

Any long, frequently used walkway in your home warrants a railing, especially if it offers assistance to someone who may need a little help walking. Railings may have other benefits as well. (See the discussion on grab bars and railings in chapter 9.)

Locked doors along a hallway can be fitted with a grab bar or smaller railing. This will maintain the continuity of the railing for the full length of the corridor but allow access where necessary.

If a railing that is attached to the wall returns *into* the wall at either end, it can prevent sleeves and other clothing from getting caught. This also provides a cue for the user that the stairs are coming to an end.

Doors and Windows

Doors and windows, besides offering views of the outdoors, are landmarks and points of orientation, provide sources of ventilation, and bring in warm daylight to cheer up the home and make things easier to see. They are sometimes opened to let warm or cool air in when the thermostat is too hard to operate or the heater or air conditioner is "not working." They also provide opportunities to exit the house.

Doors

Doors are entrances and exits to destinations. They can also be obstacles as, for example, when your loved one's wheelchair is 26" wide and the door to the bathroom is only 24" wide. (See chapter 8 for more discussion on widening doorways and accessibility.)

Make unlocked doors in the Safe Zone easy to use. For those who have arthritis or weak hand strength, round, smooth, hard-to-grasp doorknobs and thumb latches should be replaced with door levers. Door levers are much easier to operate and require a great deal less effort. Alternatively, you might install devices that convert round doorknobs to lever handles. These conversion attachments are inexpensive, easy to install, and available from numerous manufacturers. Another inexpensive product that converts a doorknob to something more easily operated by weak or arthritic hands is a Knobble. This flexible rubber "glove" fits over the doorknob. It is ribbed and requires less gripping strength to turn.

Install locks and alarms on all doors that provide access to dangerous areas, including swimming or decorative pools, ponds, balconies, and stairs. Install locks and alarms on all exits from your home if your loved one has demonstrated tendencies to wander. Remember, the alarm will only sound if your loved one gets past the lock.

Make sure your windows and sliding glass doors are tem-

Doorknob-to-lever conversion attachments:

Aids for Arthritis, Easy Street, Extend, Home Trends, Independent Living Aids, Lindustries, Maxi Aids.

Knobbles Doorknob Twisters:

Access with Ease, Knobbles, Easy Street.

You can order a tempered glass detecting kit from

A.J. Adolfi Marketing
P.O. Box 284
Washington, PA 15301
(724) 229–9740

Fake mullions for sliding glass doors or windows:

New Pane Creations.

pered glass, not dangerous plate glass. If you have any doubt, have a glass contractor inspect your glass.

Install devices on your windows and sliding glass doors that will limit how far they can be opened. As preposterous as this may sound, people suffering from delusions have been known to take desperate measures to escape from imagined intruders or to go "home," though they may be in the house where they've lived for thirty years. Simple clamps that cost as little as 50 cents at your local hardware store can be easily installed on a window or sliding door track to limit how far it can be opened. You can set them so that a door or window can be opened enough to allow a breeze in, but not a person out. Use pliers to make sure they are tight and will not slide under force. (See chapter 6 and the discussion on balconies later in this chapter.)

Make your sliding glass door as visible as possible. You don't want anyone walking into it, thinking that the door is open when in fact it is closed. Installing decals at eye level is a good idea, but may not be enough, especially for those with tunnel vision. Fake mullions may be a better idea, making the sliding glass door more visible and camouflaging it at the same time, eliminating it as a potential exit. In the case of wanderers, this may be an advantage. (See the photos on the next page.)

Windows

Windows can be sources of discomfort if your loved one suffers from delusions of people outside or people looking in at her. Furthermore, windows are reflective (especially at night), creating images on their surfaces that may not be understood and that may appear to be something or someone they are not.

Maximize available daylight, but watch out for glare. Make your home as bright and cheery as possible. Creating the opportunity to see outdoors not only will add cheer, but also may help orient your loved one as to whether it is daytime or nighttime, summer or winter.

Take note of which windows in your home face south, east, and west. These windows may let in glaring sunlight, especially

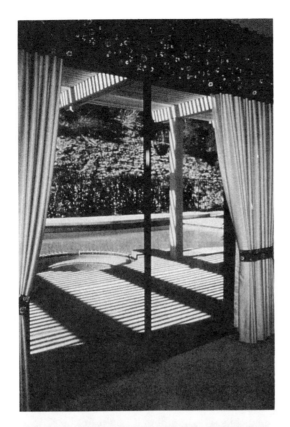

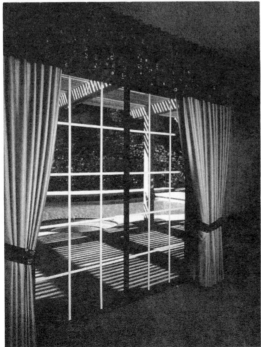

A sliding glass door may be seen as a means of escape. Those with tunnel vision may not see it at all and walk into it. Installing fake mullions solves both problems. Photos courtesy New Pane Creations.

in the morning and late afternoon. This can be very irritating during the winter when the sun is reflecting off of white snow. You may want to treat these windows to allow in filtered light yet discourage glare. To reduce glare, add exterior awnings, dark film, or window treatments such as sheer curtains, sun shields, or adjustable blinds.

Sun shields for windows:

American Health Care Supply.

Windows at the ends of dark corridors, where the light is a strong contrast to the darker indoors, can make the corridors difficult to see and understand.

Floor Coverings

Carpeting plays numerous roles in creating a forgiving and therapeutic home. It absorbs background noises and softens falls to name just a few. At the same time it can also be a problem; thick carpeting may create too much drag for those in wheelchairs or absorb odors and liquids associated with incontinence. Decisions and concessions will have to be made when deciding on carpeting or no carpeting in your home. In some areas where carpeting may play a greater role, such as the bathroom, where falls may be more likely, carpeting may be the best selection, in others it might not be.

Carpeting absorbs background noise and makes conversation easier to hear. If an older person does not appear to understand what is said to him, the problem may not be Alzheimer's. He may simply not hear you.

You have two strategies here: Identify and reduce the sources of the background noise and soften the environment. Softening the environment with upholstery, curtains, and carpeting will make a big difference, especially in areas with a lot of background noise.

Be aware of changes in flooring, such as from a smooth wooden floor to thick rugs. These require adjustments that your loved one may no longer be able to make, understand, or notice. The change in flooring thickness can be unexpected and cause a trip or fall. The change in color may also be confusing and threatening. (See the discussion on "visual cliffing" in chapter 2.)

Replace high thresholds and other "trippers" between

changes in flooring, such as carpet strips and the little metal strips that often separate carpeting from other materials. This is important, especially for those who use wheelchairs, walkers or who, like many older people, don't lift their feet when walking. This makes them susceptible to small bumps or changes in the flooring. Ask your handyman about "low-profile" carpet strips and "handicapped" thresholds that are less of a hazard.

Lower thresholds where possible. That ¾" thick marble threshold leading into your bathroom doesn't have to be that high. You can replace it with a ½" threshold tapered to make the transition easier and less of a hazard, or perhaps have no threshold at all. This will be important later on when trying to roll a wheelchair or shower chair into the bathroom.

If you need to replace your carpeting, consider a type that will help rather than hinder you. Low, uniform nap (height and thickness) carpeting creates less drag for wheelchairs and antimicrobial carpeting with nonporous backing will help with incontinence. (See chapter 7.)

Remove shag rugs. Thick carpeting can be a real problem for those in wheelchairs or use walkers, canes, or just have difficulty walking. Often elderly people walk much slower, barely lifting their feet off the ground, and eventually persons with AD need a wheelchair. Low-nap carpeting will be easier to push a wheelchair over than thick, plush carpeting.

Throw out your scatter rugs, area rugs, throw rugs, rugs with tassels, and stair runners. These villains are responsible for numerous slips and falls in the home every year. If you can't part with them, install nonslip backing to make them less likely to move or slide out from under you.

Nonslip backing for rugs:

Alsto's Handy Helpers, Harriet Carter, Home Trends, Improvements, Joan Cook, Miles Kimball, Optimum Technologies, or home improvement centers.

Replacing worn carpeting is important. I personally have been on emergency calls for victims who tripped over holes in their own carpeting, and whose feet were still caught in the carpeting when we arrived. Pay particular attention to the ends of carpeting and to stairs and other areas receiving extra wear, such as hallways. When the carpet shows signs of wear, do not try to patch it or cover holes with other rugs or cardboard. Replace it instead.

Look for carpet seams that have separated and begun to curl, creating trippers. Make sure the edges of all carpeting are secure and flat.

Shiny floors with windows beyond are the perfect formula for glare. There doesn't even have to be direct sunlight to create glare. Reflection off a white building or snow is all that is necessary to produce blinding glare. (See the section earlier in this chapter on doors and windows for ideas about reducing glare.)

The patterns and color of floor covering may also cause problems. Carpeting in a medium-toned color contrasts with most wall colors and with your loved one's shoes. A solid color will make a simpler and less confusing background. This will help people to make depth judgments and anticipate when their feet, walkers, or canes touch the ground when walking.

Patterned carpeting may be distracting and make it difficult for your loved one to understand what she is seeing. Her foot may blend in as part of the pattern or as one of the objects in the pattern. It may make it difficult to realize where the carpeting is in relation to her foot. This is especially true on stairways. Also, if anything small is dropped on the floor, such as a pill, patterns may make it impossible to find and pick up, especially if lighting is dim.

Recognizable patterns in carpeting often become objects of interest or obsession for some people with AD. It's not unusual to find a person on their hands and knees, picking at dots, flowers, or shells seen in the carpeting.

Floor coverings play a critical role in dealing with incontinence. Many caregivers insist that there should be no carpeting in a home with incontinence. However, not all of us are willing to remove all of our carpeting. (See chapter 7 for more discussion on this topic.)

Drawers, Cabinets, and Closets

Survey your home and identify those drawers, cabinets, and closets that should be kept locked and those that can remain accessible. Make sure that you provide plenty of both, as it will certainly be upsetting if your loved one cannot open any drawers, cabinets, or closets. Maximizing storage and relocating dangerous items to out-of-the-way locations will leave more drawers, cabinets and closets safe and free for your loved one to open, search, etc.

Install the right lock for the right purpose. There are locks for every purpose imaginable. Contact your handyman, local hardware store, or home improvement center. If you have a special need, contact a locksmith or a store specializing in locks. (See chapter 6 for more discussion of creative locking, which locks to use, and where to put them.)

Identify drawers and cabinets with labels and/or pictures illustrating their contents. (See chapter 2 for more discussion on ways to do this.)

If rummaging and hiding are a problem, create safe "rummaging drawers" intended to be looked through, filled with items that are interesting, removable, and harmless if lost.

Closets may be favorite places to hide things and rummage. Remove excess items stored in the closet, especially heavy items on upper shelves that could fall and hurt your loved one. The fewer things stored in there, the less likelihood there will be of an accident and the easier it will be to detect changes and discover "new" items.

To simplify your loved one's closet and make decisions on what to wear easier, remove excess clothing and items no longer worn. Take advantage of sliding doors that reveal only half the closet contents at one time, minimizing choices. Do not remove favorite items that might be missed or believed stolen, however. (See chapter 4.)

Make drawers and cabinets easy to use if they are intended to be used. If arthritis is a problem, consider replacing small, hard-to-grab cabinet and drawer handles with larger C-shaped ones that are easy to grasp and pull. On cabinet doors, install spring-loaded latches that pop open with just a push on the cabinet face, without any handles to grasp. If the absence of handles becomes a problem, use both. (See chapter 6 for some creative uses for spring-loaded latches.)

Your Home's Exterior and Yard

Consider the whole home, not just the interior. Lots of activities take place outside, so create an outdoor environment that is safe, forgiving and your loved one can enjoy.

Making Your Home Easy to Find

When preparing your home, consider everyone, not just the person with AD, but also friends, visitors, grandchildren, even emergency paramedics and doctors who may need to find your house in a hurry. There is always the possibility of an emergency, whether from a fall, an inappropriate food or chemical ingested, or some other situation.

Make sure that your address numbers are in good repair and clearly visible from the street, both day and night. In an emergency every minute counts and the sooner the paramedics can find your home, the better the chances of surviving the emergency.

Here are some ideas for making your home easier to find and identify:

Outdoor address numbers:

Brookstone, Improvements, Plow & Hearth.

- Post your address numbers in the same place on your home as your neighbors. Uniformity is a benefit, allowing those searching for your home to look in the same place from house to house.
- Post your address numbers in more than one location, making the likelihood of them being seen by friends and visitors greater. (Possibilities include over the garage, next to the door, on the mailbox, on the curb (if allowed) and on your lamp post.)
- Make sure your house numbers contrast against their background to make them visible and readable.
- Post your home's address number on the exterior with numbers that are at least four inches high (larger if your home is far from the street).
- Make sure the numbers are in a good state of repair. Numbers that are broken, have fallen off, or rotated (a 6 to a 9, for example) do little good

when someone is looking for your house, apartment, or condominium.

- If your home sits so far back from the street that the numbers on your home are difficult to see, install numbers on your mailbox and/or somewhere on your lawn.
- Remove landscaping that blocks your home's address numbers from view.
- Make sure the numbers are illuminated at night by a porch light, a post light, a street light, or a spotlight.

Make your home unique. This will help emergency personnel, as well as friends, find your home and provide a landmark to guide them.

There are adapters for your porch or front light (they fit between the socket and bulb) that will flash if you ever need to call attention to your home. Your light will operate normally until you flick the switch twice quickly, and then instead of a light that stays on you'll have one that flashes.

Yard Hazards

Few of us realize the hazards lurking in our yards until an accident occurs. This is especially true for a person with AD, who may not be so predictable. Here are just a few concerns to consider. (See chapter 9 for a more complete list and more discussion on this important subject.)

Survey all paths around your home to ensure that they are in good repair and void of "trippers," including:

- tree roots growing under pavement and cracking and lifting it
- dropped fruit or nuts on pathways
- fallen branches
- hoses and sprinkler heads
- gravel or landscaping stones
- toys belonging to children or pets.

Hallucinations and illusions are associated with AD. Eliminate

Mailbox address signs:
EZ 2C Signs

Illuminated address signs:
Home Trends, Sparkle Plenty.

Flashing light adapter:
Consumer Engineering, Radio Shack, or home improvement centers.

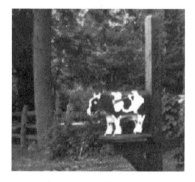

Unique decorated mailboxes make finding your home easier for visitors and emergency personnel.

"My home is the one with the cow on the mailbox."

Decorated mailboxes:
The Mailbox Factory.

potential causes by trimming landscaping around your home that creates dark areas that might be suspected of hiding strangers, that makes shapes that might be misinterpreted, or that brushes against the house on windy nights and might unnecessarily disturb your family member. Also remove yard sculptures that, with a little imagination, seem a little too real.

Remove backyard reminders of tasks that are now too difficult or dangerous to complete. This may include unkempt shrubs or gardens, the barbecue (matches and lighter fluid), swings or climbing sets for the grandchildren, pool cleaners, landscape pruning and trimming tools, etc.

Remove dangerous yard equipment that might result in injury if used by your loved one. One area often overlooked are swings, jungle gyms, etc. intended for the grandchildren. Your family member may be a little disoriented in time and feel they could be just as much fun for him or feel the need to demonstrate their use for the younger visitors, only to end up on his back in a lot of pain.

Outdoor Pleasures

The backyard is the source of so much pleasure in gardening, socializing, reminiscing, watching the grandchildren, playing with a pet, watching neighborhood activities or just enjoying the fresh air and sunshine. Maximize those opportunities.

Place outdoor furniture in a choice location in the backyard. Orient chairs and benches at 90 degrees or facing one another, rather than in one line, to make conversation easier. A good location would be a place of beauty, with something to look at, protection from wind, rain, and sun.

Make sure the chairs and benches are located where they can be seen easily from inside the house, particularly from locations where the caregiver spends a lot of time (kitchen, den, home office). It may also be important to locate the benches somewhere close by that will allow your family member to easily call or speak to you. Don't locate them near backyard equipment, such as pool pumps, air conditioning condensers, water pumps, or sprinkler pumps that make conversation difficult. Do not place portable, lightweight furniture in the yard that can be carried to the fence and used to climb over.

Take advantage of hobbies and activities that your loved one is familiar with and has performed throughout her life. Even a simple garden, if carefully planned, can provide hours of pleasure, year round, year after year. In the early stages your family member can assist in the planning, planting, weeding and watering. Once plants begin to grow, butterflies can be watched on flowers, weeds can be pulled, and vegetables can be picked. When it becomes difficult for your loved one to get outside, she can watch (and "supervise") other members of the family working in the garden. Locate the garden close to the home and where it can be comfortably viewed from favorite locations (den, porch, bedroom).

Select plants that are colorful, attract wildlife, and provide sources of pride and conversation. Imagine the pleasure you can both share when one day that tomato turns red and you both can eat it. (Several trips to the grocery store to buy more tomatoes can duplicate this pleasure, though it might involve a white lie!)

Realize that eventually your loved one may spend a lot of time in bed, so the views from the bedroom are very important. Create activity and natural entertainment for all seasons and occasions. This might include sand boxes for the grandchildren, a garden, landscaping that attracts animals and butterflies, or bird feeders and birdhouses.

Dangerous Plants

Among the problems sometimes faced by caregivers is a family member attempting to eat or taste inappropriate plants, inside and outside the home. Toxic plants include those that can make your loved one uncomfortable, as well as those that are poisonous or dangerous. They include plants whose fruit may be edible, yet leaves, stem, bark, and seeds may be toxic, and those that might contain pits that could cause your loved one to choke.

Remove toxic or poisonous plants from the house and the yard. The following are only *some* of the plants that may be toxic:

This list was modified and adapted from the Central Pennsylvania Poison Center, The Milton S. Hershey Medical Center, P.O. Box 850, Hershey, PA 17033. It is neither a complete list nor one localized for your particular part of the country.

Amaryllis
Anemone
Angel's trumpet
Apricot & peach kernels
Arrowhead
Avocado leaves
Azalea
Bird-of-paradise
Bittersweet
Black Locust
Buttercup
Caladium
Calla lily
Castor bean
Cherries
Christmas holly
Autumn crocus
Daffodil
Daphne
Delphinium
Dieffenbachia
Elderberry
Elephant ear
Four o'clock
Foxglove
Holly berries
Hyacinth
Hydrangea
Iris
Ivy (Boston, English, etc.)
Jack-in-the-pulpit
Jerusalem cherry
Jessamine
Jimsonweed
Lantana carrera
Larkspur
Laurel
Ligustrum

Lily-of-the-valley
Lobelia
Marijuana
May apple
Mistletoe
Moonseed
Monkshood
Morning glory
Mother-in-law plant
Mushroom
Nightshade
Oleander
Peach
Periwinkle
Philodendron
Plum, nectarine
Poinciana
Poison hemlock
Poison ivy and oak
Pokeweed
Poppy
Potato sprouts
Primrose
Ranunculus
Rhododendron
Rhubarb blade
Rosary pea
Star-of-Bethlehem
Sweet pea
Swiss cheese plant
Tobacco
Tomato vines
Tulip
Virginia creeper
Water hemlock
Wisteria
Yews

Some of these plants may surprise you. Many are commonly found in our homes and yards, and you may have had no idea they could be harmful.

If you have any doubt about your yard, contact your local poison control office for a list of poisonous plants common to your area. Call a local nursery or your local Agriculture Department office and ask if someone can come out to your home and check for poisonous plants in your yard and house.

Plants with thorns or spikes (rosebushes, cacti) are dangerous, especially if near a pathway where someone could accidentally fall or stumble into them. Plants that attract dangerous insects, such as stinging caterpillars, should also be avoided especially if your loved one is allergic to their stings. Check with a local nursery or Agriculture Department office to identify plants in your area that might fit into this category.

Finally, check your yard for fruit, berry or nut trees with limbs that drop their bounty on paths, creating slippery and dangerous hazards.

Wandering

Wandering can be both a constructive, healthy source of exercise and stimulation or an annoying, dangerous activity. How you plan your backyard may make the difference.

Create safe and well-planned wandering paths. Here are just a few ideas to help you start your planning process. (For more comprehensive discussion on wandering paths, what to put in them and where, see chapter 5.)

- Looped or circular wandering paths eventually lead your family member back to the beginning or to the entrance to the home.
- Wandering paths should be simple, with no side paths or dead ends requiring one to turn around to get back.
- Provide prominent landmarks at key points along the way, including at the halfway point and near the door. An appropriate landmark could be a bench, a brightly colored birdfeeder, a decorative

piece of sculpture, or a garden of brightly colored flowers.

- Trim backyard landscaping to make the entire wandering path visible and easier to travel.

Make sure your fence is high enough—a *minimum* of six feet high. Check with your local zoning department or development rules to find out what height your community allows.

"Granpa keeps asking to go home. Today he tried to go over the fence to get there!"

Fences can be climbed. It may surprise you that we warn you about this, especially when we may be talking about a frail, elderly person. Nonetheless, if your loved one does try to climb the fence, he will be neither the first nor the last to attempt this.

Make sure that your fence does not have any foot-holds on the *yard* side. (Wooden fences sometimes offer excellent horizontal or diagonal cross braces that can be used as a ladder.)

"Last week Dad climbed over the fence in the backyard. He just pushed the chair up to the fence and over he went!"

Do not store any pieces of outdoor furniture close by that can be moved to the fence and used as a ladder or step stool. Even a barbecue can be viewed as a clever (yet dangerous) boost for getting over a fence. Flimsy, unstable patio furniture or chairs and lounges that allow one's feet to go through the plastic ribs can also be a danger. Don't overreact, but do observe your family member and respond appropriately.

Gates should be locked and alarmed. To alarm the gate you might do something as simple as installing a large cow bell that sounds every time the gate is opened. Or you can be more sophisticated. Look into pool gate alarms that are designed to go outdoors and be exposed to the elements. Visit your local pool supply company for products and ideas.

Locks are better than latches. But some gates may be used more frequently or need to allow some people through and not others. A gate lock may not work for you. Outdoor gate latches usually lock automatically by either gravity or a spring. Two latches will require your loved one to operate them both simultaneously, an ability he may no longer have. Separate and locate the latches high and low, or perhaps on the outside face of your gate, beyond your loved one's field of vision. Often people with Alzheimer's do not discover locks placed in exceptional locations, making them that much more effective.

Gates can be hidden or camouflaged. Some caregivers hide gates by just hanging a sheet over them. However, hiding or camouflaging the gate is no substitute for a lock or other secure means of preventing your loved one from wandering out of the yard. Don't rely too heavily on this type of ploy. It can be figured out, especially if a walkway leads right to the gate.

Miscellaneous Suggestions

If you don't have outdoor floodlights, consider installing some. Make it as easy as possible to see real or perceived strangers that might be outside your home. Eliminate areas of darkness that could be suspected of harboring someone. Increasing the light beyond the windows also makes the glass less reflective on the inside at night, minimizing the possibility of seeing and misinterpreting a reflection.

Disconnect outdoor, automatic, motion-detecting lights that can be triggered by a dog or by someone innocently walking by the house. Pay particular attention to automatic lights visible from your loved one's room. On the other hand, if it serves you better, recognize the benefits of well-placed motion-detecting floodlights (perhaps at the corners of your home) that can alert the caregiver and point the direction of travel of a person with dementia who leaves the home at night.

Even if your backyard is safe sometimes, it may not be safe all year long. Your loved one may wander outside, into a safe yard, in the middle of winter, in the freezing cold, underdressed. You may want to alarm or place locks on doors leading even to a yard that has been safety-proofed.

Storage Sheds and Garages

Storage sheds and garages are often overlooked. We have heard countless stories of people, now deprived of their driving privileges, who have driven away on the riding lawnmower or got hurt trying to use an ax to cut wood.

Don't forget to put a secure lock on the storage shed. Both

sheds and garages are typically used for storing dangerous chemicals and tools for hobbies, pools, lawn and gardening, etc. Your loved one may no longer know what is harmful, or the proper uses for these items. Make sure that they are out of reach and that all doors leading to these areas are securely locked.

Even the simplest tools require strength, eye/hand coordination, skill, timing, depth perception, or judgment. They may be dangerous to those who no longer have these skills. This is especially true when your loved one can't admit he's having trouble. Remove reminders of tasks that are now too difficult or dangerous to complete. It is far safer to lock up tools than to deal with someone insisting on using them and perhaps hurting himself or others. Lock up or remove lawn tools, trimming tools, power tools, sharp tools, ladders, hammers, snow blowers, lawnmowers, gardening tools, etc. (See chapter 9 for more discussion on this.)

The door leading to the garage should also be locked and alarmed. Don't forget that all that it takes is the button on a remote control or a pull on the garage door to get in or out (if it is closed).

Patios, Decks, Porches, and Balconies

We all love to sit on a porch and enjoy the view or just being outdoors. However, for those with Alzheimer's disease the danger of trying to climb over the railing is very real.

Balconies are very different from porches. Porches on the first floor are usually close to the ground and relatively safe. Balconies, on the other hand, may be on the fifth, tenth, or even twentieth floor. You may realize this, but your family member (who may be recalling her childhood porch on the ground level) may not. Install an alarm and multiple locks on the doors leading to the balcony. Take steps to prevent your loved one from climbing over the railing, especially on upper-floor balconies.

There are several ways to make porches and balconies safer. Screening comes in various gauges and strengths, from fine enough to keep mosquitoes out to strong enough to keep people in. In addition, you can inexpensively and securely install additional horizontal railings to increase the railing's height, or install steel cords to provide security without hindering the view. (Check with condominium, development, or apartment authorities before making changes to the exterior of your building.)

Steel cord railings:

Feeney Wire Rope (Cable-Rail).

If there is any chance of your loved one attempting to go over the wall or railing of an upper-floor balcony, install sufficient locks on the doors and do not allow him to go out without supervision. Do not rely on additional railings or other barriers that can be overcome, no matter how unlikely or remote the possibility.

Avoid disturbing views that might frighten or agitate. Such views might include unusually loud, violent, and argumentative neighbors or dark, shadowy alleys. If fear of water is a problem this might be agitated by exposure to rain storms. Avoid porches that expose your loved one to threatening passers-by or allow them to get too close. Also avoid stagnant landscapes that may seem appealing because they are pretty, but offer no activity to watch. People here in Florida pay thousands of dollars for ocean views, but until a boat goes by they have nothing to watch.

Define personal and territorial spaces. Confused people are often threatened and intimidated by unintentional violations—people getting too close or just stopping to chat. Many are uncomfortable in social situations, and even a simple and innocent question from a passerby may be upsetting. Safe distances and lines of demarcation (such as a fence or porch railing) may create a defined and defendable space where your loved one will feel safe.

Check the edges of patios and porches. If there are drop-offs or steps that are hard to see and could result in a trip or fall, install a railing.

Inspect railings regularly to ensure that they are secure, do not wobble, and that there are no splinters. Survey your deck for warped planks and protruding nails.

Porches, decks, and patios make great areas for crafts and even for haircuts. You don't have to worry so much about spills or messing the floor, there is plenty of light, fresh air and sunshine, and lots to see.

Make your porch usable during all seasons. If your porch

is open, consider adding a roof and screening. Consider fully enclosing your porch, insulating it, replacing the screens with windows, and installing heating and air conditioning. An enclosed porch may also be convertible to a first-floor bedroom or caregiver's room at a future date. Sliding glass doors will provide a great view and can be opened in nice weather for a breeze and to allow wheelchair access.

Don't overlook the floor finish of your patio, deck, or porch. It should be smooth and the deck planks even. Canes and walkers can wobble like a table with one short leg if patio stones or sections are uneven.

Preparing your home to care for someone with Alzheimer's disease or any dementia-related disorder is difficult. Without help it can be an impossible task, reacting to crises, rather than planning for them. It takes foresight, knowledge, patience and resources. Hopefully, this chapter has introduced you to some important concerns and given you the chance to prepare.

Everybody is different. Just as the person in the mirror may be recognized, seen as a friend or a threatening stranger, each behavior and cognitive dysfunction needs to be coped with on an individual basis. There are no fixed rules.

Many of the solutions we suggest are, at best, only temporary. As the brain continues to deteriorate, the disease will eventually catch up to and surpass many of the strategies you've so carefully put in place. Your family member may outsmart a lock or pass into yet another stage, now requiring different modifications to the home. Yet many of these ideas will help and continue to help, allowing your loved one to function better in her own home environment, longer than the disease would have otherwise permitted.

The following chapters begin to deal with some of the more specific problems you may encounter. This book is in no way intended to be all-inclusive in its attempt to offer ideas and solutions, but rather to serve as a guide to direct you in looking at Alzheimer's disease with insights that are as rational as possible in an otherwise irrational world. To an experienced eye, there is often logic to this apparent madness.

2

Thinking-Related Issues

This and the two chapters that follow deal with many of the problems you and your loved one may experience with thinking, behavior, and activities of daily living. Although everyone is different and has his own unique problems, many caregivers report similar challenges. While your loved one's behavior may seem unusual, it is probably typical of the disease.

Often times your loved one is just going through a stage, and the undesirable behavior is only temporary. Some of our suggestions may solve the problems, while others may get you through long enough for your loved one to forget or abandon the behavior and go on to something else. If a specific idea doesn't work for you, a modification based on your situation and family member might. Use trial and error. Remember, what has worked for others may work for you as well.

Thinking-related difficulty (cognitive impairment) is the general disorder most closely associated with Alzheimer's disease and other dementia-related disorders. Recognizing the problems those with AD have with declining abilities to judge, reason, and calculate gives us insight into many of their unusual behaviors. Thinking-related difficulties include:

"When you've seen one person with Alzheimer's disease, you've seen one person with Alzheimer's disease."

Loss of short-term memory   Illusions
Forgetfulness   Hallucinations
Absentmindedness   Delusions

Difficulty finding things	Fear of bathing
Impaired wayfinding	Fear of water
Inability to recognize	Fear of abandonment
Difficulty completing simple tasks	Fear of strangers
Long-term memory	Fear of incarceration
Loss of self-confidence	Fear of falling
Poor judgment	Personality changes
Indecisiveness	Agitation
Difficulty reasoning	Suspicion
Inability to follow instructions	Paranoia
Impaired sense of time	Accusations
Disorientation	Loneliness
Difficulties understanding	Depression

It is sometimes difficult to separate cognitive and behavioral problems. Quite often behavioral problems are rooted in cognitive dysfunctions: Resistance to bathing (behavioral issue) may be related to the "stranger" (cognitive dysfunction) undressing them. Forgetting where a purse was left (cognitive dysfunction) may result in hiding possessions (behavioral issue) to prevent them from being "stolen" too.

Regardless, our concern here is with the home and how to modify it to help deal with these issues. Each and every one of the problems listed above is in one way or another affected, minimized, or triggered by environmental factors. Environmental factors, once recognized, can be removed and eliminated as contributors to future episodes—or you can minimize the injury or consequences when problems do arise. This book advises you of modifications, strategies, and products that you can incorporate into your own home to help you deal with Alzheimer's-related problems. The combination of good doctors, caregivers, and home modifications can, together, make caring for your loved one at home possible, safer, and easier.

Loss of Short-Term Memory

The gradual loss of short-term memory is one of the earliest and most common characteristics of Alzheimer's disease. As we investigate the problems and solutions of caring for a person with AD two basic concepts continually emerge. One is that Alzheimer's disease severs the paths of information in the brain, making it difficult to translate thoughts into actions or words. The second is that the mind seems to lose memories and information on the basis of "last in, first out." Typically in the beginning of AD only the most recent events and instructions are forgotten. As time goes by, though, information gained in the last year is lost, then in the last few years . . . eventually a lifetime of knowledge, experiences, and skills disappear.

In the early stages of AD, memory loss often goes unnoticed or is accepted as a common occurrence of aging. Some feel that Alzheimer's disease may have begun its damage as long as ten years before recognition that something is actually wrong. As difficulties surface, defense mechanisms take over: denial, attempts at covering up and hiding problems, or just blaming others. We have seen individuals very adept at the fine art of cloaking symptoms and carrying on short but relatively normal conversations with few, if any, errors. On the other hand, we have also witnessed failed attempts, though the person thought she was completely convincing.

So much of what we do depends on information learned and stored in our minds. Try to imagine what it must be like to lose your recollection of recent events: Who is the president of the United States? (To one's child) "You look familiar, do I know you?" As your family member progresses through the stages, more and more is forgotten. Products, tools, instructions—even people that have come into his life—no longer have any significance. Visits to places in the neighborhood and to friends' homes become increasingly difficult and potentially terrifying. Even rooms within one's own home of 20 or 30 years may become foreign, unrecognizable, or hard to find.

Absentmindedness

Many difficulties may center around your family member starting a project or task, then not remembering to finish it. Tasks involving the stove, smoking a cigarette, or even forgetting to

"Dad gets up at night and after washing his hands forgets to turn off the water."

Water Wand:

International Environmental Solutions, Sammons Preston.

turn off the sink faucet can lead to serious injury or damage. It is a good idea, for example, to seek out appliances and devices that turn off automatically. (See chapter 9.)

This may sound relatively harmless and insignificant until you consider the damage that might occur if the water were to spill over the sink and onto the floor. Carpeting could be ruined, and the water could go through the floor to rooms or apartments below, resulting in thousands of dollars of damage.

There are numerous products designed for other purposes that might serve you well. One of the easiest to use is the Water Wand. This inexpensive device (designed for people having difficulty turning knobs) screws into the end of a sink faucet and extends about three inches down. You leave the water turned on all the time, but nothing comes out until you push the wand, ever so slightly. When you remove your hands, the water turns itself off. You simply cannot forget to turn off the water! It works in the kitchen, too.

When using devices such as the Water Wand, however, make sure that the water cannot get too hot. Most of us are accustomed to turning on the water by rotating the hot and cold water handles. With the Water Wand, all you have to do is touch the wand—the water is already adjusted and turned on, just not flowing.

Taking extra precautions to avoid scalding is a good idea. Your family member may not realize that with the Water Wand

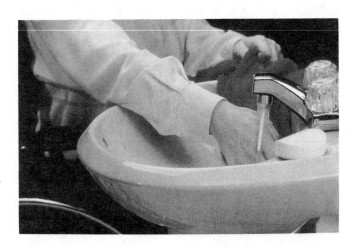

The Water Wand automatically turns the water off, eliminating the possibility of an absentminded user causing a flood. Photo courtesy International Environmental Solutions.

there is no need to turn the knobs to turn on the water. He may inadvertently change the temperature settings. Hot water may come out. In this case, the best safety precaution might be to turn the thermostat on your water heater to its lowest setting, so that the water cannot possibly get too hot.

Another possibility is a faucet with an electric eye that senses a person's hands in front of it and turns the water on and off automatically. Some electric eye faucets can be set to deliver water at a preset temperature, with adjustments made at the valves below the sink, or with a single knob on top. You may have seen these in airports or other commercial bathrooms; they are available for residential use, as well. Discuss this with a contractor who can coordinate both the plumbing and the electrical work. (Some electric eye faucets are battery operated, requiring no electrical work.)

Electric-eye faucets:

Access One, Bradley, Kohler, Speakman, Toto Kiki, plumbers, or plumbing supply stores.

Whenever possible, it is wise to incorporate multiple safety steps, looking at all the possibilities to prevent damage or injury. In conjunction with an electric eye faucet or a Water Wand, for example, consider using a flooding alarm, an inexpensive alarm that notifies you if water is detected on the floor. (See the picture on page 59.) These are commonly used in laundry rooms and basements where leaks or flooding are more likely to occur. They plug into the wall and have a remote sensor on the end of a wire that lies on the floor. If this sensor comes in contact with water, an alarm lets you know.

Flooding alarm:

DTE Edison America, Home Trends, Improvements, Independent Needs Centre, The Safety Zone, or home improvement centers.

Often problems associated with absentmindedness involve forgetting just one step in a series of steps, such as not using protective mittens when taking a hot pan from the oven. So simple, you would think—but not for a person with dementia.

Your loved one may become dependent on maps of the home and neighborhood and lists for the most common daily routines, making sure that not even the tiniest step is forgotten.

Recognize these lists and other adaptations for what they are—your family member's attempt to adapt to difficulties she is having. If she feels these reminders will help, they might be important clues for the caregiver. Take advantage of them. For example, directional signs in the home ("To the Kitchen," "To the Bathroom," "Evelyn's Room") might help when your family member is having difficulty finding her way around the house.

Difficulty Finding Things

"Mary just can't seem to find any-thing. She loses her glasses all of the time and blames everyone, claiming they were stolen."

The cause of problems with finding things isn't always Alzheimer's disease. As we age, some of our "parts" become worn and develop problems. This is especially true with our vision. It's not uncommon for vision to be the problem rather than forgetfulness. AD complicates the problem: Mary's defense mechanism may be to blame the occurrence on others, rather than on her eye problems.

Designate a place for storing glasses (or jewelry and other commonly lost items), such as a special bowl on the table. Make sure the color of the frames contrasts well with the color of the bowl (as well as the table and bedspread) to make them easier to see. Also increase lighting, and provide spare sets of glasses to replace those that get lost.

For items that repeatedly disappear, like glasses, keys, or remote controls, make sure you have spares. In the meantime, you can use the spare until the original is found.

The Smart Key Tracker, a device that attaches to your keys and beeps when you clap your hands: Brookstone.

There are also unique products, like the Smart Key Tracker, that attach to key rings and "beep" when you clap your hands. Just follow the "beeps" to find the lost keys! For larger items, like a purse, insert a battery-operated, remote doorbell—it has a longer range and it's louder. Just make sure you don't lose the doorbell button.

Signage

"Mom can't find anything in the kitchen—even things like dishes that have been in the same place for twenty years."

"Yes, my granddaughter did these for me. Aren't they precious?"

Label doors, drawers, and cabinets with pictures (and/or signs) illustrating their contents. A great source for these pictures is catalogs for general merchandise stores. They sell everything from dishes to pots and pans. What better source of pictures? Cut them out, then tape them to the outside of the cabinet or drawer. If it works, apply this principle wherever it might help, such as on bedroom drawers. This can be a great project for young grandchildren or the entire family. Instead of a necessary cue, present it as a conversation piece, a source of pride.

Consider large helpful labels on products as well . . . toothpaste, shaving cream, orange juice, milk, etc.

Alzheimer's disease blocks the neurological pathways of information traveling in the brain. This oversimplified description alludes to the remarkable ability the mind has to adapt to even severe difficulties. When one pathway does not work, the brain tries others. Your loved one may not recognize the bathroom door, but he may understand the sign next to it reading "Bathroom."

For some people with Alzheimer's disease, the ability to read and understand written words lasts way beyond their ability to reason and follow instructions. This is contradictory to the condition of aphasia that often accompanies Alzheimer's disease; we offer no rational explanation. Aphasia is the inability to recognize, comprehend, and understand words. Those who suffer from it are unable to associate the word with the actual object. It affects one's ability to read, understand signage, and communicate. Have you never desperately searched for a word that was on the tip of your tongue? With AD, however, it can affect everyone differently, and at different stages of AD. Some retain the ability to read and comprehend signs and labels long into the disease, whereas others lose this ability earlier. Some caregivers have told us that signs and labels simply do not work; others swear by them! Some individuals with AD have even made their own signs and lists.

With this in mind, remember that you may (or may not) be able to successfully direct your loved one with signage. If it helps, use signs and other environmental cues as part of a redundant cuing plan. Remember, too, that lack of success with signage may not be due to aphasia. Poor lighting or sign locations, missing glasses, or other obstacles may also affect one's ability to see and read the signs or labels.

If you do use signs or labels make sure:

- the lettering is LARGE and BOLD enough to read;
- the letter styles are simple and easy to read;
- there is plenty of light for reading;

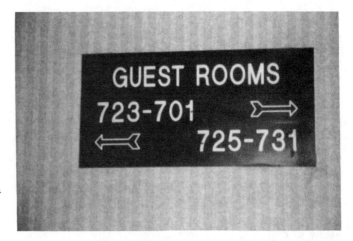

This hotel sign does not give clear information about which way to go. Make sure your signs are understandable.

- signs are located logically and where they can be seen;
- the letters contrast to the background (black letters on white or yellow background);
- the message is simple and brief; and
- the message is clear and understandable.

Good Lettering
Good Lettering
GOOD LETTERING
Bad Lettering
Bad Lettering
Bad Lettering

Including your family member's name in the sign makes it more personal and effective, making the point that the sign is intended for him.

Eliminate intermediate interpretive steps that may or may not be successful. For example, photographs of plates and dishes on the appropriate kitchen cabinet may work well, while pictures of plates and dishes drawn by your grandchildren may

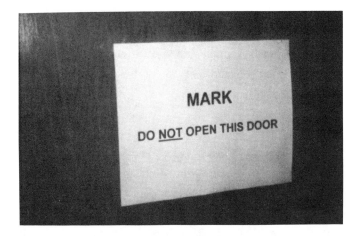

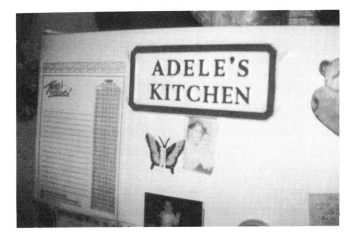

An effective sign is clearly lettered. Adding your family member's name to a sign tells him that the message is for him.

be more difficult to understand. It's better to use pictures that require little, if any, interpretation. Be direct and clear with signage, be it for the bathroom, identifying your loved one's bedroom, or directing him to the dishes and plates.

If appropriate, try using terms from the past. For someone who is relating to her childhood more than to the present this might mean "Potty" rather than "Toilet" or "Bathroom." Or it might mean words from a second language; for example, someone who spoke Spanish in his earlier days may relate to "Baño" more easily than "Bathroom." See what works!

Use redundant cuing—that is, multiple cues, rather than just one. For example, identify the bathroom not with just one sign, but with several. Leave the light on to emphasize the room and so the toilet can be seen through the open door.

Hang colorful bathroom towels where they can be seen from outside the room, add a sign next to the door that reads "Bathroom." You might try adding a symbol of a toilet or a picture of a child using the bathroom next to the door, *and* paint the door trim a different color to make it more apparent.

Placing a sign on the door may not be enough. If the door happens to be open, the sign may not be visible. Signs should be placed on the wall to one side of the door, preferably on the side from which the room is normally approached. (You may want to place signs on the door *and* next to the door.)

Do not put labels on doors, cabinets, or drawers that are locked or out of bounds. The absence of a sign or label can also be a signal, saying: "Don't open this door. There's nothing important in here." Or just make it less noticeable (when all the others have labels).

Organization

Use clear, plastic storage containers and open shelving. This allows your family member to see the contents, making them easier to see and find. It also helps caregivers who may not be familiar with where things are stored in your home. This is especially important at critical times when attention needs to be focused on your loved one, not on searching for soap or where you keep the towels.

Consider removing doors from some of the cabinets, revealing the shelves and items stored on them. Alternatively, replace cabinet doors with doors that have decorative wire screens or clear plastic panels, rather than opaque wooden panels. Avoid glass panels that can be broken and cause serious injury.

Shelf steps:

Get Organized, Home Trends, The Safety Zone, Hold Everything.

Step shelves, too, can make cans and boxes on shelves easier to see, each row of items elevated a little higher than the one in front. (Some caregivers have made their own step shelf by simply cutting a 2" × 4" piece of wood to fit inside their cabinets.)

Group kitchen utensils and ingredients according to their use. For example, put ingredients necessary for a bowl of cereal together (except the milk, maybe) so they will be convenient and

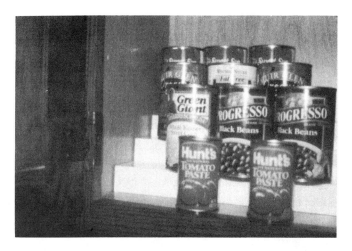

Step shelves make the entire contents of a shelf or cabinet easier to see—for the person with AD and the caregiver.

easy to find and no one item will be forgotten—box of cereal, spoon, bowl, and sugar. (This will also be a gentle reminder of *all* the ingredients necessary for the successful completion of this task.) This may also be helpful to an outside caregiver unfamiliar with where ingredients are stored in your home.

Hang utensils, pots, and pans on the walls to make them more visible and easier to find. This may also act as another cue to help your loved one identify and recognize the kitchen. Furthermore, by taking advantage of available wall space for storage, you may gain valuable, accessible storage space elsewhere in the kitchen.

Trial-and-error is a valuable tool. Hanging utensils on the wall may be a great idea for some, but if your mother has been accustomed to looking for the big spoon in the drawer for years, she may not think to look for it on the wall, or recognize it hanging there. Furthermore, what worked yesterday may not necessarily work today.

Difficulties with Multi-Sequential Tasks

The home is full of multiple tasks that we have to perform simultaneously: from preparing meals to adjusting both the hot and cold water knobs at the sink. Even carrying the groceries into the house may require one to open and close the car door while carrying the packages.

People with Alzheimer's disease often have trouble performing simultaneous, multi-sequential tasks. You might want to take advantage of this difficulty when denying access. For example, gate latches often close by gravity. Placing two on a gate requires the user to operate both at once, since if you open one, then let go of it to open the other, the first will just lock again.

Even doing the dishes requires more than one sequential task. You've got to fill the sink with water, add the detergent (just the right amount), then wash, remove, and dry the dishes. Making this a team effort and giving your mother only one of these tasks, such as drying each dish as you hand it to her, may allow her to continue to share in this satisfying family responsibility.

"Mom loved to do the dishes. She did them every night, but now she has stopped and you can tell she misses it."

Long-Term Memory

Much of your loved one's life may eventually become forgotten—her accomplishments, interests, skills, and even the personality that she has developed over the years. However, long-term memory often remains remarkably intact. Events, people, and occurrences from long ago are often remembered down to the smallest detail, while instructions just given are already forgotten. Your mother may not be able to tell you what she had for lunch only a few moments ago, or even that she had lunch, yet miraculously she can tell you how much change she received on a purchase made 40 years ago or what she was wearing that day. It is not unusual for seniors who came from another country, but have not spoken their native language for many years, suddenly to revert to speaking *only* in that tongue.

Take advantage of what *is* remembered and remains familiar. If familiarity brings comfort, then pictures, books, and other reminders of past events, people, or places are worth cultivating. Seek out photographs, articles, items picked up at a flea market, and paintings relating to earlier careers, hobbies, accomplishments, neighborhoods, cities visited, etc. Even magazines and related items may remind your loved one of memories or stimulate interesting conversations. Sometimes people with AD are better able to relate to periods long past than those that are more recent.

Preserve the life your loved one had before. Decorate his

Reminiscence Magazine is full of pictures and articles from years gone by; (800) 344–6913.

Reminiscent products:

Nasco.

favorite spaces with memorabilia. Unless it results in agitation, display your loved one's personal collections where he can enjoy and talk about them. Each item will probably have its own story, stimulating hours of conversation and pleasure.

Display awards, trophies, honors, and photos of events involving your loved one and his accomplishments. These will serve as conversation pieces, allowing your loved one to relive events over and over again.

Try using photographs of your loved one from years ago, rather than recent photographs. Your loved one may not be able to recognize herself as she looks now, but may be able to recognize herself as a child, teenager, or young adult.

This is a golden opportunity. Find a book on horses at the bookstore, flea market or at a garage sale. She can enjoy it over and over. You might cut out some of the pictures, insert them in frames, and hang them on the wall to become conversation pieces Grandma is bound to enjoy. Create an environment that surrounds your family member with pleasurable memories.

Add labels to photographs (especially pictures of family members, places, and events) to help your loved one remember who or what is pictured. Adding labels stimulates conversation and provides information, encouraging stories that your family member may enjoy sharing over and over with anyone and everyone willing to listen. For the visiting caregiver, these insights will also remind them of the wonderful and colorful person your loved one is, rather than just a patient.

Locate conversation pieces where they can be seen. As Alzheimer's progresses, your family member may eventually spend much of his time in his bed or a favorite chair. What can he see from his bed? What can he see when lying down? Give those items offering the greatest pleasure the most precious locations in the room, where they can be easily seen from the bed, lying down, such as on the night stand and most visible walls.

"Dad no longer recognizes himself in recent photographs, but he does seem to recognize himself in photos in his 1945 Army uniform."

"Grandma used to love riding horses. She just loves to listen to stories about those times."

Self-confidence

People afflicted with Alzheimer's often realize that there is something wrong much sooner than the spouse or family. Over the years, they may become very good at covering up and making convincing excuses for their absentmindedness—but eventually the disease wins. When this happens, forgetfulness, lack of judgment, and inability to make decisions may be replaced with anxiety and loss of self-confidence. Cognitive disorders may manifest themselves in behavioral disorders.

Poor Judgment, Indecisiveness

As Alzheimer's develops, decisions become more and more difficult and frustrating. At first, choosing from several items is tough, then even selecting one of two items may become too much. There may be fear and embarrassment about making the "wrong" decision. Out of anxiety making no decision may be safer than making a "wrong" one.

Activities that are easy and successfully completed may be repeated again and again. Eventually, only those decisions that are simple and safe remain in the repertoire.

Consider the advantages of sliding closet doors. Open, overlapping sliders reveal only half the closet and half the clothes to choose from, making the decision of what to wear today easier and simpler. If you feel this will help (and not confuse your loved one more), organize the closet accordingly, and remove clothes that are no longer worn or are out of season.

Group kitchen utensils and products according to their use. For example, put all the ingredients necessary to make coffee together so they will be convenient and easy to find. They'll also serve as gentle reminders of *all* the ingredients necessary for the successful completion of this task. This may also be helpful to a visiting caregiver unfamiliar with where ingredients are stored in your home.

Simplify the Environment

This concept holds no greater value than in its ability to contribute to understanding and navigating the home environment, making decisions, and finding things and places. It will be more possible for your loved one to find something familiar (and maybe help himself out of an otherwise hopeless situation) if there is less clutter, simpler and clearer pathways, and fewer distractions to confuse him. In a room with less furniture, there will be less to confuse your family member, making it more likely that he'll see the way out of the room or choose the right direction to go. On the other hand, if your family room looks like a gift shop, with knickknacks everywhere, strewn with small pillows, magazine racks, and decorator items, it will foster greater confusion and difficulties.

Create a Therapeutic Environment

As the mind deteriorates, many of the normal information paths break down. But the brain is remarkable—if it loses one way to send or receive information, it will try to come up with another. Maybe one that is not quite as good, but another, just the same.

We should help wherever possible. Incorporate subtle cues and landmarks in the home, to offer additional or new mental paths for information to travel. For example, a sign on the door and on the desk of the offiice created at home for Mr. Smith reads:

Art no longer recognized his office at home. Though he saw the books on the shelves, his desk and favorite chair, he wasn't able to make the association between them and the office he once used every day.

Art Smith
Vice President

Use redundant cuing. Add labels and signs to doors, drawers, and cabinets. If the labels don't seem to work, add pictures of the items illustrating their contents. Use multiple landmarks to orient and guide, including subtle cues that may work as substitutes for cues that are more apparent, but less successful. (See chapter 8.)

Create an environment that encourages the successful completion of tasks. This avoids both the embarrassment associated with wrong decisions and reminders of the disease that may accompany them. Taking steps to encourage the successful completion of tasks will help your loved one succeed in an environment that is making less and less sense to her. The more successful behaviors that can be positively reinforced, the better her day and the caregiver's day will be.

Encourage independence by creating opportunities for activities your loved one enjoys and can perform safely and successfully by himself. If backyard birds are entertaining, provide

Irene couldn't find her way back inside when she went in the yard to work in her garden. She would walk and walk until she had to sit down and rest. So we decided to place a chair next to the door. Now, when she gets up, she just opens the door and comes in.

a safe and comfortable place to watch and feed them. If crafts or other table activities are preferred, create a safe, maintainable area with plenty of light, views of surrounding activities, and close to supervision.

Create special places to satisfy the needs or habits of your loved one as they develop. These special places also contribute to the safe and successful completion of tasks, such as simple crafts. For example, a special place might be created in the den, in front of the sliding glass door where there is plenty of daylight (with additional lighting for evening activities). The laundry room might include a special place for your family member to sit and contribute (folding and sorting) out of reach of dangerous items. A special place in the kitchen might even allow your family member to prepare some of his own meals and help prevent delusions that "the family is trying to poison me."

Successful communication is important. As we get older, few of us are fortunate enough to be affected by only one age-related problem. Many of us have to contend with several. For example, your family member may be dealing not only with Alzheimer's, but also with difficulty hearing. If you suspect this, certainly have her hearing checked, take steps to improve acoustics, and minimize background noise in your home. This is especially important for those special places in the kitchen or laundry that may be close to the dishwasher, sink, washer, dryer or other sources of background noise that could interfere with hearing or understanding. Apply this concept to visual impairments, as well, and the importance of light, glare and furniture arrangements. (See chapter 9.)

Any and every upsetting episode that can be avoided should be avoided.

Create an environment that minimizes opportunities for accidents and embarrassments. Do not locate items of interest where your loved one may have trouble reaching them or close to other objects that can be knocked over or broken.

Remove dangerous power tools, especially for men who may have used them for a good part of their lives, either professionally or as a hobby. Quite often people with Alzheimer's don't realize that their judgment is impaired or that they can no longer use certain tools safely. These tools may represent something familiar, something that gave them a sense of pride and accomplishment. Certain tools (pruning shears, axes, wheelbarrows, etc.) require special skills, hand/eye coordination, timing, and strength that your family member may think he still has but actually does not. He may persist and try to use them regardless. The same goes for cooking appliances and sewing equipment. It's great to encourage independence and independent activities, but not if they are dangerous. (See chapter 9.)

Disorientation to Time and Place

As the mind declines, orientation may become affected, concerning time, place, and people. Your family member may lose track of time, get the days of the week confused, or not realize if it is winter or summer. Eventually he may not remember what year it is. As time goes on, your family member may not recognize his own home and may incessantly ask to go "home," even though he may have lived where he does now for twenty or thirty years. Eventually, your loved one may not recognize the caregiver, close friends, his wife, or even his own children. Although love is a strong bond and seems to be a mighty warrior in this battle, the disease usually wins.

"Uncle Mel never knows what day it is. He now calls the operator and asks her—several times a day. My wristwatch shows the day, date, and time. Are there any wall clocks available that show them also?"

Your family member's brain, though declining, is still a powerful organ. When faced with problems, it will often come up with solutions on its own. Opportunities exist, even in the most seemingly futile situations. Creativity, trial and error, and your loved one's individual strengths are some of your best tools. Keep an open mind. Look for possibilities.

Sense of Time

Alzheimer's disease often impairs the ability to recognize the correct day of the week or time of the day. This may develop into seriously inappropriate actions at inappropriate times, such as attempting to walk outside or leave home in the middle of the night.

If your loved one is no longer able to read a clock with hands, try changing to a digital one that doesn't require that intermediate step of translating the hand positions to the time

Digital clocks that display the time, day of the week and date:

American Health Care Supply (digital), Chicago Clock & Gifts (digital), Crestwood (w/ hands), Get Organized, Linden.

Large-faced and talking clocks:

Bossert, Easy Street, J. C. Penney Special Needs Catalogue, Lighthouse Enterprises, Lighthouse of Houston, LS & S, Maxi Aids, McKesson, National Federation for the Blind.

Talking calendar:

LS & S.

Talking watch:

Bossert, Easy Street, Independent Living Aids, Lighthouse Enterprises, LS & S, Maxi Aids, McKesson, TFI Engineering.

"Uncle Al goes outside in the middle of winter without putting on his coat. We are afraid he will catch pneumonia."

"Mom is always asking us to take her home. She has been living in this house for 23 years, yet she doesn't realize that she is at home."

"Ida thinks she is still living in her old hometown of Parma, Ohio (though she's really living in Florida). Every year her brother sends her a big envelope of autumn leaves—which just delights her."

of day. There are also digital clocks that display the time, day of week, and date. Some caregivers encourage the use of talking clocks that announce the time of day at the push of a button. Talking clocks are available in English and in Spanish.

Impairment of judgment, one's inability to tell right from wrong, appropriate from inappropriate is characteristic of dementia. Most of the time there is no rational explanation for wrong behavior or inappropriate decisions. But every once in a while, an environmental factor is interfering and offers some rational explanation. Removing the environmental factor may solve the problem.

With this in mind, avoid environmental contradictions. A poster of a summer scene on the wall in the middle of winter or two clocks in the same room with different times can be confusing.

"Take Me Home . . . I Want to Go Home"

Given the frustrations and disappointments that naturally accompany this disease, your loved one may be seeking the warmth and comfort of a previous time, place, or lifestyle when she was protected and comfortable. She may be seeking another, previous home, occupied by parents who nurtured and took care of her.

Another possibility is that your mother is living farther and farther in the past and that, with more recent memories gradually disappearing, she no longer recognizes her present home. No amount of logic will convince her that this is "home." For where she might be, it may not have come into her life yet.

Take advantage of items that your loved one *does remember* and *can relate to:* his name, familiar furniture, pictures that he recognizes (maybe from days gone by), and whatever else is working for him, including precious pets or pictures of grandchildren that may seem to break through the memory barriers on their own.

On the other hand, if "take me home" becomes a problem, you may have to remove items that remind your loved one of the home he used to live in and other places where he may want to return. Pictures of the old neighborhood may cause unpleasant memories. Briefcases, suitcases around the house, shoes at the door, car keys, hats on the hat rack, and other visible reminders of traveling may remind your family member of leaving for "home" (or the office).

Place appropriate cues where they will serve a purpose. For example, if your loved one wanders out the front door and then turns around to come back inside, she may not recognize her home and be hopelessly and suddenly lost. A sign at the door (Mary Jones's house) or in another noticeable location might help. Use the name she remembers. Some women may no longer relate to their married name, but rather their maiden or childhood name. Whatever name she recalls and responds to is the name to put on the sign. Though it doesn't happen often, English may not be the language that she now recognizes, especially if she spoke another language as a child. Experiment, be creative, and find what works for you.

Take advantage of items that attract your family member. If animals are something that he is drawn to, place a ceramic animal in plain sight, outside, near the door. If color is attractive, place planters filled with bright red geraniums on either side of the door and paint the pots a bold color.

Make your home as warm, comfortable, and inviting as possible. It is certainly possible that your loved one is confused by being unfamiliar with his surroundings. No home can ever replace the sense of familiarity now gone due to the disease. But an unfamiliar environment can at least be cozy. Introduce features that he likes best: favorite colors, music, paintings. What are his preferences for decorating? Does he like pictures of flowers or animals, sports, children, or Paris?

Realize also that seeking "home" could be a reaction to something else: loss of control, loss of freedom, or upsetting situations (for example, the cabinets now locked for your loved one's own safety). "Home" may represent a place where she didn't have these problems, a place of fond memories rather than restrictions and rules she cannot understand. If she were "home," she would regain this control.

Don't overlook the possibility that "home" may represent something completely different.

When I volunteered in nursing homes every Wednesday, one of my favorite people to visit was Freddy. Freddy was 76 and had suffered a stroke and two heart attacks. He was usually found sitting in his chair in a catatonic state, white and motionless. I would walk up to Freddy and tell him who I was and that I would come back in a few minutes to see how he was doing. Invariably, I would see a very slight flicker of his eyebrow, acknowledging me and my promise. When I returned 10 minutes later, Freddy would be full of color and full of life, ready for a conversation. Freddy used to tell me two things, "I'm waiting for Wednesdays and going 'home.'"

"Bessie watches the television and thinks the events on the screen are occurring right outside our living room. To her the television is nothing more than a window, and violent movies and news broadcasts are all too close to home, upsetting her to no end. Yesterday she was horrified, thinking that people were being killed in our front yard, and all day she wanted to call the police."

"Arthur swore people were coming into his nursing home room at night. As it turned out, his room was next to the kitchen, and he was hearing the staff arrive early in the morning. To him they might as well have been in his room!"

"In our home there's a portrait of my stepfather. He passed away several years ago, but we still have his picture hanging in the dining room. It looks so real that you can't look at it without waiting for him to say something! His eyes follow you around the room as you walk. It's quite disturbing for anyone, especially for someone who may be confused."

"Mom, those bugs are terrible. Let's go somewhere safe, where they won't bother us."

What Freddy, like many other depressed people, meant when he spoke about going "home" was dying. If other signs of depression point to this possibility for your loved one, consult with appropriate medical professionals.

Misinterpretations, Hallucinations, and Delusions

Misinterpretations (or illusions) are inaccurate interpretations of real objects or occurrences. For example, a breeze moving a curtain may be misinterpreted as a man hiding behind it. Sounds from war movies on television can be mistaken to mean "There's a battle going on—*right outside.*" A shadow may be misinterpreted as a deep, dangerous hole. Hallucinations are objects, sounds, smells, or experiences created and residing entirely within a person's mind (but sometimes triggered by things that are real). For example, imaginary bugs crawling on you are hallucinations. They are not real or seen by others, yet they truly exist to those experiencing them. Delusions are stories based on inaccurate, but solidly adhered to, beliefs. They result in paranoia, fears and suspicion: "Those people are after me," "He's trying to kill me," "They're beating me," etc.

Misinterpretations, hallucinations, and delusions are common with AD. Some may be caused by nothing at all, other than what is going on in your loved one's mind. Others may be triggered or caused by environmental stimuli that can be identified and eliminated: portraits that are just a bit too realistic, voices from an unseen radio or answering machine, the fan blowing the curtain interpreted to be a human stalker.

Misinterpretations and hallucinations can be experienced by all the senses: touch, hearing, vision, smell, and taste. Most commonly hallucinations are seen or heard, yet complaints of nonexistent smells (smoke), tastes, or things touching people with dementia are not unheard of. Imaginary bugs crawling on someone may be felt, as well as seen.

Look for things around the house that might trigger hallucinations or reinforce in your loved one's mind that they are real. For example, designs in wallpaper can be interpreted as bugs, suggesting to a person with AD that bugs are crawling on him, also. If your family member is constantly picking imaginary lint off clothing, maybe the white spots in nearby carpeting, upholstery, or wallpaper are the source.

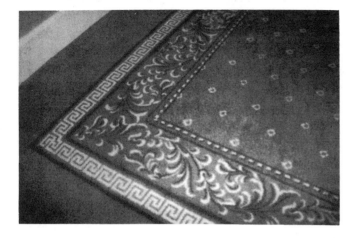

Certain designs and patterns can trigger hallucinations in the person with Alzheimer's. Can you see the white "pieces of lint" in this carpeting?

Realize also that true hallucinations may have no trigger at all and no amount of detective work will reveal their source. But you could create a special place for your loved one where she can feel safe, comfortable, and relaxed, where you can take her to get away from the hallucinations.

Examine pictures and paintings on your walls. Paintings, lithographs, photographs, portraits, or prints can be invitations for misinterpretations or even trigger hallucinations. For example, photographs and portraits that look real might be understandable sources of discomfort. Your loved one may be frightened, or want to stop and talk to them. At night, faces in pictures may be misinterpreted as people in the room. Photographs and paintings of still-lifes may appear so real that your loved one may want to touch the flower or take a bite out of the fruit.

Wallpaper should be simple with conventional patterns. Avoid designs with flowers, figures, or animals that your family member may want to talk to or pick. Even wallpaper patterns composed of repeated objects, such as boats or teapots, may be confusing and your loved one may try to touch them. Vertical stripes may suggest jail bars that might reinforce delusions of being trapped or held against her will.

"Henry goes to bed at about 9:00 every night. I used to enjoy staying up a little later to watch television until, awakened by the noise, he got upset insisting that there were people in the house— the voices from the TV. Our solution was to invest in a TV with a headphone jack. Now I can watch and listen to television using headphones as late as I want."

Headphones or wireless personal listening devices for televisions:

Deaf Products, General Technologies, Hammacher Schlemmer, Harris Communications, Hear More, HITEC, Maxi Aids, McKesson, National Flashing Signal Systems, Potomac Technologies, Radio Shack.

"Dad tells us amazing stories of being robbed, aliens, and events that he claims happened to him that very day, though I know he hasn't left the house. We eventually realized that he was just repeating what he saw on TV, as if it had happened to him."

Check your air vents and ceiling fans. Poorly directed vents that blow air on curtains or blinds can cause them to move and give the impression that someone else is in the room. Vents or fans that blow pieces of paper off a desk or table can trigger other explanations (ghosts or thieves).

Television is a common source of misinterpretations. As a person becomes more confused, it becomes increasingly difficult to recognize what is real and what is not. Quite often events on television are thought to be occurring inside or right outside the home, as if the television were a window. It is not uncommon to hear reports of mysterious people in homes that turn out only to be voices from the television or radio.

Remember that even when short-term memory is failing, long-term memory can remain remarkably intact. Imagine the fear and confusion that a veteran might experience seeing news clips of battles taking place in foreign countries! Perhaps a black-and-white television may be less realistic and easier to understand than a color set.

Misinterpretations, hallucinations, and delusions can also be caused by hearing difficulties or hearing aids. One gentleman kept complaining of radio signals in his head and people eavesdropping on his conversations. The problem turned out to be his hearing aid. Another gentleman we know kept hearing inexplicable buzzing sounds in certain areas of his home. These turned out to be the noises coming from the ballasts inside his fluorescent lights, picked up and amplified by his hearing aid. Replacing the fluorescent lights with incandescent bulbs solved this problem on the spot.

Shadows are often misinterpreted by people with AD.

Any dark place where someone "could be hiding" is an invitation for concern. Don't you remember, as a child, being afraid of the monster under the bed? There was never one under there, but I remember always checking *several* times before going to sleep.

It's a good idea to leave lights on in dark areas suspected of harboring people. Add more lights where necessary. Direct light upwards to reflect off the ceiling, distributing it more uniformly, and resulting in fewer shadows. (See chapter 9 for more discussion on lighting.)

Paranoia is a delusion characterized by irrational suspicions, feelings of persecution or mistreatment. They can range from thinking you are the devil to an unreasonable and inexplicable hatred of you or everyone. Your loved one may scream that you are trying to kill her and feel that she needs to protect herself. It's difficult to look at your loved one, a loving mother or wife of countless years, and see someone so confused that she may hurt you or someone else in the family, with little or no remorse or realization of what she did.

Observe your family member carefully and, if necessary, take precautions to protect yourself and the rest of the family. If paranoia becomes an issue, it is critical that you seek medical advice to get your loved one's delusions under control.

We don't want to advocate converting your home into a personal prison, but we don't want you waking up to find your loved one standing over you, either. If you are in danger, it is up to you to take appropriate action.

Be creative. Something as simple as a lock, a sign ("Andrew and Sally's Room"), and a wireless doorbell outside your bedroom door may allow your loved one to still find you, yet prevent unexpected visits.

If you think you may be in danger:

- Remove any and all items that can be thrown or used as weapons to locked storage areas. Survey and safety-proof your home with this concern in mind.
- Consider installing locks on bedroom doors and using them at night.
- Install motion-detecting chimes to notify you of nocturnal activity. (See chapter 5.)

Visual Cliffing

"Visual cliffing" is the misinterpretation of changes in colors as differences in depth, elevation, or planes. The dark brown area rug on the light beige floor may appear to be a deep hole.

One lady insisted that every time she walked down her hallway someone was following her. As it turned out it was only her shadow, caused by one poorly placed light fixture that created a shadow next to her every time she went by.

"Grandpa is afraid of the closet. He is constantly telling us that there is someone in there, and sometimes he even talks to them."

"Last night Arthur got out of the house and ran next door. He begged to use the neighbor's phone, claiming that we were trying to hurt him, and then called 911. When the police came, he had forgotten all about it."

"Uncle Phil has a terrible time walking in the kitchen. He thinks all of the colored squares on the floor are holes that he might step in."

The black strip of tile decorating the kitchen floor may be seen as a trench.

For someone unstable on his feet, getting past such perceived obstacles may be threatening or impossible. He may try to jump or step over the "holes," walk around them, or refuse to proceed altogether. Visual cliffing can be a hazard or a tool. (See the discussion of passive barriers in chapter 6.)

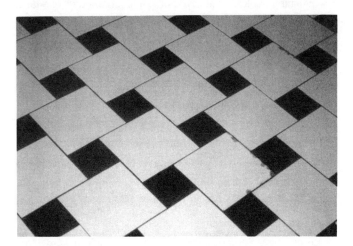

Visual cliffing causes the person with AD to perceive the dark tiles in this floor as holes.

Eliminate obstacles, *real* and *imaginary.* Dark tiles *in the path of travel* can be painted with water-based paint or covered with contact paper, which can be removed later without damaging the floor. Replace dark floor mats with lighter ones. In rooms where the problem cannot be removed or covered, install a gate to prevent unassisted access, thus preventing potential falls.

Floors don't have to be different colors to be misunderstood. Shadows can also appear to be very real obstacles. Good, uniform lighting can go a long way toward eliminating shadow obstacles. Examine your home and make sure that lighting is well-placed and sufficient to prevent shadows.

Shiny waxed or tiled floors may be mistaken as slick, slippery, or icy surfaces. Marble floors are especially a problem. Shiny, reflective flooring may cause difficulty with depth perception and judgment, making it hard for your family member to tell when her foot will touch the ground. This may cause her to fear the "slippery" floor. She may just stop and refuse to walk on it.

Mirrors and Reflections

Some suspected hallucinations may actually be misinterpreted reflections. People with Alzheimer's are often not able to recognize their own image in the mirror. Many misinterpret this "strange" person as someone on the other side of the mirror watching them (a departed spouse, brother, or sister) or a stranger in the room.

As part of my research I ride with Fire Rescue, not only to observe accidents in the home and what might have been done to avert them, but also to observe emergencies involving people who may be confused. Quite often callers report strangers in the house. More often than not, these "strangers" turn out to be misinterpreted reflections in bathroom or bedroom mirrors.

People react differently to the "person in the mirror":

- The image may be a source of fear—a stranger or a long-departed loved one. Your family member may become protective or hostile, throwing things at the person in the mirror or maybe trying to hit him. If this happens, take immediate action:
  - remove the mirror,
  - place something in front of it,
  - turn it around,
  - cover it with contact paper, or
  - paint it with water-based tempera.
- The image may become a concern. Sometimes the person in the mirror becomes someone who "requires care," often in the form of food. This food may be removed from the kitchen or hoarded at dinner time and then hidden for the person in the mirror. Often times this food is found later, long forgotten, when the smell gives its location away. Remove or cover the mirror, and the "friend" should go away, and so too the need to steal food for him.
- The image may become a friend and confidant. You might consider taking no action at all, as this newfound friend may be a source of comfort and stimulating conversation.

"Jorge won't go to the bathroom. He doesn't want to pull down his pants. He sees his own reflection in the mirror and thinks there is someone in the bathroom with him."

One lady insisted that a ghost was in her bathroom. Fire Rescue arrived on the scene and found the lady alone in her house. Even in front of them she would go into the bathroom and emerge quite upset, insisting that her TWIN sister (who had died several years ago) was in the bathroom!

"Aunt Betsy talks to the lady in her bathroom mirror. She steals food from the dinner table to feed her. It's only her reflection, but we can't convince her of that."

Often, the image people with Alzheimer's have of themselves is one of several years or even decades ago. Anything more recent may be completely unfamiliar and unrecognizable . . . a stranger.

Full-length mirrors can be particularly alarming since they show the entire figure of the "stranger," making the image that much more believable. Even a momentary glimpse of a figure in the mirror can be cause for alarm. Many institutions for those suffering from dementia disorders eliminate mirrors entirely from bedrooms, beauty parlors, and other areas.

Your family member is probably unaware of most of her behaviors. If she knew she was doing certain things or looked the way she does, it might be disturbing to her. For example, if your loved one looked in the mirror and saw herself ruminating (a muscular disorder that appears as a continuous involuntary chewing behavior), it might be alarming and upsetting.

Mirrored walls can be confusing. It is not unusual to hear stories of someone unable to find his way out of even a small bathroom where there appear to be several doors, some of them reflections of the real one. Especially confusing are mirrors facing one another and creating the illusion of infinity, and mirrors on abutting walls creating an illusion similar to images found in fun houses.

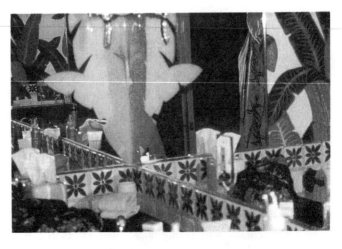

A mirrored wall can be very confusing for the person with Alzheimer's, who cannot distinguish between the real room and the reflection.

Occurrences that are normal, common, and understandable to you may be terrifying for someone who is confused. For example, your loved one's own reflection in a window at night might appear to be someone looking in from the other side.

Windows can reflect images of people in the home (for example, people walking in the hallway). Provide shades or curtains to block these images, as well as to calm fears of being watched from outside. Window treatments (curtains, verticals, venetian blinds or sheers) can serve multiple purposes: beauty, minimizing glare during the day, and eliminating reflections in the glass at night.

Images on television screens, lights, or numbers from digital clocks can be reflected in glass, both day and night, to the surprise of even those of us who have no cognitive impairments. I have also heard stories where a person's bedroom door was left open at night and the reflection of people walking outside their door was seen in the television screen and thought to be ghosts! Reflected images can easily be misinterpreted by a confused person and the event be mistaken by a caregiver for a hallucination. Take steps to recognize and eliminate potential misinterpretations that will avoid stress for both your loved one and the caregiver.

Even the glass used to frame photos and lithographs can be a source of disturbing reflections. Using nonbreakable nonreflective Plexiglas (available at local framing stores) to frame photos and paintings will prevent injury from accidental breakage. It will also eliminate the reflection of images that may be misinterpreted when your family member looks closely at the pictures.

Fears

It's hard to imagine a world so surrealistic that no one and nothing is familiar, where things as simple as a fork or a set of keys have no understandable meaning or significance. Where everyone is a stranger, and they all keep telling you that you know them, but you don't. Where "strangers" undress and bathe you, whether you want to be bathed or not—a world run by someone else's rules that you just do not understand. And what we don't understand, we naturally fear. Is it any wonder that some people

"Dad gets extremely upset at night. He is convinced that people are outside his window, looking in at him!"

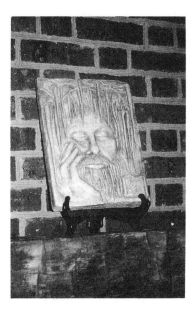

A piece of sculpture like this could be both frightening and confusing to a person with AD, who might interpret it as someone else in the room or even possibly stuck in the wall.

One lady lived in a very fine Alzheimer's care facility. Understanding her strong love for her family, and especially for her grandchildren, the staff encouraged her to put pictures of her grandchildren up on the wall. The family became involved and one day brought pictures of all of the grandchildren, blown up to make them easier to see. They sat down with her and cut out the faces of the children and pasted each of them on the wall in her room. Soon incessant blood-curdling screams and crying came from her room, but no one could figure out why. Finally, someone realized that the faces (only), cut out and pasted on the wall, appeared to her to be her own grandchildren "stuck in the wall," with only their heads protruding!

with Alzheimer's get frustrated to levels of violence and agitation? That there are such things as catastrophic reactions?

Fears may manifest themselves in unusual ways. For example, jealousy, accusations, or the need to know whom the caregiver is talking to on the phone may represent a loved one's fear of abandonment. A need to pick imaginary lint, dust incessantly, or rearrange things around the home may express the fear of no longer being needed.

After all, what we don't understand we naturally fear. For someone with dementia there may be much that is not understood: overwhelming environmental stimulation, people and rooms that are no longer familiar, objects that no longer make any sense. Look around your home. Many of us sacrifice logic for what we think is beauty.

Fear of Bathing

Fear of bathing is common for people with Alzheimer's disease. Bathing is not a simple task, but rather a series of multiple tasks: undressing, adjusting the water temperature, washing, drying, etc. Furthermore, being no longer in control or allowed to make decisions about when, how, or why to bathe adds to confusion and frustration. The natural reaction is resistance. As the disease progresses, a lack of familiarity and understanding of surroundings may be the final straw to transform misunderstanding into fear. Consider this partial list of potential bath and shower-related fears:

- fear of the loss of privacy
- fear of losing control
- fear of water
- fear of an unfamiliar room or place
- fear of being abandoned in the bathroom
- fear of being burned or scalded
- fear of falling or slipping (see chapter 8)
- fear and confusion caused by bathroom noises (flushing toilet, fan, open windows)
- fear of the water's depth (some people with AD cannot accurately perceive depth)

- fear of being bathed by a "stranger" (though it may be a spouse of 40 years)
- fear of showering (some older people may never have taken a shower before or in their youth, only baths).

Don't overlook life experiences. Some older adults are survivors of wars and concentration camps, where showers represented something very different. These far away images are well-seated in their long-term memory, and may surface just enough to create some very real fears associated with the shower or bathroom.

What might "that room" and being forced to bathe in it represent for Esther? As mentioned earlier, Grandma Esther had once been in a concentration camp, where showers were recognized as places of death and torture.

For this lady, the answer was to sit her mother on a seat in an empty tub and bathe her with a hand-held showerhead. No longer forced to enter a pool of water, she had nothing to fear. To add a little extra security a grab bar was installed, so she always had something to hold on to, even standing in the shallow water collecting at her feet.

These are not typical examples, but they show how important the past is, and that you may need to do some detective work to understand what is going on in the mind of your loved one.

Another issue might be fear of the bathing process itself or loss of control. Many caregivers feel that fears are based on what the caregiver might do with the water (splash it, get it in her eyes, etc.). Perhaps she is living in her past and it is traumatic to violate parental "voices" telling her not to get her hair wet. Maybe your family member is concerned about having her hair look just right and is anxious that it will be ruined by the water. Some individuals get upset when they are unable to escape or control the water spraying from the showerhead. As you can see, there are many possible reasons.

There may also be a fear of water. Almost every researcher, caregiver, and gerontologist has his or her own theory on this subject. Some speculate that it might be based on a fear of the

"Grandma Esther hates her showers, grasping everything within reach to stay out of 'that room' and holding on for dear life."

Another caregiver found no rhyme or reason for her mother's fear of water, which she had for fifteen years. After further discussion, the daughter mentioned that her mother had almost drowned as a child. Apparently, the problem was only partly due to Alzheimer's, and partly to a previous experience, embedded in her long-term memory.

"My husband won't get into the tub. He says it's too deep and he won't be able to get out."

water's depth (helped along by failing depth perception), others point to concerns over:

- being scalded
- being immersed
- drowning (based on a childhood experience)
- getting water (or soap) in the eyes
- getting one's hair wet (or face or bandages)
- the force of the water coming out of the faucet
- falling into the water and not being able to get out
- splashing and noises (shower spray or the bathtub filling)

Some caregivers explain that it's the water's lack of tangible features that makes it difficult to understand (your hand goes right through it), thus fear of the unknown. Others theorize that the anxiety comes from the sounds of the water or an inability to understand where it is coming from.

Whether there is actually a fear of water, or what might be done with the water, is hard to determine. Fear of water may just be fear of water. Sometimes it is impossible to apply a rational explanation to an irrational concern.

Make your bathroom as comfortable and homelike as possible. Provide soft towels, plenty of light, and warm colors—things we associate with comfort and home. Add cute pictures of children bathing that reinforce the purpose of the room and reflect good feelings. (See chapters 1 and 4.)

Make the Bathroom as Safe as Possible

Anticipate resistance, agitation, and even violent behavior. (See chapters 4 and 9.) Your bathroom should include grab bars, non-slip or slip-resistant floor finishes (in the shower and tub and on the floor in front of them), a shower or bathtub seat, and a hand-held shower head. These measures won't guarantee a perfectly safe bathroom, but they are a great start.

Softening the bathroom environment will absorb some sound. Providing carpeting on the floor, towels on the wall, and curtains on the windows will also help. Consider installing sink and bathtub cascading faucets (available at your local plumbing supply or home improvement store) that don't splash, but rather slide the water into the tub, gently and almost silently. If there appears to be a concern about getting into the water, provide a bathtub seat so your family member won't have to sit in the water. (See chapter 4.)

Smaller, darker bathrooms seem to be more frightening. Darker rooms appear smaller, the more light you introduce into a room the larger it miraculously appears. The colors of the walls, towels, and flooring can all play a role. Adding a light, especially in the shower or over the tub, can help as well. Do you have a larger, brighter bathroom somewhere else in your home that would be more comfortable for your family member?

Your loved one may not be able to perceive the bottom of the tub. This may be particularly true for darker-colored bathtubs, since darkness is associated with distance and depth. Install a light-colored, slip-resistant tub mat that will help define the bottom of the tub and bring it closer.

If your loved one is afraid of being immersed in the tub, maybe a bathtub insert will be helpful. A bathtub insert is either a full or a half tray that fits on the tub and allows your loved one to sit and bathe higher, rather than down in the bottom. A half tray is similar to a bath seat, and a full tray runs the full length of the tub. (See chapter 4 for more discussion of bathtub inserts and their benefits.)

However, if your loved one is afraid of the tub, consider converting your bathtub to a shower. Talk to a local contractor to see how viable this option is for you and how much it might cost. If you go to the trouble of converting your bath to a shower, we strongly recommend that you consider a wheelchair-accessible, roll-in shower. There are companies that offer conversion kits to replace your bathtub with an accessible shower. (See chapters 4 and 8.)

Offer More Control

Install grab bars that allow your family member to control his rate of descent and offer something to grasp when standing, sitting down, or getting up in the shower or tub.

"Cousin Bert used to be in the Navy. He spends hours telling us stories of his voyages to the Orient and South America. But when it comes time for his bath he won't go near the tub, screaming loudly that we are throwing him overboard!"

Bathtub inserts:

Clarke Healthcare Products, Diversified Fiberglass Products.

Roll-in wheelchair-accessible shower kits:

Aqua Bath, Clarion, Concept Fibreglass, Fiberglass Systems, Invacare Continuing Care, Kohler, Lasco, National Bathing Products, Swan Corporation, Tub-Master, Universal-Rundle, Warm Rain.

"Grandma Marilyn goes crazy the minute she sees the bathtub full of water. We can't get her to take a bath. What can we do?"

Bathtub seats:

Activeaid, AdaptAbility, Aids for Arthritis, Easy Street, ETAC USA, Frohock-Stewart, Graham Field, Guardian Products, Invacare Continuing Care, Judson Enterprises, Lumex, McKesson, North Coast Medical, R. D. Equipment, Sammons Preston, Sears Home HealthCare Catalogue, St. Louis Medical Supply, Wheelchair Warehouse, and home medical supply and home improvement centers.

Hand-held showerhead assemblies:

Access with Ease, Alsons, American Health Care Supply, Guardian Products, Jalco, Lumex, M.O.M.S., Sammons Preston, Sears Home HealthCare Catalogue, Shamrock Medical Equipment.

Install a bathtub seat. This way Cousin Bert or Grandma Marilyn can enter a dry bathtub, sit down, and be gently showered rather than stepping into a pool of water of unknown depth or a raging spray of water. Your loved one can enter a dry bathtub and have the water gently fill while sitting there.

Look for hand-held showerheads (which your loved one can hold herself and control) that have a pause or on/off control on the hand-held head itself. These showerheads also have other advantages. You can bathe your family member partially, protecting bandaged areas or a woman's hair from getting wet. You can also better control the water and check its temperature. A hand-held showerhead also allows washing private areas without requiring your loved one to stand and turn around.

Fear of Abandonment

The fear of being left alone or abandoned is also common among Alzheimer's sufferers. Shadowing, or following the caregiver like a puppy, is a possible indication of this concern. Though a delusion, it makes perfect sense. Alzheimer's robs people of their cognitive abilities, yet they many retain some insight into and concern about their condition. They may further be concerned about being a burden to their caregiver and about the possibility of him or her leaving as a result of "being so much trouble." Imagine how frightening it might be to realize, even for brief moments, that you can no longer take care of yourself, that nothing makes any sense anymore, and that there's perhaps only one person that you recognize and can rely on for help. What would you do without that person?

Difficulties with short-term memory add to the problem. There may be no true sense of time. Your disappearance for only a few seconds may seem to have taken hours or perhaps feared permanent. Simply walking out of the room can trigger this fear, and there is no argument in the world that will convince your loved one that you left the room for only a second. (See chapter 3.)

Eliminate the need to leave your family member alone—even for only a few minutes. Maximize storage in the bathroom, den, and favorite rooms around the house to prevent having to leave your loved one to go get something. Remove furniture that blocks or restricts views from favorite chairs. Provide an intercom in the bedroom next to the bed allowing you to answer calls from other locations in the house, such as the kitchen or your bedroom.

At night, to help your family member find you, close the doors leading to other rooms and leave your bedroom door open. Adding a hallway night light may also help by serving as a beacon. (See also chapter 5 for notification devices to notify you of nighttime activity.)

Wireless intercom:

Radio Shack, The Safety Zone, Solutions, or home improvement centers.

Fear of Strangers

Not all strangers are feared. Workers that come into the house and loved ones that are no longer recognized may or may not be feared. In fact, they may become newfound friends.

Fear of strangers and the inability to recognize a family member, even of twenty or thirty years, is not uncommon. Though we cannot offer any suggestions on improving the recognition of "strangers," we can make suggestions for avoiding or dealing with the resulting behavior.

What environmental needs would *you* have if *you* were threatened by a stranger? One thing you would need is your own space, providing a safe distance or buffer zone between you and the "intruder."

Create definable space and lines of demarcation, distinguishable features of the environment that, if passed or violated, mark an intrusion on one's personal space. As long as these lines are not crossed, the intruder is respecting your loved one's space and "keeping his distance." Features such as the porch railing or fence in the yard create lines of demarcation separating your family member from those who walk past your home. Inside your home lines of demarcation can be defined by room boundaries or the way the furniture is set up within a room. They can also be created by applying colored electrical tape to the floor.

Personal space can be violated by anyone. Children playing, traffic paths within the home, pets, even caregivers can get too close. Create space for your loved one by arranging furniture or locating his chair so that he can observe from a safe distance and

"To my father, everybody's a 'stranger.' He no longer recognizes Mother or us. When real strangers, like the TV repairman, come into the house he panics and becomes hard to control."

The most precious territory you possess is your own space.

not feel violated. This will be important to the success or failure of special places that you create for your loved one.

One way to allow your family member private space in her own room and still allow her to see what is happening outside is to replace the bedroom door with a Dutch door. A Dutch door is cut in half horizontally in the middle to create two independent sections, a top and a bottom. When the top is open and the bottom closed, it provides a necessary barrier to protect personal space and at the same time allows your loved one to see and hear everything going on outside her room. (Dutch doors are also a kind means of confinement and restraint.) An alternative to a Dutch door might be a child-proof gate in the doorway or even a screen door. (See also chapter 6 for more discussion of Dutch doors.)

Don't isolate your loved one. He needs socialization as well as personal space. Make your changes based on current concerns, balancing his needs for personal space and socialization with his fears and behaviors. Realize, too, that environments can be changed as soon as the "strangers" leave, to make it possible to again interact with friends and family.

Fear of Incarceration

Freddy was clearly upset by the mullions on the windows in his room. As it turned out, in his youth he had been in jail. The horizontal and vertical "bars" (actually the wooden mullions) on his windows triggered unpleasant memories of this experience—he thought that he was in jail again.

In some cases, behavior is triggered by environmental cues that caregivers may not be able to anticipate. Personal history is a big factor.

Imagine how your loved one might react to this wallpaper if he once had a bad experience with imprisonment. As attractive

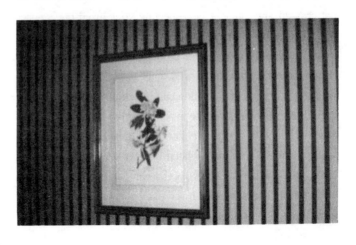

Striped wallpaper can reinforce the delusions of incarceration.

as the wallpaper is, can you see how vertical stripes might be interpreted as bars of a jail cell? Imagine how upsetting they might be to one who suffers from a delusion that he is being confined against his will or trapped in an unfamiliar place.

Suspicions and Accusations

As mentioned earlier, thinking difficulties often manifest themselves as behavioral difficulties. The *thinking* problem of forgetting where one put one's false teeth may result in *behavioral* accusations that the caregiver has stolen them. Look for environmental clues. If you can discover a possible cause that can be eliminated, modified, or controlled—perhaps you can eliminate a trigger that may be causing the problem. (See also chapter 3.)

Often a person with Alzheimer's will hide something, then later discover it is missing. Not remembering that she hid it herself or where it is hidden, she is likely to blame someone else. This does several things: It takes her off the hook, contributes to her story of denial, and allows her to avoid responsibility for her forgetfulness. Unfortunately, this scenario often leads to becoming fixated on the missing object so adamantly that delusions and agitation result.

Accusations are often a form of denial, of avoiding the recognition and acceptance of any cognitive impairment or of the disease itself. It is far easier to blame someone else than to accept the fear and terror of a progressive, mind-robbing disease. Allow your loved one this dignity and look for ways to minimize the episodes. (See the section on hiding and rummaging in chapter 3.)

Install hooks on the wall clearly displaying valued clothing, your loved one's cane, etc. These are items frequently thought stolen.

Buy duplicate items. When an item, such as your mother's favorite red dress, is repeatedly believed to be stolen (and is actually at the cleaners), consider having more than one red dress. Hang one in plain view so it cannot be said to be stolen—and if it is, you can simply point to it: "Mom, it's right over there," or "Mom, you're wearing it."

"Aunt Rody calls almost every day, begging me to come get her and help her escape. She says that they (my cousins) are forcing her to stay there and she wants to go home. (She is at home.)"

"My red dress has been stolen."

If your loved one mistakes his own reflection in mirrors for a stranger in the house, this may reinforce the idea that there is someone in the home who might be stealing things. It gives her further reinforcement to hide things (for safekeeping) that won't be found later, which will reinforce the "stolen red dress" story still further. (See the sections earlier in this chapter on reflections and mirrors.)

"Uncle Ed locks himself in his room and dials '911.' He claims that people are trying to hurt him."

In this case it would be a good idea to disconnect or remove the telephone from Uncle Ed's room and change the lock on his bedroom door to a passage lock (one that is not lockable from either side). Also notify your local 911 emergency system that your loved one has Alzheimer's and is confused. If the system is advanced enough, this information can be added to its database.

Many suspicions become delusions (stories created to rationalize confusion). Almost all delusions bear some bit of truth. A curtain moving in the breeze at an open window is real, but not so the story of people coming through the opening and stealing the remote control. Once recognized, such a problem can be easily resolved by closing the window.

Isolation and Loneliness

The kitchen in many homes is a hub of activity, where meals are cooked and eaten and the day's activities are discussed. In other homes this hub may be the dining room, family room, den, or living room. Everyone wants to be included in family activities. No one wants to be excluded or left in the back bedroom while the rest of the family is enjoying themselves, discussing the days events or working together, including those who may be confused. Make it possible to include your loved one in family activities. (See the discussions earlier in this chapter on special places.)

Encourage socialization with friends and family. There is a reverse correlation between socialization and depression: the more contact and interaction with people, the less despair.

Make socialization and communication as easy and comfortable as possible. Be aware of background noises (air conditioners, radios, televisions, even kitchen sounds) that may hinder conversation and interfere with hearing the other person. Organize your furniture to invite conversation by arranging chairs and sofas to allow people to sit facing each other. That way they can see the subtle facial expressions and body gestures that contribute to hearing and understanding a conversation. Even people who are confused can be receptive to body language.

Depression

Patient Depression

As any caregiver will tell you, positive mental attitude goes a long way, not only in avoiding depression and catastrophic reactions, but also in helping the caregiver, and sometimes miraculously improving the medical condition of your loved one. The opposite is true as well: Depression and negative mental attitudes can have detrimental effects.

Depression is a common problem with 25 to 30 percent of people with Alzheimer's disease. Some observers feel that depression is a reaction to the disease and your loved one's realization that he is no longer able to complete normal everyday tasks or the realization of what the future may hold. Others conclude that depression is a result of the deteriorating brain.

People with Alzheimer's are often found crying, tearful, or seemingly depressed. Ask them why, and the response is often "I don't know" or "I'm just not the person I used to be." Agitation and hostility, too, can be signs of depression and concern. Depression can also give rise to agitation, thoughts of suicide, combativeness, and resistance to guidance and directions, further complicating the tasks of the caregiver.

Depression should be dealt with by qualified medical professionals. (Ask your doctor, or contact a local chapter of the Alzheimer's Association for more information.) However, the environment can play a role in helping your family member and caregiver cope. Creating a more caring and pleasant en-

"Daddy used to be an engineer, now he gets terribly depressed at not being able to assemble a simple puzzle."

"Mom won't let anyone do anything for her."

"Grandmother sits in her chair most of the day clutching a doll, as if it was her baby."

"George used to sit in his favorite chair in front of the window for hours at a time. He rarely said anything and seemed to be perfectly content doing absolutely nothing. He was one of the happiest men I knew. Depression was the farthest thing from his mind."

Music from the "good ol' days":

Collectors' Choice, Elder Books, ElderSong Publications, Hammatt Senior Products, HeartWarmers, Nasco, Potentials Development, Senior Products, Sound Choice, Wireless.

Video Respite Tapes:

Barbara Jacob Productions, Cross Creek Recreational Products, Innovative Caregiving Resources.

vironment will go a long way toward helping your loved one maintain her dignity and self-respect for as long as possible.

Things are not always as they appear. Though your loved one may be staring out of the window for hours at a time, he may not be depressed, but involved in life review. This may appear to outsiders to be stagnant inactivity, when in fact your family member may be actively and pleasurably engaged in reminiscence.

What makes your loved one smile?

- Pictures, phone calls, visits or simply discussions involving the grandchildren?
- Watching children playing outside or walking by the house?
- Pets? Feeding backyard animals?
- Discussions of her past?
- Familiar music?
- Favorite colors, smells, and sounds?
- Reminders of the "good ol' days"?

A note of caution: Some caregivers have reported that music, though well-intended, has caused their family members to become distraught over not being able to remember the words to favorite sing-a-long tunes. More often than not, however, the words and pleasures found in these older songs lie deep in their long-term memory and surface with the familiar melodies.

Create a bright, cheerful home that wards off depression. Use pleasant colors, paintings, and pictures of happy subjects (children, puppies, kittens, humor, sports, and personal favorites). Put up pictures that reflect joyful times and people having fun, such as scenes of musicians or children playing. Pictures reminiscent of your loved one's career and accomplishments may be particularly interesting and stimulate hours of conversation.

Dark homes can cause depression, eye strain, and fatigue. Bring plenty of sunlight into the home (but be careful of glare). Some researchers have suggested that too little sunlight or a dark home may even cause "sundowning" (agitation or depression that consistently occurs for people with dementia in the later part of the day). Increasing the level and quality of lighting in your home can do wonders for everyone's attitude. This may be more true in the winter months when days get shorter, providing less light per day.

Provide more flattering lighting in your home. Few of us are lucky enough to grow more beautiful as we age, and as we age most of us would probably prefer not to be reminded. (If this were not true the cosmetic industry would certainly be in a lot of trouble!) With this in mind, install the most complimentary lighting possible, particularly in rooms with mirrors. Use full spectrum light bulbs or incandescent bulbs (rather than fluorescent ones) that are higher in the warmer colors (yellows and reds, rather than blues or greens), especially in the bathroom and anywhere else where there's a mirror. Also avoid clear light bulbs with harsh, glaring filaments.

How you look influences how you feel. Lighting can have a significant impact on your appearance and mental attitude. The better we look, the better we feel—about our appearance and ourselves. Make it possible for someone who is still concerned about her appearance to look as good as she possibly can.

Further complications arise when people with AD do not picture themselves as they really are, but rather as they remember themselves from years ago. If your loved one is living in the past, his image of himself may not correspond to his reflection. He may not perceive himself as old and therefore may not recognize the man in the mirror. Poor lighting will only make matters worse by presenting an image even harder to recognize.

Alternatively, if the reflection in the mirror is too depressing to your loved one, it may be worth removing or covering mirrors. Reminders of aging and a frightening condition can cause people to feel glum.

Bring in the outdoors! Eliminate any dark, closed-in feelings in your home. Open curtains and raise shades to bring in more sunshine, make the home's interior brighter, and allow better views of the outside and entertaining activity.

Once you have maximized the view of the outdoors, give your family member something to look at. Install birdfeeders

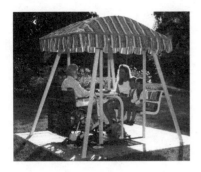

Rocker gliders allow one or more to comfortably sit and rock outside. Options may even include platforms for wheelchairs. Photo courtesy WhisperGlide.

Rocker Gliders:

Broda Enterprises, Outside the Ordinary, WhisperGlide.

and plants that attract wildlife: birds, squirrels, chipmunks, butterflies, etc. Consult your local nursery to determine what plants are most successful in your area. If there is a local chapter of the Audubon Society in your area, call them for their suggestions.

Invite the grandchildren to come to Granpa's and Granma's house to play. Install a sandbox or other safe play structure. Locate it in the backyard in clear view of Granpa's or Granma's favorite chair or bed.

Create a garden project for the family with flowers and vegetables selected by Granpa and Granma. Maybe a waist-high garden could be built that would involve everyone from planting to picking the flowers. Consider selecting plants that benefit not only the human family members but also the local wildlife—choose plants that produce berries and attract birds (for hours of pleasure watching and enjoying the fruits of your labor). (See the list of suggested reading at the end of this book for resources on accessible gardens.)

Surround your loved one with reminders of his greatest accomplishment: his family. Make collages of family photographs. Work with your loved one and the family to pick out the photos to go into the collages. Display them where they can be seen and discussed. (Don't forget to put labels on pictures of the people, pets, and places in the pictures.)

If they cause a problem, remove pictures and photographs of *departed* loved ones. Portraits of deceased family members may require caregivers or friends to explain over and over that these people have died. This may create unnecessary, repeated episodes of mourning and sadness, as their passing is experienced and re-experienced. It may also cause discomfort to your friends, visitors, and outside caregivers who may not realize that the people in the photos have passed on or who may not be accustomed to dealing with people with dementia.

Failure is upsetting. Create an environment that is conducive to success. Make it easy to find things. Open-faced cabinet doors, stepped storage of shelf items, and labels on doors and cabinets make contents more visible and offer subtle reminders for those who have difficulty remembering or finding things.

Loss of one's ability to maintain her home can also be depressing. Simplify your home's environment. Less clutter, fewer objects on tables, and fewer pieces of furniture give the home a cleaner, simpler, less intimidating appearance. It will also be easier to keep clean and may make it possible for your family member to do some of the tidying herself.

A person must continue to believe that she is serving a valuable purpose. Modify the home to help her perform everyday activities. Often for women, two key rooms are the laundry room and the kitchen. If these rooms cease to be user-friendly, affecting her ability to carry out "family responsibilities," then her contribution and value to the family may be perceived to be significantly diminished.

Provide whatever is needed to help her maintain self-confidence and her ability to perform daily activities, even if they are only folding laundry or drying dishes. In the laundry room, for example, make it easy to find things by storing safe items on open, accessible shelves in plain, easy view. Label boxes of detergents to make them easier to understand and harder to use improperly. In the kitchen, labels on cabinets and food containers may also help. And lighting is always a factor. If you have trouble seeing, you are obviously going to have trouble performing tasks that require you to see, not to mention reading the labels.

Take steps to minimize accidents and resulting injuries. Every accident and forgotten event may be a reminder to your family member of his condition. It doesn't matter if the accident was unavoidable or the forgotten event was one that any of us might have forgotten. To him it may be a depressing reminder of his disease.

"An active mind is a healthy mind." I don't know who originally said this, but it holds truth even for those with Alzheimer's disease. Provide your loved one with activities and choices that keep her mentally active and challenged. Boredom is sometimes a cause of depression.

Keep your loved one physically active. Keep him busy and provide opportunities for exercise. There is less depression when one is involved in enjoyable and thought-provoking ac-

No one wants to be or perceive himself to be a burden to someone else.

For some the vision of growing older and realizing declining abilities is cause for depression.

tivity. Create a path in the backyard or around the house and walk it with him each day. Place interesting landmarks along the way. This can become a daily routine that you will both enjoy. Be sure to make the path wide enough and safe. Watch out for "trippers" and other hazards along the way. (See chapters 5 and 9.)

Simplify the environment and safety-proof your home. Remove unnecessary furniture and items that can be knocked or tripped over and cause accidents—potentially depressing symbolic "failures." (See chapter 9.) Locate cleaning supplies close by that help in minor emergencies, such as spills, incontinence accidents, small items that get broken and have to be swept up, etc. Being able to clean up accidents quickly may make the upset easier to forget, minimizing the trauma.

If your loved one finds them depressing, remove reminders of activities, hobbies, and projects that are too difficult or dangerous to continue to perform, such as sewing, knitting, needlepoint, carving, building model airplanes, or barbecuing in the backyard.

Caregiver and Family Depression

Those afflicted with Alzheimer's disease are not the only victims of depression. While not all persons with AD realize they have a problem, their family and caregivers are usually devastated. They get depressed as well, sometimes severely. Perhaps as many as two-thirds of all caregivers are affected by depression. Don't overlook the well-being of the caregiver and family regarding depression and efforts to modify the home.

With this in mind, the Respite Zone in your home is that much more important. Make sure that all family members have spaces of their own and ways to be by themselves, grieve, be alone, take care of personal matters, or enjoy brief, but valuable, periods of normalcy. Many families work in shifts. When you're off, you need to be remote and isolated from the problems you wish to escape. (See chapter 1 for a discussion of the Respite Zone.)

Suicide

Suicide, though rare, is a subject of much controversy regarding Alzheimer's and other dementia-related disorders. In the early stages, when planning and carrying out a plan is still possible, a few people with AD may have commited suicide, maybe to avoid what they felt the disease would bring or the burden they might impose on their family. Some caregivers, empathizing with their suffering loved one, may even assist and then take their own lives. Whether true or not, it is well worth mentioning and taking the appropriate steps to prevent.

This book describes numerous steps that you, as a caregiver and family member, can take to lighten the heavy load that Alzheimer's places on your loved one and family. By making it possible for your loved one to remain at home, you may make this period in her life a lot more endurable. We hope so.

If suicide is a possibility, discuss it with the appropriate medical professionals. Bring it up in your support group and take precautions around the house, such as removing all weapons (and ammunition), keys to the car, and any medications that could be dangerous if taken in excess.

The Joy of Pets

Pet therapy is common and well recognized. Many institutions seek out and hire people to bring in pets for residents to hold, talk to, and play with, recognizing the immeasurable benefits of a friendly, furry pet.

Pets also can be the surrogate objects of maternal or paternal responsibility that may fit the period in which your loved one may be living. You certainly cannot re-create her baby, but you can introduce a warm, cuddly, furry surrogate. A call to your local veterinarian or animal rescue organization may be all that it takes to find a new-found love and companion that is already trained and house broken.

Taking care of someone else—a child, spouse, or pet—is an important factor in one's self-image. It is also an important part of one's life; a responsibility and source of pride for per-haps many years. The loss of a loved one can be soothed, or a reversion back in time can be successfully indulged by sub-stituting a cuddly pet for the child or spouse. (A common sight in geriatric institutions is an older lady refusing to give up her doll or "baby.")

A conversation doesn't have to make a bit of sense to be pleasur-able. Maybe that's one of the ad-vantages of talking to pets!

Pets make great friends. A dog or a cat will sit in your family member's lap for hours listening and enjoying his com-pany, asking no questions, and requiring no explanation, no matter how little sense his conversation makes. Furthermore, your family member can't be embarrassed about anything he says to a cat or dog.

In countless facilities I have watched smiles appear on oth-erwise smileless faces, created only by the appearance and feel of a furry cat or dog. I have personally witnessed a man's loving, devoted pet bring him out of catatonic states, consis-tently, when no one else could. Just the feeling of the small dog running up and down this man's rigid body brought a smile to his face. The puppy didn't care if he drooled or said anything. The smell of his master and the sheer pleasure of just being with him was sufficient for the two of them.

Another benefit that a dog might offer is its keen nose and ability to find food hidden in your loved one's room. This might be the key to eliminating food hoarded and hidden in the bed-room. (Talk about being turned in by your best friend!)

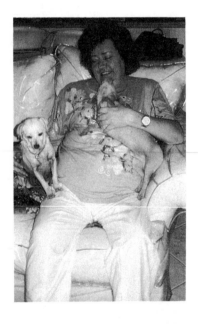

Pets can be wonderful therapy—they don't ask questions or make correc-tions. Photo courtesy Barbara Cusano.

Playing with and walking a dog may be good exercise for both your loved one and the dog. If you do decide to get a dog, at least in part for this reason, be prudent in your selection. Do not get one that is too big and could pull your family mem-ber or cause a fall. Avoid pets that are too frisky. They can overwhelm your loved one, who may not know how to deal with so much energy. Also be sure the dog that you get has a good disposition.

Be sure your pet is healthy (and has all of its shots). If you are worried about taking care of the pet, call your local veter-inarian. Some actually make house calls for older customers who may have difficulty bringing their pets to the clinic.

Make it as easy as possible to take care of the pet. Needless to say, a family member who has difficulty getting around should not be needlessly burdened by taking the family pet for a walk. Select your pet carefully. A puppy or overactive animal may be too much for your loved one and cause more problems than solutions. A fenced backyard and a pet door may be all that is necessary to resolve this problem. Remember also that smaller pets make smaller messes and require less food!

Pets make great diversions. Who can turn away from a warm, soft cuddly animal, even in times of agitation? The purring, loving cat or snuggling, devoted dog is a friend who asks no questions and shows no favoritism, even to those who are confused.

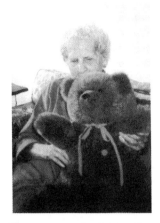

Photo courtesy the Spinoza Company.

Many housing developments will not allow pets. If your loved one can't keep a pet, consider a stuffed animal or even putting up pictures of puppies or kittens. In the absence of a live pet, you may be able to substitute a doll or stuffed animal. They don't have to be real—they can all bring smiles and comfort.

Finally, don't forget wildlife—or stuffed animals. We have heard stories of caregivers who have attempted to encourage animals and wildlife by putting up birdfeeders, *unsuccessfully*. When the birds didn't come, they placed fake, stuffed birds in the feeder that were then always there when their family member went to look for them. It wasn't exactly honest, but the pleasure gained made up for the chicanery. (The same holds true for ceramic squirrels, frogs and turtles that can be placed in the garden.)

The soft, cuddly Spinoza Bear, which contains a cassette player and comes with prerecorded tapes:

Nasco, the Spinoza Company.

This chapter offers a lot of suggestions. You certainly do not have to incorporate all of them. Some will be appropriate and helpful, others may not apply to your situation at all.

Remember, support groups and day care programs are vital tools for keeping your loved one at home. We strongly urge you to seek them out. Contact your local chapter of the Alzheimer's Association or Area Agency on Aging to find out about meetings taking place in your area.

3

Behavioral Problems

"All behavior has meaning." This statement has been repeated by numerous experts in the field of aging. Behavioral problems are often related to cognitive issues. Your family member may hide his "valuables" because when looking in the mirror, he saw someone else, a "stranger"—the very "stranger" who has been hiding all those items now missing, or who may steal his possessions. Hoarding may be triggered by recollections of childhood memories (such as the Depression) that have no relevance at all today. His present home, full of hard-to-understand rules—times for meals and baths, enforced by "strangers"—may no longer be comfortable or represent what a home is supposed to be, so the more familiar "home" (recalled in his long-term memory) may be sought.

Potential behavioral problems are many. Here just a few:

misplacing items	withdrawal
hiding things	declining social skills
hoarding	eating inappropriate items
rummaging	abnormal sexual behavior
shadowing	wandering
dependence	repetitive actions
resistance	repetitive questioning
aggression	picking at things

combativeness   leaning

"sundowning"   "stalling"

catastrophic reactions

Rummaging, Hiding, and Hoarding

Rummaging, hiding, and hoarding are common activities among those with dementia. Rummaging is the constant searching for things. Once found or collected, these items may be either hidden or hoarded. Hoarding is the constant collecting of articles, much like the proverbial squirrel putting food away for when it might be needed.

Almost anything perceived as valuable can be hoarded or hidden. Rarely is there any *apparent* logic for the items of choice. Money, saved under the mattress in earlier days, may find its way there again. Food is commonly put away for "safe-keeping." Unfortunately it often gets eaten or discovered long after it's edible.

Hidden or misplaced articles may reappear anywhere. Checkbooks may be stored in the refrigerator, or keys in the sugar bowl. The TV remote control can wind up under the sofa cushion, food put away in bedroom drawers or a zippered pillowcase (now a purse). More often than not, both the act of hiding and the hiding place are forgotten. Upon discovering that something is missing, your family member may accuse you or others (real or imagined) of stealing.

"Uncle Sam hides the mail (checks, bills, packages, etc.), forgets, then says the mail never came."

Hiding can result not only in accusations, but also denial. This might be a cover-up for your loved one's condition, having forgotten where he put something, or a failure of his short-term memory. It is a lot easier to accuse someone else than to accept responsibility for having forgotten where you put something—a reminder of this dreaded disease. Denial is a lot easier than acceptance.

The stealing delusion may be connected to a concern that "people" are in the home and taking things. Misinterpreted reflections in mirrors may reinforce the belief that there *is* someone else in the home performing this mischief. Your loved one may even have conversations with these "strangers."

Rummaging and hiding may also be an effort to mark and protect possessions, in reaction to your loved one's inability to recognize people around him. If everyone is a "stranger," he may feel the need to hide his valuables. Ironically, however, the more things that continue to disappear, the more necessary it may become to hide and safeguard remaining possessions!

Items may disappear for days and all kinds of suspicions may arise, only to end (temporarily) when the "lost" item is found in Uncle Sam's drawer, in the wastepaper basket, or under a "secret" cushion in the living room. Some caregivers report their loved ones removing the burners on the stove and hiding their caches in the cavities below. Other dangerous yet favorite hiding places include the garbage disposal, the kitchen sink drain, the trash compactor, and the toilet.

Hiding may also be unintentional, a symptom of the disease. For example, the milk may have just been put away in the dish cabinet by mistake. Such innocent slip-ups can be avoided if you minimize the number of wrong locations that are available. Locks on some cabinets and drawers can reduce the number of remaining locations to misplace items. Simplicity and organization within rooms can make misplaced items more noticeable.

Rummaging, on the other hand, is scrounging and searching for things (of "value" or "need"), logical or illogical. It often takes on obsessive characteristics and becomes a chronic daily activity. Items of choice often make no sense to you whatsoever (hangers, cardboard boxes, rubber bands, paper napkins, paper towels, toilet paper, plastic bags, etc.), but all the sense in the world to your loved one.

Rummaging and hoarding, if not controlled, can get out of hand. Often hoarding becomes an obsession, with extraordinary quantities of similar items collected and stored, as if the world were running out of Oreo cookies. We have heard stories of people who rummage in garbage day after day, collecting useless trash and storing it in their homes, until there is literally no room for them to live. Their houses become filled with boxes, garbage, and other unsanitary items. People with Alzheimer's disease often lose their ability to tell the difference

"Our neighbor goes out each day and rummages through the neighborhood dumpsters, bringing anything made of cardboard home. Her house is filthy, filled with boxes (some with rotting food in them) in every room."

One lady collected pens and pencils. Every drawer was filled with them. When asked why, she would simply respond, "Just in case I ever need a pen."

"Mildred goes through the closets and cupboards collecting hangers and cookies and packing them in her suitcase."

between items that should be kept and those that should be thrown away—therefore *everything* is kept.

In some cases hiding, rummaging, or hoarding may have "logical" explanations. Food may be hoarded or hidden away for imaginary people, seen as reflections in the mirror, hallucinated, or on the television. People who have gone through such trying events as the Holocaust or the Depression may be recalling (in their long-term memory) the value and scarcity of even the simplest of items, such as scrap metal (paper clips) during the war or crusts of bread when those around them were starving. Rummaging may be an attempt to find items that were previously hidden, now discovered missing.

Respect your loved one's right to rummage. Recognize the pleasures and satisfaction that may be gained from it. Rummaging, hoarding, and hiding, though hard to understand, do provide some sense of well-being for your loved one, as if she has properly prepared for some imagined future trip or future need. Sometimes hoarding, rummaging, and packing things in suitcases accompany requests to "go home." Your loved one may be packing for the trip!

Hiding, rummaging, and hoarding can have serious consequences—or they can be meaningful and constructive sources of *controlled* and *supervised* activity when normal activities are beyond your loved one's abilities and interest. As the disease progresses, the number of activities your loved one can successfully perform will gradually diminish. If hiding, rummaging, or hoarding seems to provide enjoyment, satisfaction, or other benefits for your family member, it may be in everybody's best interest not to discourage it, but to passively permit it under careful, possibly clandestine supervision.

Hiding, rummaging, and hoarding cannot be cured by modifying the home. However, their detrimental effects can be minimized.

Our home modification strategy for hiding, rummaging, and hoarding includes five steps:

- Protect your valuables.
- Make it easier to discover when items are missing.

- Make it simpler to notice changes and find hiding places.
- Create places where it is okay to rummage and hide things.
- Eliminate the dangerous and bad places to hide and rummage

Protect Your Valuables

Protect your valuables and items that if taken would be truly missed. Don't overlook seemingly unimportant items. Even *your* toothbrush may need to be put away, out of sight and reach. For those who have managed family finances or office books in the course of their lives, receipts, checkbooks, and bills may take on a disproportionate importance. Your family member may find a few of these around the house and feel that they need to be stored in a "special" place for safekeeping (never to show up again).

Survey your home for items that cannot be replaced. Put them in safe locations, such as a lockable cabinet, drawer, or in a locked room. If your family member has delusions of strangers coming into the house and stealing things, this may give you a justifiable reason to buy an inexpensive safe or lockable cabinet to protect everyone's valuables.

Protect such items as:

bills and receipts	computer disks
checks	telephone messages
medical records	important books
birth certificates	children's homework
warrantees	memos and notes
tax records	mail
product instructions	work-related reports
insurance documents	purses
jewelry	cash
licenses	important letters
school books	remote contols
credit cards	keys
valuable photographs	wallets or billfolds
schedules	checkbooks

"Grandpa is forever going through our drawers looking for things. When he finds what he is looking for it disappears, sometimes for days."

"Uncle Phil spends a lot of time outside. Our yard is fenced and he can't get out, but the mailbox is inside the fence and the mail is always disappearing!"

Locking mail box:

Alsto's Handy Helpers, The Safety Zone, Trail Side Mailbox.

Relocate your mailbox to outside the fence, or install a lockable mailbox.(The mailman won't need a key, since the mail can be inserted through a slot.) The mailbox is a popular place to hide, rummage, and remove mail, including important documents, such as bills and arriving checks.

For those small items that keep disappearing (keys, remote controls, etc.), provide dummy replacements that will not be missed and are okay for your family member to remove and hide. (Mark the fake keys and remote controls with small dots of nail polish to distinguish them from the real ones.) Ask your local hardware store or locksmith (anywhere they make keys) for a handful of keys that may have been cut wrong and are destined for the trash can or return to the factory.

Be sure to have spare keys, backed-up computer disks, and replacements for items that, if lost, would result in considerable inconvenience.

Make It Easier to Find Lost Items

Eliminate clutter throughout the house. This will make it easier to find things that "disappear" and hiding places as they develop. A home in which everything has its place makes it that much easier to find things that are out of place.

"Uncle Earl is forever hiding my car keys, and the TV remote control is constantly disappearing. Yesterday, after missing for over a week, we found the remote inside one of the shoes in his closet."

Minimize the number of available hiding places and discover the favorite ones. This will help when your family member announces that she has lost her glasses or someone has stolen her false teeth. These are two good preliminary steps, but now let's look at some ways to reveal those items that have disappeared.

Face it, you're not going to teach Uncle Earl not to hide your remote control. Two minutes after you explain in detail why this is inappropriate, your explanation will probably be forgotten and soon your remote control will again be missing.

Smart Key Tracker:

Brookstone.

There are products, such as the Smart Key Tracker, that attach to your key chain and beep when you clap your hands, making it easier to find missing items.

To help you find the TV remote control that keeps disappearing, you can replace your little one with a LARGE universal remote control. This will make it a little more difficult to hide or lose.

For larger items that tend to disappear, attach or insert a battery-operated wireless doorbell (for example, inside purses). The button can be attached to a wall more permanently (so it too won't disappear). Its bell is louder and its range is considerably greater. These devices will lead you to the hiding places as well as the articles hidden there.

Finally, if hiding becomes a serious problem, consider installing a surveillance camera somewhere in your family member's room. Surveillance cameras are less expensive than they have ever been. Some people use them to see who is at the front door or to look out for babysitter child abuse. You can use them to find out where your loved one is hiding food in her room!

There are several types on the market, including wireless cameras that require no expensive household wiring and transmit to small TVs that you can take with you to different locations in the home: the kitchen, the laundry room, etc. Some companies offer cameras disguised as teddy bears and others so small that they can be hidden in the room so that no one will recognize them.

You may be able to use your own television to view your loved one, by hooking it up to the surveillance camera. This can also help late at night when you suspect she is up and about or when you want to make sure she hasn't fallen out of bed. Just turn on your bedroom TV to the correct channel and your mother's a new guest on the *Tonight Show!* Check the product's instructions and discuss your plans with the sales representative.

Create Places for Rummaging and Hiding Things

Do not put locks on *all* drawers and cabinets—leave some that are okay to search. Provide safe, accessible places to rummage. Finding a drawer that he can open might help to calm the frustration of not being able to get into another, more dangerous drawer.

These safe "rummaging" drawers, boxes, closets, and cabinets are for harmless but interesting items such as gloves, wash

Large universal TV remote controls:

Alsto's Handy Helpers, Dynamic Living, Independent Living Aids, Mature Mart, Sammons Preston.

Surveillance cameras:

surveillance or security stores, Alsto's Handy Helpers, Canwood Products, Crest, J. C. Penney Special Needs Catalogue, Kids Club, Radio Shack, The Right Start, The Safety Zone, Vivitar, or home improvement centers.

cloths, eyeglasses, or junk mail, intentionally placed there to be discovered, removed, and hidden. These articles should be selected on the basis of safety and your loved one's changing interests. One week packets of sugar may be the article of choice, next week it could be rubber bands. (A visit to a local garage sale can turn up lots of interesting items. Your loved one might even go with you and pick them out herself.) When items are found they can always be returned to the "rummaging" drawers (to be removed and hidden again), continuing to provide your loved one with feelings of accomplishment and satisfaction, as well as harmless, constructive activity.

Make the cabinets and drawers that are okay for hiding and rummaging more attractive than the others. They should be interesting and alluring to divert your loved one's attention from storage areas that are off limits. Do this with color and choice of handles. Knobs that contrast with the color of the drawer are easier to see. Drawers of different and brighter colors will attract attention and be easier to recognize as drawers. Drawers that are more accessible are also more attractive. Larger, C-shaped drawer pulls are more appealing because they are easier to grasp.

Now that you have created safe sources for rummaging, create safe hiding places: drawers, closets, trunks, boxes, etc. Make these hiding places prominent and attractive. The more hiding places that you know about, the more likely you will be to find what is hidden in them later.

Provide reachable space on closet shelves for articles to be stored or hidden. Make things easy to see. Don't confuse your loved one (or make it difficult for you) by overfilling the closet with too much clutter stacked on shelves that might fall. Check these hiding places on a regular basis for dangerous, spoilable or missing items of value.

Motion detector light adapter:

Alsto's Handy Helpers, BRK Brands, The Safety Zone, and home improvement centers.

Provide a light in the closet that automatically goes on when the door is opened or motion is detected. This will make the closet easier to use, more inviting, and less intimidating. Visit your local home improvement center for adaptors that turn the closet light on when motion is detected.

Designate a special room in your home for your family member, where only she is allowed to go. Look for behavioral clues as to what rooms may be preferred over others, where she is already hiding things or feels comfortable. This room can be her safe and protected area, where no one else may invade or trespass. Provide accessible drawers, niches, cupboards, and cabinets that can be checked when your family member is not likely to find you "snooping" in her private room.

Buy a lockable chest, safe, or cabinet for your family member and *turn the keys over to him.* Make sure that you have extra keys to replace the originals when they become "lost" or hidden. This is a form of "validation therapy," buying into your loved one's perception that others are responsible for the items' disappearance and the need to provide a safe place to store his valuables.

Lockable trunks: Hold Everything.

If these plans work, items that need to be protected or hidden will go somewhere in this special room or in your family member's cabinet. You can retrieve them later when you are sure you won't be caught. You may feel this to be a violation of your loved one's privacy—but it will make it possible to ease his and your concern about losing precious items.

Creating a room of his own and providing safe hiding places may also eliminate more dangerous hiding places, such as the disposal in the kitchen. It will narrow your search area as well, and may prevent losses.

Eliminate Bad Places to Hide and Rummage

Eliminate bad places to hide things by discovering them and taking the appropriate action. For example, if your family member likes to hide things in the bathroom trash can, simply remove it.

Place locks (and alarms) on doors leading into dangerous closets and rooms. Install locks on appropriate drawers and cabinets to make them out of bounds. Remove trash cans, especially those in the kitchen, that might be favorite targets for rummaging, containing rubbish or other items inappropriate for consumption or hoarding.

Change is difficult for those with dementia, but it can be used to your advantage. Once discovered, trash cans, and waste baskets used as hiding places can be relocated to places equally convenient for the caregiver, but no longer available to your family member.

People, though confused, can still be very creative. You may find food or missing items hidden almost anywhere: in pillow covers, under the stove burners, in the clothes dryer, or in the dishwasher. Garbage cans, waste baskets, and trash compactors are also popular hiding places that could result in a valuable item inadvertently thrown out or crushed.

You can be just as creative! Child-proof locks can be used on the dishwasher, refrigerator and virtually any kitchen appliance. Trash cans can be placed in remote cabinets and child-proof locks then applied to the cabinet doors. Your local baby supply store and home improvement center are other good sources of child-proof locks and accessories that you may find helpful in making dangerous hiding places inaccessible. (See chapter 6.)

Sink drains are sometimes used to hide small items of "value." Besides substituting inexpensive costume jewelry for the real jewelry, replace drain screens that have large holes or slots with screens that have smaller holes (that won't permit rings or earrings to pass through). Visit your local hardware store, home improvement center, or kitchen supply store for replacement drain screens. If you have an unusual sink, contact the manufacturer or the local representative for custom drain covers or inserts.

For the disposal hole (larger than the regular sink drain) buy a *disposal* strainer and insert it in the drain hole. Disposal strainers are designed to fit in the large sink hole to the disposal. They are available at most home improvement centers and from plumbing supply dealers. (This is not a substitute for disabling your disposal.)

Check to make sure that you have a drain trap under the sink that is accessible in case small articles are dropped down the drain. Know how to remove it and what tools are required. If you have any questions, contact a local plumber. He can show you how to use the drain trap, or install one if yours is missing, inside the wall or in some other inaccessible location.

In the shower and other floor drains (the laundry room, for example), make sure the cover has only small holes. If the

Child-proof locks:

Alsto's Handy Helpers, Brainerd, Fisher-Price, Gerber Products, OFNA Baby Products, Perfectly Safe, Rev-A-Shelf, Safety 1st, The Safety Zone, The Right Start, The Woodworker's Store, and baby supply stores. For more secure locks, contact a locksmith.

"Mom is afraid someone will steal her jewelry so she tries to hide it in the bathroom drain."

Home improvement centers should have several types of drain covers from which you can choose, or discuss this with your plumber.

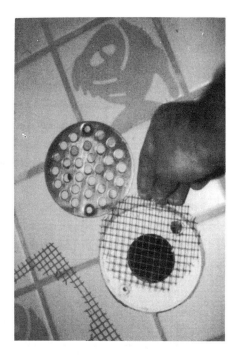

Inserting a piece of metal screening beneath the drain cover prevents someone from trying to hide things in the hole below.

holes are too big, allowing items to be hidden down there, replace it with a drain cover with smaller holes. Or you could buy a small piece of heavy-duty screening (metal fabric), cut it out to fit, and insert it beneath the drain screen.

At least one company offers a shower mat intended to go over the shower drain, thus hiding it from view. It is slip-resistant and has small holes allowing the water to drain. (The same concept may be effective over the sink drain and disposal in the kitchen.)

Disconnect the trash compactor. Given its attractiveness as a hiding spot and its ability to crush and destroy valuables, it is wise to disconnect the trash compactor and minimize it as a potential vehicle for losing precious articles. You can still use it as a trash can if you make sure there are no valuables in it before throwing out the garbage. (You may also want to install a child-proof lock on the door.)

Disconnect the garbage disposal. In addition to eliminating the disposal as a hiding place, eliminate it as a potential source of danger, as well. Your loved one may no longer have any idea of the relationship between the switch on the wall that turns the disposal on and the curious hole in the sink. Disabling the

Shower mat that covers the drain: The Safety Zone.

"Last night I woke up and found Ernie in the kitchen with his hand in the garbage disposal hole fishing for something. I don't even know what he was looking for."

disposal could avert catastrophe if someone goes looking for something in that hole and, needing more light, turns on the *wrong* switch.

You may be able to disengage the garbage disposal easily by unplugging it. If there's no plug, your disposal may have its own circuit breaker in your electrical panel which can be turned off. We don't recommend this as your sole effort to safety-proof the disposal because it is too easy for someone to inadvertently turn it back on. If you do use the circuit breaker option, it's a good idea to place a sign on the electric panel reminding yourself and informing others in the house *not to turn it back on.* (See chapter 9 for more suggestions.)

Another popular and dangerous hiding place in the kitchen is underneath the stove burners.

"Mom hid some papers underneath the burner coils in the stove. We discovered them while preparing dinner."

To solve this problem, you could replace the coiled burners with solid burners. Solid burners are less likely to be removed, since the cavity below is not visible, plus they don't look like something that is removable.

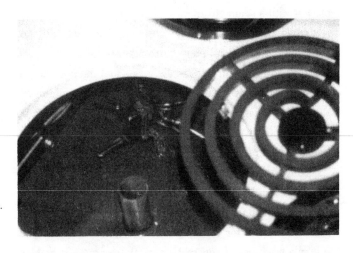

The cavity underneath stove burners is a dangerous, but common, hiding place.

Solid burner replacement coils:

Improvements, appliance dealers, the manufacturer's representative for your stove, and home improvement centers.

Continuous ceramic cooktops are available through most appliance dealers.

Some stoves, such as those manufactured by Jenn-Air, have modular plug-in units. You can simply replace the entire panel of coiled burners with a panel of a different kind, such as solid burners or a smooth glass-top unit.

If it's time to replace the stove, consider a continuous ceramic cooktop or an induction cooktop model. Both have continuous, smooth surfaces with no burner coils or inserts that can be removed. An induction cooktop offers the additional advantage that it only heats metal pots and pans, not the burners, so your loved one is far less likely to get burned (or catch his sleeve on fire). Also, nonmetallic items placed on the burners, even if the burners are turned on, will not get hot or catch on fire. (One warning, however: If anyone in your home has a pacemaker, check with the manufacturer of the induction cooktop to make sure the unit is safe and won't affect the pacemaker.)

If the stove is being used at night when everyone is asleep, your loved one may be putting everybody at risk. You might choose to deny access to the kitchen by installing a door and locking it. Some caregivers have had success with installing "saloon" doors with a latch (or multiple latches). They are easy to install, look good, and are simple to lock. (See chapters 5 and 6.)

To discourage hiding and rummaging in certain drawers, paint them the same color as the cabinet, making them blend and disappear into the background, less visible and less inviting. Drawer pulls that are smaller and the same color as the drawer may be difficult to see and grasp, thus deterring use of those drawers. Another way to discourage the use of certain cabinets is to camouflage them. Apply the same wallpaper to the cabinets and door faces as on the wall behind them. (See chapter 6 for more ideas.)

"Out of sight, out of mind" can be an effective strategy to eliminate places to hide and rummage. Being able to see a cabinet, yet not open it is cause for upset. Free-standing cabinets can be removed or turned around. Others may be hidden perhaps by placing a sheet over them.

Induction cooktops are a relatively new item: General Electric, Jenn-Aire, and check with appliance dealers.

Agitation, Combativeness, Aggression, and Resistance

Anger and aggression can be caused by anything, and you certainly don't have to be confused to become angry. Alzheimer's disease just adds to the list of potential causes. Regardless, the following section illustrates a few of the causes that are related to the disease and how you might address them.

We all have our own stress threshold! It may just be closer and easier to reach when you have Alzheimer's disease.

It must be inconceivable to live in a world that is impossible to understand, where everyone is a "stranger" and you have to follow rules that you cannot even remember. You may have lived for 60, 70, or more years free to do anything and go anywhere that you wanted, yet now every freedom seems to have been taken away. How would you react to this?

Your loved one may not be able to understand that she doesn't understand! The inability to perform the most common everyday tasks and depending on someone else for every little thing may be a foreign concept to her. She may not understand dependency. Imagine what it must be like, after a lifetime of being a family leader and provider, finding yourself helpless, unable to perform even the simplest, most common task. This may not be easy to accept, and she may be fighting it.

In the earlier stages of the disease many realize that something is wrong. It's not unusual to hear stories of family members doing something very inappropriate (such as urinating in a hallway), then suddenly realizing what they have just done, becoming quite upset. Their embarrassment may culminate in frustration, then lead to hostility . . . or just sadness. Making it as easy as possible to find and get to the bathroom may help to avoid episodes like this.

Environmental Pollution

Aggression may be triggered by environments that are overly confusing, noisy, or irritating. Constant noise from the television or conversation may result in frustration. A room overly cluttered with too much furniture and busy decorations may result in your loved one becoming confused, then aggravated, re-directing his feelings at the caregiver. A cold and uncomfortable bathroom may provoke violent attempts to escape, appearing to be defiance of the care being offered there.

Imagine driving down the highway and being expected to read and comprehend *all* of the billboard signs on both sides, at the same time. Worse still, everyone else around you is able to do it, without difficulty. Now apply this concept to your loved one sitting at a busy dining room table with conversation taking place on all sides, the baby crying, and kids fighting, or trying to walk through a room with flowered upholstery, patterned carpeting, and complicated wallpaper designs. Your family member might feel overwhelmed.

Be aware of other factors or equipment outdoors that may be distracting or disturbing: loud noises such as an air conditioner starting up, neighbors arguing, dogs barking, traffic horns, sirens, and car backfires. Noises, people, and everyday occurrences that we take for granted may be confusing and annoying to your loved one. (Refer to the discussion later in this chapter and chapter 4 on difficulties hearing and seeing.)

Even the colors and subjects of certain paintings in your home can make your family member uncomfortable. You'll want artwork that is colorful, yet calming. Soft, pastel colors may be far less upsetting than art featuring violent, vibrant colors.

Keep these paintings simple and understandable, but not too realistic. Historical scenes depicting battles or Japanese paintings of frightening theatrical masks, for example, may upset a person who is having a difficult enough time just trying to comprehend ordinary things. Abstract or surrealistic paintings may cause discomfort as well. Surrounding your loved one with subject matter that is familiar and understandable and reinforces good feelings can create a friendlier, less agitating, environment.

In a home environment for someone with Alzheimer's disease, artwork can serve a valuable purpose: to remind your loved one of happier, more familiar times or of activities that are appropriate for that room; or just cheer up someone who may be a little sad.

Loss of Freedom and Access Denial

Aggression can also result from losing the freedom to roam and enjoy the entire home. A person's house is sometimes her most valuable possession. She has spent many years paying for it, building it and turning it into a home. Doors and cabinets discovered locked may not be understood. Explanations that the locks are for her safety and well-being may be understood only momentarily or not at all. When confronted with locks and gates, it's not unusual for people with AD to use persistence and brute strength to defy and overcome them. Some have become so irate and determined that they have actually knocked doors down in their efforts to get through them or climbed over fences or out of windows.

Relocate knives and dangerous items to locked drawers that are out of the way or in other safe rooms, allowing as many remaining drawers as possible to be left accessible. If you provide some accessible drawers among those that are locked and off-limits, you might be able to thwart the frustration, rage, and persistence directed at defeating a locked drawer.

To reduce some agitation, remove cues that suggest unsafe activities, reminding your loved one of things he is no longer allowed or safely able to do. For example, the hat rack (clearly in sight by the front door), the dog's leash on the doorknob, or car keys hanging on a hook where they have been stored for years may all be reminders of leaving the house, going for a daily afternoon walk, to the office, or driving—pleasures, habits, and liberties that may no longer be safe for your loved one.

Rational and Irrational Fears

Your loved one may have some reasonable concerns. People are not always kind. Someone may really be harassing your loved one (innocently sitting on the porch) with comments, by violating his personal space, or with body language. This could happen when your loved one is alone outside, unable to understand, or deal with it rationally.

"Uncle Jesse used to love sitting outside on the front porch during the summer. Now we take him out there and in just a matter of minutes he becomes agitated and we have to bring him back inside."

Aggression may be the direct result of perceived danger or discomfort. For example, people no longer recognized, even loved ones, may represent a threat and trigger an unreasonable defensive response. Care needs to be taken to ensure your loved one's space is protected and definable, so he won't feel violated by "strangers."

Even though your family member may have irrational fears, they are fears just the same. Maybe he is afraid of being left outside, abandoned. Maybe the backyard has become a "strange" place, no longer familiar. Consider moving your loved one's chair or bench closer to the house, allowing for continuous conversation, a safe distance from perceived dangers, and a reassuring view of you.

Catastrophic Reactions

Catastrophic reactions are extreme emotional responses. They can sometimes escalate to violent behavior, including screaming, flailing, self-mutilation, throwing objects, grabbing things and not letting go, or using items within reach as weapons. A catastrophic reaction can be triggered by almost anything, logical or not, real or perceived, present or past. Usually the episodes are soon forgotten, though the damage remains.

"At bath time Mom gets terribly violent. She screams that we are trying to rape her or kill her baby!"

They may be caused by real concerns. Your family member may have just surpassed his limits of tolerance, now venting his inability to understand or follow directions. Maybe he desperately wants to tell you something important, but is unable to do so. After a lifetime of verbal eloquence, your family member may not even be able to tell you something very simple.

Realize that communication may be difficult and words or behavior may only be symbols. "Flower" may mean the painting on the wall or "red," the dress. Translation may be cryptic and only your patience and clever detective work will lead to successfully solving the puzzle.

Some episodes of agitation may be substitutions for your loved one's inability to communicate discomfort, especially serious or extreme problems. For example, she may be in pain from bed sores or other age-related conditions. She can't say, "Honey, I have some terrible sores on my back that really hurt." She may not even know where she hurts or why she hurts. All she can do is either sit there and suffer or become irritable and irate.

Be extra sensitive to what makes your family member comfortable and uncomfortable. Does she have arthritis, osteoporosis, or other reasons causing pain and discomfort—that she cannot explain? Conditions as simple as room temperature, glare, reflections in a window, a draft from a ceiling fan, or noises can create an uncomfortable environment.

Or maybe he is reacting to imagined experiences: delusions, such as beliefs that people are out to get him.

What has the environment got to do with these outbursts? When these difficult times occur, try to step back and observe from a distance. Of course, the cause may have nothing to do with the surroundings, but consider *every* possibility. Look for both logical and seemingly illogical causes. Are there voices coming from the television that could sound like a plot? Is the bathroom too cold? If you become more aware of how the environment can contribute to discomfort, you may be able to avoid some of the resulting problems. For example, softer, pleasant colors, fragrances, and music may help to create more calming surroundings and reduce agitation in the bathroom.

"Last night Dad got so angry that he threw an ashtray at Mom. He hit her in the head and we had to take her to the hospital."

Protect *everyone*, not *just* your loved one. Sometimes agitation is very difficult to deal with, possibly even violent. Your loved one may attempt to hurt people close to him. You may need to remove small items that can be thrown or used as weapons. Lock them up, put them in an inaccessible room or cabinet, take them out of your loved one's reach.

Create the safest environment possible, one that passively averts or minimizes injury in situations when control is difficult. This applies to all Safe Zones that your loved one is free to use, and especially those areas where episodes of agitation repeatedly occur, such as in the bathroom.

Non-breakable lamps:

American Health Care Supply.

Put away valuable and breakable objects. Replace fragile lamps with non-breakable ones. Soften sharp, hard edges of counters and tables that, if struck by a flailing arm, could cause a bruise or worse. Provide grab bars or railings to hold while your loved one settles down and make sure floors are slip-resistant to prevent falls while attention is focused on rage, not safety. Pay particular attention to those areas where problems frequently or typically occur, such as in the bathroom or at the dinner table. (See chapter 9.)

Sundowning

"Sundowning," or sundown syndrome, is a phenomenon characterized by agitation, heightened confusion, or unusual behavior occurring in the late afternoon or early evening. It is a relatively new subject, and little information is available, but theories abound. Some researchers feel that for some women, who have spent a lifetime caring for their families, the anxiety of preparing dinner meals late in the day makes them more irritable. In nursing homes, afternoon changes in staff shifts may be noticed and trigger agitation. Another theory is that sundowning is actually related to the sun and declining light at the end of the day. This theory suggests that it can also occur on cloudy days, in rooms with few or no windows, or more often during the winter when the days are shorter and often more dreary. (In other words, it may be related to seasonal affective disorder, SAD.) Finally, logic tells us that people are naturally more tired at the end of the day and that might be a contributing factor. The true cause of sundowning is not yet known.

At present there are no proven steps to prevent sundowning. You may discover factors in your own home that trigger these occurrences. Closely observe *your* family member and *your* home surroundings. Look for consistencies in his behavior and misbehavior. Does he seem to be happier in certain rooms and less happy in others? Are those rooms brighter or darker? Can you detect any repetitive patterns of location and time? How can you brighten up your home?

Some researchers have tried to modify interior lighting. Shades or screens have been used on the windows during the day and interior lighting increased at night to create a more uniform, 24-hour lighting level. To the contrary, others have increased the light in the home to bright levels during the day and dimmed it at night to enhance and simulate sunlight cycles. Some caregivers also suggest placing certain lights on timers to go on at dusk to make the transition easier and more subtle.

Since sunlight plays a key role in our ability to distinguish between day and night, modifying lighting cues may cause your loved one to become further confused and not able to determine the correct time of day, especially after waking from a nap. We often wake up a little disoriented. Modified lighting may only add to the confusion.

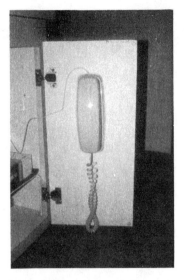

A fake telephone or battery-operated doorbell can divert your family member's attention at difficult moments.

"Hello."

"Mom, it's Judy calling to see how you are doing."

"Hi, Judy, how are you?" (as you wash under her arms)

"Oh, Mom is just great." ("Rinse off here, Mom.")

"Is that the baby I hear in the background?"

("Mom, turn so I can wash your back.")

"Okay, I guess you have to go." ("Let's rinse off a little now.")

"I'll tell Mom that you called. Bye, bye."

"Mom, that was Judy. She is thrilled that you are doing so well. She wanted to talk to you, but the baby was crying. She's going to call you later. Now give me your foot."

Some caregivers report that daily periods of sitting outside in bright sunlight and pleasant surroundings result in calmer, happier family members. Pick out a perfect spot in the backyard for a bench, located so that you can supervise her from inside the house, and providing a view of interesting activity. (See chapter 1 for more ideas that will help you create that special place in the backyard.)

Fatigue is also a possible cause for agitation occurring late in the day. After all, it takes a great deal of effort, both physical and mental, to deal with the difficulties associated with Alzheimer's disease. And when else would the cumulative effects be more likely to manifest themselves than later in the day? Places to sit and relax may prove to be very beneficial. Provide them both inside and outside.

Diversions

Once it has been determined that there is no real or serious cause for discomfort or agitation, re-directing your loved one's attention to more pleasant thoughts or activities may be one of your best solutions. Diversions and distractions are sometimes the best strategies for handling irate, irrational behavior. Your home environment can provide plenty of opportunities. Caregivers have suggested numerous techniques to divert a loved one's attention at difficult times, giving him time to cool down or forget the cause of his frustration.

One caregiver we spoke to installed a fake telephone in the bathroom cabinet and a secret button on the underside of the sink base cabinet. Whenever the situation got difficult (usually due to bathing) the phone would mysteriously ring, and everything would stop while she answered the phone. (Note the conversation that took place.)

How about a remote doorbell with the button cleverly located nearby in the bathroom? Imagine if, rather than a ringing telephone, the doorbell rang right when your mother was furious that you were going to get soap in her eyes or get her hair wet? You wouldn't even have to leave the room, just take advantage of the re-directed train of thought.

Some episodes of agitation will be unavoidable. They just happen. Where room allows provide a comfortable chair for either you or your loved one to just sit down and "regroup." You could also take your family member to the special room or area that you specially prepared for her to feel safe and calm, far from agitation and cause of discomfort. Often the confused or disheartening thought is simply forgotten and the problem resolved.

Music can be great therapy, both calming and diverting. There are several excellent categories of music or tapes to select from:

- calming music (New Age music, calming nature sounds)
- music that one can join in and sing along with
- music relating to happy times in your loved one's life (maybe childhood) that bring back pleasant thoughts and memories
- patriotic songs
- religious or gospel music.

Calming and soothing music can also be helpful for getting a good night's sleep. Some caregivers use it to drown out agitating nighttime noises and lull their loved ones to sleep.

What else catches your loved one's interest? The next time the grandchildren come over, film them playing in the yard. How about a video of a trip to the zoo, the kitten playing, or the puppy performing tricks?

These are but a few of the potential diversions that you can create in your own home for special situations. We also suggest that you join a support group and attend lectures on Alzheimer's disease to not only discuss your problems, but to learn other ways that caregivers have dealt with similar situations.

Picking at Things

"Picking" is the inexplicable fixation to touch, handle, or work at and remove small items bit by bit, such as peeling paint. Items of choice may be real, real-like (for example, flowers in

Music from the "good ol' days": Elder Books, Hammatt Senior Products, Nasco, Potentials Development, Senior Products, Sound Choice, Wireless.

Patriotic music from the 1940s: Wireless.

Favorite hymns and spirituals: Nasco, Potentials Development.

"Recently all Mom seems to be interested in is her beloved Cleveland Indians. So we taped the World Series and now when she gets agitated, we stop what we are doing . . . because it's time for the game. Her upset disappears and she is thrilled each time they win!"

upholstery patterns or objects in paintings or photographs), or imaginary, visible only to your family member (such as invisible bugs or lint on a person's clothing). The activity may be occasional, triggered by environmental factors, such passing by the interesting wallpaper, or it can be compulsive.

Picking at things is a common behavior among people with dementia. Items of choice include:

- hallucinations—imagined bugs, spots, lint, etc., visible only to your loved one
- peeling paint or fuzzy fabrics
- edges of wallpaper curling or detaching from the wall
- objects in photos or paintings so realistic that they beg to be touched
- carpet and upholstery patterns, particularly those with spots resembling lint or small patterns (paisley, for example)
- objects or figures in wallpaper patterns
- spots in fabrics and materials.

Also look for patterns in your home that might suggest dirt or bugs that can be transferred or interpreted as crawling insects or lint on your loved one or on people he encounters. If "bugs" are a problem, perhaps there is flowered upholstery nearby that "may attract bugs." Are there designs in the carpeting that appear as spots or lint? After all, doesn't it make sense that if it's on the floor it's probably also on your clothing? Look around for clues on wallpaper, upholstery, carpet patterns, etc. Your solution might be as simple as slip-covering a chair to cover the problem-causing pattern.

Observe your loved one and discuss the problem with *her.* She might, in fact, tell you what the source of the problem is and all you have to do now is remove or cover it.

If picking is not harmful, you might not want to discourage it. It may provide an activity that is safe and that allows your family member to feel that he is serving a useful purpose (removing the lint, be it real or not).

On the other hand, if paint peelings are eaten or contain

lead, then picking could be dangerous. In that case, have an expert inspect your home and take the appropriate action.

Shadowing

Shadowing, or clinging to a caregiver or loved one, may be a desperate attempt to compensate for a fear of being helpless, left alone, or even abandoned. Time may no longer be clearly understood. Being left alone for only a few seconds may seem like an eternity. Or maybe your loved one is reliving her responsibility as a child to follow her mother and remain right by her side.

"Grandmother follows me all around the house, like a puppy dog."

Shadowing or clinging can be burdensome on the caregiver. You can't go to the mailbox, the bathroom, or even your own room for a few moments of peace. The minute the caregiver is out of sight, the person with AD panics. He follows you everywhere you go, clinging to a form of security: the only person familiar to him, who knows his needs, and can understand him. After all, who wants to be left alone when frightened and confused?

Open up your home to make yourself easier to see as you move from room to room and go about your daily activities. Select your special areas with this in mind. You want not only to make it easier to observe and supervise your loved one, but also to make it possible for her to see, talk to you, and watch what you are doing. Provide chairs in the kitchen where she can sit, watch, or help. Make it possible for her to be with you whenever possible and maybe you can eliminate some of those times when caregiving seems difficult or burdensome.

Remove doors or keep them open to make it easier for your loved one to see you. Replace certain doors in your home with Dutch doors, which allow the lower half to be closed and the upper half to remain open, allowing for security and views at the same time. Rearrange furniture that may block views. You may be surprised by the difference that moving a few bookcases, the china cabinet, or wall shelving can make. Consider getting rid of larger pieces that noticeably block views.

When you can't be in visual sight, take advantage of inexpensive intercoms (that you can carry with you), available at

Wireless intercom:

Radio Shack, The Safety Zone, Solutions.

"Last week I went out to get the paper. No sooner was I out the door than Mom went out right behind me, down the street, and disappeared. If it weren't for the neighbors, we might have never found her."

"Bessy follows me everywhere I go, all day long. I can't get a minute to myself, even if I have to go to the bathroom!"

electronic and home improvement stores. Though your loved one may not be able to see you in the laundry room, you may still be able to talk to him and reassure them that you will be right back.

Stories like this one are numerous—you go out the door for a paper, get into the car, or just go into the garage. Suddenly you turn around and there's your family member, having silently followed you. You didn't even know she was there. She could just as easily have kept on going right down the block, and you might not have realized it until it was too late. This is called tail-gating. It's potentially a serious problem and a major concern for caregivers. (See chapter 5 for further discussion on tail-gating.)

Your bathroom may be a good candidate for a privacy lock. A privacy lock is lockable only from the inside. Most bathroom doors already have one. If your loved one locks himself in there, a special key or even a wire coat hanger can be inserted to release the lock. Another possibility is just installing a secret lock (or hook and eye latch) in the bathroom door, high above or way below the normal location for a lock, where your family member is unlikely to discover it. Check your local hardware store or home improvement center for a selection.

Repetitive Behavior

Your loved one may live in a world where only a few tasks remain safe and can be completed successfully. Is it any wonder that these few activities may be repeated, again and again? If this is satisfying to your loved one, why discourage it? Instead, create a special place where he can enjoy them, perhaps a favorite chair, on the porch or at a table in the den by the window. Repetitive behavior may be a blessing in disguise. Some may be worth encouraging for everyone's benefit. Take advantage of it where possible.

Some caregivers ask family members to help with the household chores—sorting laundry or silverware, folding napkins, etc. Upon completion, the basket of folded napkins is then taken out of the room, disheveled, and brought back as yet another basket of napkins that needs sorting. The result is hours of activity for the family member that makes her feel as if she is fulfilling a much-needed family role. (See chapter 4 for more suggestions.)

This trickery makes some caregivers feel guilty, though your loved one feels that she is contributing, and it is making her happy. If it works, use it. Some caregivers have a name for this—deceptive therapy. Continue this crafty, yet constructive, loving caregiving, and create a comfortable place in the kitchen, den, or bedroom where the task can be easily and enjoyably performed.

Realize that repeated questioning—questions asked over and over—is typically part of the disease. If your loved one no longer has the benefit of short-term memory, events that occurred only moments ago just disappear and there is nothing we can do architecturally to change that. On the other hand, problems such as hearing impairments or background noises can contribute to repeated questioning—and these problems can be corrected.

When persistant phone calls tie up your phone line, consider putting in a separate line for your friends and family to use. Call your local telephone company to see what it will cost and how to get it done.

"Mom calls me 30 to 40 times a day. Sometimes my kids can't even get through to talk to me themselves."

Eating Inappropriate Materials

Sometimes people with AD will attempt to eat inappropriate and perhaps dangerous items. Your loved one could ingest something poisonous or have difficulty swallowing a piece of candy. Given the problem of dysphagia (the inability to chew or swallow properly), the result can be choking, and your loved one may not be able to alert you. Almost anything that will fit in a person's mouth can wind up there. Care needs to be taken around the home to remove toxic or small items. (See also chapter 9 for a partial list of potentially dangerous common household items.)

Unsupervised trips to the kitchen or refrigerator can wind up with your family member eating (or drinking) inappropri-

Small, compact refrigerators:

American Health Care Supply, Koolatron,* Igloo Products,* Intirion, Marvel, U-Line, or appliance dealers. (*Make sure you ask for the converter that allows you to plug the unit into a wall outlet.)

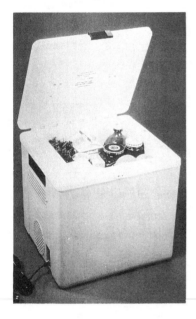

Medications and potentially dangerous foods can be stored in a compact refrigerator located in a locked Danger Zone, preventing them from being mishandled and leaving the kitchen refrigerator a much safer place to visit. Photo courtesy Koolatron.

"Dad keeps trying to eat the little balls of soap in the guest bathroom."

ate or uncooked items, such as raw chicken, uncooked pasta, pickle juice, or medicine (stored in the refrigerator). This is obviously a problem you want to avoid.

Possible solutions include placing a child-proof lock on the refrigerator, installing a door with a lock leading to the kitchen, camouflaging the refrigerator so that it is no longer recognizable, or removing hazardous items from the refrigerator. For those items that require refrigeration yet need to be kept out of harm's way, purchase a small, compact refrigerator and locate it in a safe, locked room.

Remove medications and other dangerous items from *all* unlocked medicine cabinets in the house. It's not unusual to go into the home of a person caring for a loved one with AD and discover that they have taken all the right steps in their family member's bathroom, yet forgotten about other bathrooms. Lock *your* bathroom and medicine cabinet also. Check the guest bath and powder room, anywhere trouble might lurk.

Manufacturers intentionally package their products to attract attention. Brightly colored detergents, shampoos, and cleaning products, often formulated to smell like fruit, and packaged with pretty, happy people on the label, are appealing, but misleading. Such packaging may be particularly attractive to someone who is confused, looking for the slightest suggestion to reinforce her incorrect judgment. It's not unusual to hear of someone with Alzheimer's misinterpreting this information and trying to drink or eat a pretty, but toxic, product. (See also chapter 2.)

Some items around the house look edible but aren't, including decorator soap in the shape of small colorful balls, fruit, or flowers, and plastic fruit that may look so real that anyone would be tempted to take a bite. Your loved one too may be convinced and try to eat them. Look around your home. Remove products that appear to be something they are not.

Grocery stores sell liquid soap dispensers that can be placed on any sink counter, so you don't need to have little balls of soap lying around. If the problem occurs in the shower and bath you can install a wall-mounted soap or shampoo dispenser. These offer other advantages as well—less clutter, and you won't have to bend down to pick up bars of soap or a bottle of shampoo that drops on the floor.

Your family member may attempt to eat anything, including dirt. Dirt itself is not dangerous, but the germs it contains can be. For potted plants, use sterile, "soil-less" dirt substitutes, such as Pro-Mix or Sunshine Mix. Although these peat-based mixtures are not edible, they are a lot cleaner. This is not to suggest that you should allow your loved one to eat dirt. If discovered, do have your family member spit it out and remove the source.

With Alzheimer's, almost anything is possible. Make continued awareness, caution, and home surveys a common practice, especially if your family member begins to display this kind of behavior.

Soap and shampoo dispensers:

American Health Care Supply, Better Living Products, Improvements, Independent Living Aids, The Safety Zone, Tubular Specialties Mfg.

"Sometimes we find Aunt Rose eating the dirt right out of the flower pots. She hasn't gotten sick yet, but I'm afraid that she might. What do I do?"

Inappropriate "Sexual" Behavior

What appears to be inappropriate sexual behavior can actually be related to the environment. For example, Judah Ronch, in his book *Alzheimer's Disease: A Practical Guide for Families and Other Caregivers,* describes a man who occasionally walked through his house holding himself, fully exposed for all to see. Those who saw this assumed it to be a sexual gesture, but in fact, as the author explains, this behavior was his way of reminding himself why he had gotten up and where he was going—to the bathroom!

Perhaps if it had been easier to find the bathroom, this man would not have needed to take such drastic steps to "remind" himself where he was going. People with AD can be remarkably creative when it comes to finding temporary solutions to their problems. (Recall the discussion in chapter 2 on preparing lists and maps.)

Organize your home and furniture to make important routes obvious and direct. Move his favorite chair a bit closer to the bathroom, or outline the path to the bathroom on the floor with colorful electrical tape. Provide cues to help direct him. (See chapter 8.)

Similarly, incorrect or incomplete dressing (resulting in

exposed underwear or parts of the body) is often due to one's inability to remember the proper sequence for dressing. (See chapter 4.)

"Esther keeps taking her clothes off and walking around the house naked."

Undressing in public might be a reaction to uncomfortable temperatures, perhaps caused by your loved one fiddling with the thermostat. The house may be too warm for her, and she may not be able to explain this. She may not even understand why she is uncomfortable. Her solution may be simply to remove extra clothing.

If undressing is a problem, check the room temperature and the thermostat (someone might have improperly adjusted it). Older people are often very sensitive to room temperatures. Remember also that your idea of a comfortable room temperature may not be the same as your loved one's.

Just as you might take off a sweater if you are too hot, your family member might take off his clothing, or put on additional or inappropriate clothing if he is too cold or feels a draft. It might help to hang an appropriate housecoat, sweater, or warm blanket in plain sight to cue her to the proper clothing in the event that she is cold.

Spontaneous Vocalizations

Spontaneous vocalizations or involuntary screams can be frightening and hard to understand.

"Granny Ann sometimes just starts screaming. She used to utter only a few sounds, now she yells for several minutes. I'm afraid the neighbors will hear her and call the police."

The most obvious and immediate reaction may be to close the doors and windows to contain the sound. A better approach may be threefold: Talk to your neighbors to let them know what the problem really is and how you're handling it (not with torture as they might suspect), soften the environment to absorb some of the noise, and try, if possible, to discover the cause.

People with Alzheimer's may attempt to verbalize discomfort any way they can, and that may mean screaming. Look for pain, frustration, and unresolved concerns. Maybe the television is giving her delusions of discomforting events that she perceives as a real threat to her or her family. Try to imagine yourself in your loved one's position and see if you can discover any possible outside causes.

Use diversions and pleasant input, such as music, outdoor views, bright and pleasant rooms, family activities, or stories on tape to distract your loved one from whatever might be distressing her.

Recognize that there may be no answer. After all, Alzheimer's is a disease of the brain, and the causes for her concern may reside solely in her mind.

Stalling

"Stalling" is the inexplicable action of walking and then suddenly stopping. Often the feet stop, but the momentum continues, causing your loved one to fall in a forward direction. It often happens at door openings, upon entering a larger space, or at the end of a stairway.

One caregiver suggested creating a definable path through the room by applying strips of colored tape to the floor or carpeting. Your loved one may then focus on the pathway, rather than on whatever it was that triggered his stalling. Go into any hardware store and ask for colored electrical tape.

If stalling repeatedly occurs at one particular location, ask yourself what is different there. What is different between the area to come and the area just past? Is he going from a dark area to a brighter one, or vice versa? Would an additional lamp help to equalize the lighting? Does the flooring material change in texture or color? Could there be a "visual cliffing" problem, where the darker color floor is seen as a hole or step? Does he perceive one area as more hazardous or harder to navigate? Do railings in the hallway suddenly stop? Did he just go through an opening or past something? Is this the end or a recognizable point in an unusually long path or route?

Try to discover why your family member makes a distinction between these areas and suddenly stops at this particular juncture. Maybe creating a sense of continuity with a railing, to round the corner and follow into the next area would help. Use trial and error.

If your loved one continues to stall and a fall is likely, give her a better, safer reason and place to stop. Place a soft, stable chair there, where she can rest. When she gets up, the cause for the stalling (possibly exhaustion) may no longer matter.

Behavioral problems are traumatic for everyone involved. The extraordinary change in someone so close to you, the realization that this person is just not who she once was, must be a hard reality to face. Dealing with a former family leader who is now totally dependent on others for the simplest of tasks or trying to discourage dangerous behavior of a determined person is understandably upsetting. The home may not be able to solve these problems, but it is our contention that preparing your home, as best you can, will eliminate the triggers, causes, and the consequences of many.

4

Activities of Daily Living

Activities of daily living are the typical day-to-day tasks and basic functions necessary to live independently, sustain, and care for oneself: eating, dressing, bathing, toileting, ambulation, and continence. For our purposes we will also consider secondary tasks, not necessary for survival, but part of everyday life: cooking, laundry, housekeeping, bill paying, banking, etc. These are referred to as instrumental activities of daily living. Thirdly, our lives are composed of many other activities, important sources of pleasure that are well worth noting: socializing, reminiscing, gardening, doing crossword puzzles, neighborhood walks, religious affairs, and walking the dog, just to name a few. Autonomy includes being able to continue these pleasures, as well. You will want to create an environment that supports and encourages all of these types of activities.

We will also look at activities of daily living in terms of both the person with AD and the caregiver. Alzheimer's disease gradually hinders peoples' abilities to perform activities of daily living. In some cases, the activity is conducted by your family member, in others the caregiver assists, taking on much of the burden. So home modifications will need to assist both the person with Alzheimer's and the caregiver, accordingly.

There are four stages that we will consider:

- activities that can be performed by the person with AD,
- endeavors that require assistance for completion,
- tasks that can no longer be conducted by your loved one, and
- substitute tasks for those activities that can no longer be completed.

The home should not be an obstacle to the successful completion of any task your loved one attempts. This chapter also offers clues, insights, and strategies to assist your family member to perform favorite activities, household and personal responsibilities for as long as possible; often longer than the disease normally permits.

In the early stages of Alzheimer's disease, your loved one will still be able to perform many activities of daily living and family responsibilities, despite occasional accidents or episodes of forgetfulness. As time goes on, more and more of these activities will require assistance. As a caregiver, you will need to simplify tasks, slowly begin to join in and assist, then carefully remove the tools and reminders of those responsibilities when they become too difficult or dangerous.

People with AD are creative and adapt in so many ways. They have been known to take incredibly clever steps to cover their mistakes and adjust to inabilities. For example, secret lists may become essential tools to help your mother remember every step involved in preparing a simple meal. So too are maps that illustrate the trip from bedroom to kitchen, or from home to the grocery store, only a block away. Take note: These maps and lists may be important clues, clearly indicating steps that work for your loved one.

"Elsie made the best cakes in town. But even with her lists, she would forget to add some of the ingredients. We thought it would be best to just 'run out' of flour and put away the sugar. Now we buy the cakes and she thinks she made them. Everybody's happy."

Caring for yourself and your family are important responsibilities that contribute to self-esteem and perceived value. Losing these abilities can be devastating and depressing. It may be possible to offset the trauma by enabling your loved one to contribute in other ways; perhaps by teaching you how to make her pie, supervising in the kitchen, or just assisting. The importance of feeling needed remains well into the disease. As long as she feels she can contribute, she will continue to enjoy the accompanying satisfaction. The more satisfaction, the greater the likelihood of having a good day.

Your father may no longer be able to build a garden, but providing him with a safe, comfortable place on the porch to watch and supervise may remain a valuable way for him to participate in the project. Or perhaps you can think of other tasks to substitute for those that have become too difficult.

Provide socks to sort, papers to file, yarn to role into a ball, leaves to rake, towels to fold, plants to water, etc. Create opportunities whenever and wherever they present themselves. Your home is a gold mine of possibilities, some cleverly devious, yet rewarding, just the same.

Create an environment conducive to the successful completion of tasks. Simplify choices. Plan activities so that all decisions are the "right" decisions. Recognize the triggers and causes for failure. Perhaps you can replace a jigsaw puzzle of 100 pieces with one of only five or ten. Consider how this approach might apply to all sorts of activities in your own home.

Throughout all this, embrace the rewarding contributions that your loved one is still able to make. People love to help, and there remains an inherent, lifelong desire to feel needed. Take advantage of this concept whenever possible and create opportunities where you might need your loved one's assistance, whether it's helping in the kitchen, watering the plants, sorting the silverware (that you mixed up just for the occasion), or dusting with a feather duster. Even going through catalogues to help you find a special gift or item can result in hours of constructive, purposeful entertainment. We all want to provide worthwhile contributions. Your loved one is no different. Many a caregiver has discovered the magic in these few words: "Thank you, Mom."

Toileting

Toileting includes not only using the toilet, but cleaning oneself or helping your loved one clean herself upon completion as well. Assistance with toileting is without question one of the

"Grandma can no longer cook safely, so we placed a special chair at the kitchen table for her. From there she supervises Mom preparing meals, baking pies, etc. Grandma seems to accept her inability to cook, but enjoys ordering Mom around and making sure she didn't forget the cinnamon for the pies—over and over and over!"

Puzzles with only a few pieces: Nasco.

"My wife, Arlene, can no longer trim the hedges or do the yard work. We once had the most beautiful yard in the neighborhood, all due to her. Now we help her trim some of the flowers, and then take her to the mall for a few hours, while our yard man comes in and finishes the job. When she returns she doesn't realize that someone else did all the work, and we go on and on about what a wonderful job she did and how beautiful the yard looks. Then she spends hours sitting on the back porch admiring her beautiful yard!"

"After a lifetime of caring for others, Mom is having a difficult time being cared for herself, especially when she needs help using the toilet and properly cleaning herself afterwards."

Hand-held toilet bidet/sitzbath:
North Coast Medical, Sammons Preston.

"Uncle Ivan can't seem to urinate into the toilet. He goes all over the floor."

"My wife just won't sit down on the toilet seat. If I try to force her she gets angry, then hostile. The last time she stormed into the den . . . and soiled herself."

Soft toilet seats:
Sammons Preston, home improvement centers, or home health care supply stores.

"Ted is afraid to sit down on the toilet seat. He's concerned he won't be able to get back up."

most difficult-to-accept of all caregiving tasks. It's unpleasant for both the caregiver and the care receiver, yet we are continually amazed at how many caregivers accept this responsibility with love and compassion. (See also chapters 1, 7, and 8.)

Even as dementia robs people of their memory, the need for privacy and self-esteem remains. How can you preserve privacy, dignity, and comfort in these awkward circumstances? Recognize the problems and minimize the consequences as best you can. For example, replacing the bathroom door with a shower curtain might preserve privacy, yet allow access, if immediate assistance is needed. Or how about installing a hand-held cleansing device to make it easy for your loved one to clean herself, or the caregiver to offer assistance?

Difficulty in the bathroom takes on many forms. Maybe Ivan is having trouble seeing the toilet. This is common for seniors with visual problems, as well as those with dementia, especially if your bathroom is all one color, with white toilet, floor, and walls. To solve or minimize this problem, make the toilet easier to see and reach, and to clean up. (See chapter 7 for more ideas.)

Perhaps the toilet seat is uncomfortable. As we grow older, muscles and fatty tissue between the bone and skin atrophy. Many people lose their built-in comfort cushion, so when they sit down on the hard toilet seat, skin rubs directly against bone. The only way your loved one may be able to react or communicate this discomfort is to resist sitting on the toilet seat. Uncomfortable toilet seats, however, can be replaced with soft, cushiony ones.

Quite often toilet seats are too low, making it difficult and painful for those with arthritic joints or weak muscles to stand or sit down.

Fears associated with toileting are not always of toileting itself, but related concerns. After a long life of being totally independent, Ted may resent depending upon someone else. He may feel guilty that he has become a burden or possibly afraid of being dropped while being assisted. There are as many possible causes as there are solutions. (See chapters 7 and 8.)

Could your loved one be afraid of falling off the toilet? Consider installing wall/floor mounted or fold-down grab bars on both sides of the toilet to prevent her from falling to either side. (Some bars even have a toilet paper holder attached!) Fold-down bars are especially good because they can be easily lowered when needed and raised when not. They are also helpful when a wheelchair comes into play, since the bars can be lifted out of the way for transferring from the chair and then lowered for support and security once the transfer is complete.

Fold-down grab bars:

American Health Care Supply, ASI, Barclay, Basco, Bobrick, Carex, DSI, Elcoma, ETAC USA, Frohock-Stewart, Häfele America, HEWI, Invacare Continuing Care, Lumex, McKesson, Otto Bock, Sammons Preston, Tubular Specialties Mfg., or home improvement centers.

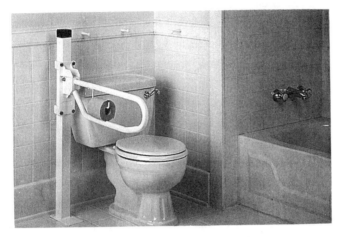

Fold-down grab bars next to the toilet not only provide a secure support when standing up but also prevent one from leaning and perhaps falling over while sitting. Photo courtesy Sammons Preston, a BISSELL® Healthcare Company. Reprinted with permission.

Maybe your loved one is afraid of being left alone or abandoned in the bathroom. People with dementia often have unrealistic concepts of time—seconds may seem like hours, a day, or even a week. With short-term memory impaired, she may not be able to recall how long you have been away. People with AD, though confused, may also be concerned about being a burden. She may fear you will give up and leave her to fend for herself.

Consider all the possibilities. Recognize that the causes can also be irrational.

Is your loved one afraid of the water in the toilet? Then remove the water. Though this may not sound like a very pleasant solution, *it is a solution.* Try turning off the valve below and flushing the toilet twice, removing the water from the bowl and the tank. Once she is finished, turn the valve back on so the tank will refill and the toilet can be flushed again.

Some caregivers have told us that they have had success with adding toilet bowl tablets to the tank. The water turns blue and becomes an item of interest rather than fear.

The bathroom may be a scary or uncomfortable place. Even if your family member has used that same bathroom for the last 30 years, it may now be unfamiliar. Worse still, the bathroom may be uncomfortable—too cold, too warm, too institutional, too drafty. Reinforce the cues that suggest an appealing bathroom, one that would make anyone comfortable. (See the section on bathrooms in chapter 1.)

"Uncle Ron knows that he has to go to the bathroom, but when he gets there he just doesn't know what to do."

If this is a problem, try providing pictures as gentle reminders. Look for humorous artwork of children in the bathroom. Maybe a tasteful picture of a child sitting on the toilet could go on the wall directly in front of it. (Visit your local framing company to look through their catalogues of pictures and artwork.)

Toilet bidet devices:

Access with Ease, AdaptAbility, American Health Care Supply, Enrichments, Hygiene Specialties, J. C. Manufacturing, Lubidet, Maddak, McKesson, MNO Sales, North Coast Medical, Sammons Preston, Toto Kiki.

For those who have difficulty cleaning themselves, bidet devices can be added to your toilet. These devices produce a water spray for cleaning the user. Some attach to your toilet, with hoses that extend either to the sink or to the valve below the toilet. Available options on the more expensive units include heated toilet seats, heated water, and water pressure adjusting controls. Some even provide drying fans!

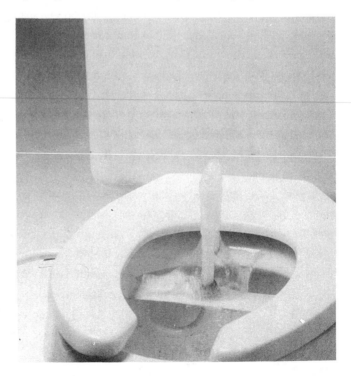

A bidet device is recommended if your family member has difficulty cleaning up after using the toilet. Photo courtesy Sammons Preston, a BISSELL® Healthcare Company. Reprinted with permission.

Some caregivers feel strongly that the sound and feel of water stimulates urinating. They suggest using a bidet that introduces the sound and feel of warm water to help the person urinate (while sitting on the toilet).

The three situations here involve vessels that could have been mistaken for a toilet. Have you never inadvertently and absentmindedly done something inappropriate, like throw a wadded-up piece of paper in the hamper by mistake? Your loved one's mind is impaired by disease, so more and more mistakes like these are likely. He may even recognize the error afterwards and be embarrassed. (See chapter 2 for discussion on cues and signage that may help avoid these types of errors.)

Note the similarity of a hamper to a toilet with the lid up. Try using a laundry bag or child-proof hamper, or replace your hamper with one that has less resemblance to a toilet and might require more skill to open. Add some color and decoration to minimize the resemblance, recognizing the fact that some white hampers with openings may also look like urinals.

Remove the opportunities for confusion. If your father uses the wastepaper basket or hamper for a toilet, remove it. Put it in the cabinet, close the door, and if necessary lock it up.

Alzheimer's gradually takes your loved one back in time. Your family member, as a child, may have been taught not to flush toilet paper down the toilet because of inadequacies in the plumbing system. Just as people with AD may revert to languages they spoke as a child, they may also revert to practices that were appropriate then.

Perhaps here too it might be best to remove the alternative vessels, leaving only the correct one behind. Or you might try a sign reading "Flush Used Toilet Paper Down the Toilet." You can always use the excuse that the sign is for the grandchildren or visitors, not your mother!

"Dad goes to the bathroom in the wastepaper basket."

"Mom went to the bathroom in her purse today."

"Granpa just unzipped his pants and peed in the flower pot. Why?"

"My husband keeps going to the bathroom in the hamper."

Child-proof hampers:
Safety 1st.

"I went into the bathroom after Granny was done. There was a terrible smell. Instead of flushing the toilet paper down the commode, she had thrown it into the trash can!"

Bathing and Showering

Bathing and showering are basic activities of daily living, but as AD progresses, priorities change. Hand-in-hand with a possible decline in the senses of smell and vision, the priorities of bathing, grooming, cleanliness, and appearance may be neglected. Your family member may not realize that he smells bad or that he is dirty—he may even think he just took a bath.

Your loved one may feel so strongly about this that her defense mechanisms add to the problem. Delusions may contribute to her resistance to bathe and "stories" created to justify her fears. Whether a ploy to avoid that dreaded bath or as a result of the disease, your family member may not realize she has a problem with hygiene. (See also chapter 2 for discussion on fears associated with bathing.)

"I already had my bath today!"

"I just took a bath."

"I don't need a bath!"

Maybe as a young girl your mother only bathed once a week, perhaps on Sunday before going to church, or when the bed sheets were changed. These may be the standards, rooted in her long-term memory, which she is now recalling. Suddenly every day is bath day. She has no control over when she bathes, who bathes her, or even how she bathes. How might you react to this situation? Or perhaps the bathroom is just uncomfortable—too warm or too cold. (See chapter 1.)

Loss of Control

Loss of control of the bathing process can be a major cause for agitation and avoiding the bath. Allow your loved one as much control and as many choices as possible. Make decisions safe and easy. For example, a shower seat and grab bars offer the options of standing or sitting. A safer bathroom allows minimal concern for danger or accidents. A hand-held showerhead (with an on-off control) lets your family member control the water. Extra wash cloths allow your family member to wash himself or hold one as you wash him. Plenty of towels allow him to help dry himself. You may need to create additional storage space in your bathroom to make these items available when you need them. (See chapter 1.)

Privacy

Though it may be difficult to provide the privacy your loved one insists on, you can create the illusion of privacy or provide some minimal privacy while maintaining the supervision necessary to ensure safety and adequate bathing.

This one is actually easy. You have several options:

- Bathroom door knobs are usually privacy locks, lockable from the bathroom side only. To solve Aunt Myrna's problem, keep an emergency key close by. Usually, a straightened coat hanger or any tool that you can insert into the hole in the outside knob will do—push it and simultaneously turn the knob, and the door should open. For more information on what might serve as an emergency key for your particular lock, call a local locksmith.
- Replace the privacy lock with a passage lock (that has no locks). (For your own privacy install a hook-and-eye latch in a location where Aunt Myrna is less likely to discover it—either high or low, beyond her normal range of vision.)
- Consider replacing the bathroom door with a heavy shower curtain or folding door to allow both privacy and quick access.

Perhaps a call button next to the toilet will help. Or a wireless intercom could be installed, so that you can listen for calls for help. Intercoms also make it possible for you to conduct a two-way conversation, with no effort required by your loved one, yet still maintaining privacy and dignity. There are several sorts of pagers available; or a simple bell could be used to summon help.

Safety

In addition to common falls and bathroom accidents, people with AD are also at risk for unpredictable reactions and outbursts. These can result in hostile attacks on the caregiver, irrational displays of panic, or persistent resistance to bathing. Your loved one may do anything to defend herself or to escape this "terrible" task.

One winning combination for safety and caregiving in the bathroom is:

- Shower or bathtub seat
- Grab bars

"Aunt Myrna locks herself in the bathroom and then can't figure out how to unlock the door."

Passage locks are available at home improvement centers or from a locksmith.

Wireless intercom:

Radio Shack, The Safety Zone, Solutions, or home improvement centers.

Bell to jingle:

Graham Field.

Personal pager:

Access with Ease, AdaptAbility, Brookstone, Crestwood, Enrichments, Harris Communications, Hear More, LS & S, Sammons Preston.

Personal pager worn on wrist:

J.C. Penney Special Needs Catalogue.

- Non-slip floor and tub surfaces
- Hand-held showerhead

A hand-held showerhead is a removable, replacement showerhead on an extension hose. It attaches to your existing showerhead, the wall, or a vertical rod, allowing it to be adjusted or moved to any height. Look for hand-held showerheads that have a pause or on/off control on the spray head.

Hand-held showerheads offer several advantages:

Hand-held showerhead assemblies with pause and on-off controls at the handles:

Access with Ease, Alsons, American Health Care Supply, Care Catalogue, Carex, Guardian Products, Jaclo, Lumex, M.O.M.S., McKesson, North Coast Medical, Inc., Sammons Preston, Sears Home HealthCare Catalogue, Shamrock Medical Equipment.

- The caregiver can aim and direct the source of water, avoiding the need for your loved one to stand up, twist, and move around to get wet or rinse off soap.
- Your family member can remain sitting while showering, minimizing the risk of a fall.
- Water can be directed to clean difficult spots, such as the anal or genital areas, which might be soiled due to incontinence.
- The flow of water can be controlled. If your loved one becomes upset, the caregiver can easily turn off the water or allow him to hold the showerhead.
- The caregiver can bathe only certain areas and not others, protecting bandaged areas, the face, or hair.
- Your family member can shower without being forced to sit under a continuous rush of water.
- A hand-held showerhead makes it possible to redirect the water if it is too hot or cold. In a small, confined shower your family member might be unable to escape scalding or freezing water from a fixed, wall-mounted showerhead.
- If necessary, the caregiver can conveniently check and adjust the water temperature.
- Your family member can feel the temperature of the water before getting into the shower. He can be gently introduced to the shower, rather than forced into a rushing surge of spraying water.

See chapter 8 for a discussion of shower seats and other ideas to help getting in and out of the shower or tub.

Bathing Alternatives

There are many other products and devices helpful in the bath and shower. As the disease progresses and changes your loved one, you will need to make changes also. As your family member has more difficulty walking, certain modifications will be helpful. You may eventually need a tub or shower that is wheelchair accessible. If fear or resistance to bathing becomes an issue you may want to consider alternatives. (See also chapter 8, where I discuss bathtub seats and transfer seats, inserts and even bathtubs with doors.)

In the later stages of Alzheimer's disease your loved one will likely become bed-bound, unable to walk or visit the bathroom. Bathing will be difficult. Here are two products that might help:

- A sponge bath may be one answer. You can use a washcloth and warm water, or a packaged product called the BagBath, a soothing cleanser in a non-woven cotton cloth.

- Another option might be giving your loved one a real bath, *in bed,* using an inflatable bathtub called the E-Z Bath. Your family member rolls on his side, allowing the uninflated tub to be placed under him. A special wet/dry vacuum cleaner (provided by the company) inflates the tub walls, sort of like a child's inflatable pool. Hoses run from the inflatable tub to

BagBath:

Incline Technologies.

E-Z Bath and E-Z Shower:

HomeCare Products, McKesson, Sammons Preston. Ads we saw included a 25-foot hose, the vacuum cleaner to inflate the tub, and a hand-held showerhead. Make sure you discuss your situation with a customer service representative and get all of the accessories you need when ordering.

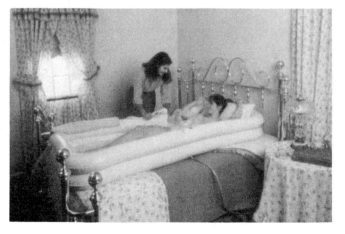

The E-Z Bath allows you to bathe your family member even if he is bedbound. Photo courtesy E-Z Bath.

Anti-scalding devices:

Accent on Living, AdaptAbility, Joan Cook, Independent Living Aids, Keeney, Memry Corporation, or home improvement centers.

Anti-scalding showerheads:

Accent on Living, AdaptAbility, Brookstone, Independent Living Aids, Keeney, Lighthouse Enterprises.

Anti-scalding device for the bathtub faucet:

Keeney.

Pressure-sensitive temperature-limiting bath and shower valves:

Delta, Kohler, Moen, Price Pfister, plumbing dealers.

the bathroom for water and drainage. Ordinary garden hoses can be used to extend the lines if the bathroom is far away. There is also an E-Z Shower, which uses a bag of water overhead for a gentle shower, in bed.

Adjusting Water Temperature

Judgment and hand/eye coordination are skills that gradually disappear with AD. With their loss come inherent dangers throughout the house, dangers that require constant awareness on the part of the caregiver. In this case, however, you actually have at least three alternatives:

- Install anti-scalding devices.
- Replace your hot and cold mixing valves (in the shower and tub) with pressure-sensitive, *temperature-limiting* valves.
- Turn down the thermostat on your water heater.

Anti-scalding devices should be installed in *all* faucets in bathrooms, the laundry room, and kitchen, as well as in showerheads. These inexpensive, easy-to-install devices fit on or in the faucets and protect you and your loved one from getting scalded. (For more information refer to the chapters 1 and 9.)

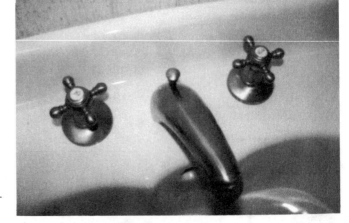

Old-fashioned X-handled faucets might be easier for your loved one to recognize. Photo courtesy Miller's Fine Decorative Hardware, Inc.

A single-lever or single-handle faucet may be difficult for those who are confused. Remember that people with dementia often retreat back into their past, when life was different. Single-control faucets were not available decades ago and may not be recognized now. Many are also difficult to grasp and turn.

Consider replacing your single-lever handle with a more conventional, old-fashioned model, which really is a simple job for a plumber or handyman. Visit your local home improvement center or plumbing supply store to select from a variety of models.

Dressing

Dressing and grooming are essential activities of daily living. They are no less important for your loved one, though she may no longer possess all the skills necessary to successfully complete these tasks or make the right decisions. At first, the problems may be as minor as misplacing stockings or a favorite sweater. As time goes on, the amount of clothes in the closet may become overwhelming. Fear of making the wrong decision may result in no decision at all.

What to Wear

When something is discovered missing, it is common for people with AD to accuse someone else of stealing it (though the dress or pants may be at the laundry or in the hamper). To avoid Barbara's reaction, try having two red dresses or two pairs of green pants, hanging the spare on a hook or hanger in a visible location. One of the two red dresses will always be visible or being worn. When the accusation is made, it can easily and quickly be resolved. Devious, yes—and often successful.

If Barbara insists on wearing the same dirty red dress, let her put on the "same" red dress. Only you will know that you have switched it with its twin—a clean red dress.

If you can't duplicate the red dress, consider purchasing a small, compact washer/dryer. Locate it upstairs, near the bedroom or bathroom. If Barbara insists on putting on the same dirty red dress, let her—but wash it first, maybe even asking

"We've got one of those single-lever faucets in the bathroom, but Martha can't figure out how to use it. She puts the handle in the middle and when the water comes out warm she says the water heater is broken again."

"X"-type hot and cold water knobs:

Renovator's or home improvement centers.

"We just gave Barbara a shower and she insists on putting on the same red dress. It's so dirty, but she is so adamant that we either give in or face World War III."

Combination washer/dryer that requires no venting:

Bendix, Equator Corp.

Stacking washer/dryer:

Maytag, Westinghouse. Also check with appliance dealers. Many offer small, compact washer/dryers for apartments.

her to help. (See chapter on 7 for more discussion on compact washer/dryers.)

Decisions are difficult for those with dementia. Often people will simply choose the same article of clothing over and over. It's the safe thing to do: Why chance making a wrong decision by choosing a different pair of pants? Again, two or three pairs of the "same" green pants will make it possible for Uncle Ernie to be able to wear the "right" pair of pants for every occasion. Why question his choice if it makes him happy?

"Uncle Ernie wants to wear his green pants every day. He's only got one pair. What are we to do?"

Simplicity and organization are essential for people in the middle stages of Alzheimer's disease. The simpler the closet is organized, the less intimidating it will appear. In addition, it is far easier to choose from two or three items of clothing than it is to choose from a full closet.

Take advantage of sliding closet doors, which reveal only half the closet's contents at a time. Organize your family member's closet so that half the shirts and pants are on one side and half on the other. When it's time to select a pair of pants, slide open the closet door, revealing only three pairs of pants to choose from, rather than six. (If he's fond of that pair of green pants, have one on each side!) If the pants (now on the other side) are discovered missing, all that is necessary is to slide the doors to reveal the pants in the other section.

(An advantage to your family member's preference for wearing the same-colored clothes each day is that if he ever wanders out of the house, it will be easier to describe what he is wearing to the police.)

"Dad goes into his closet and puts on his lightweight pants—in the middle of winter."

Get rid of excess clothing, and relocate off-season clothing somewhere else. This, too, will minimize the number of choices in the closet.

Organize your father's closet so that only appropriate clothes are available. You might also try cuing him to the correct season with a calendar on the wall displaying pictures of snow-covered landscapes in winter and sunny fields of blossoms in the spring.

Remember that older people need two to three times more light than they did when they were younger. Sufficient light makes it easier to tell the difference between the blue, brown, and black socks and to distinguish light pinks from off-whites and other pastel colors. Provide more lighting in your family member's room, especially in areas where it is most needed— near the closet, dresser, and mirror.

Dressers, Drawers, and Closets

Try finding a magazine or catalogue with pictures of underwear (shirts, socks, etc.), cut them out, and paste them on the appropriate drawer. Another possibility would be to store a few pairs of underwear, socks, and shirts on open shelves in the bedroom. This would make them more visible and easy to find.

"Allen can never find his underwear. He gets so embarrassed. But he is charming and just says he knows they are here somewhere, the underwear fairy has been here again!"

Putting Clothes On Correctly

Again, simplicity and organization are key. You can organize clothes so that they demonstrate the order of dressing. Use two or three grab bars or towel rack accessories that provide multiple rods. Hang the clothing in layers, so that each layer hides the one beneath it. Display the clothes in reverse order. The underwear goes on top, then the shirt, and at the bottom are the pants. To get to the next level of clothing your loved one will have to remove the layer on top. If he puts them on in that order your plan will work.

Free-standing towel bar unit:

Improvements, Unison Metal Products.

"Mom keeps putting on her underwear outside of her pants. It is so humiliating. She's always been so careful of her appearance and what she wears. Now she can't seem to do anything right. Yesterday she just sat down and started crying."

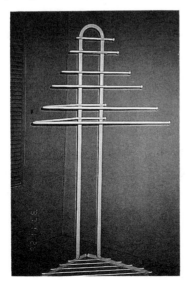

With a multi-armed rack, you can hang your family member's clothing in layers, encouraging him to put them on in the right order. Photo courtesy Unison Metal Products.

"We bought a cut-out paper doll at the store with all the accessories. We pasted these figures on Mom's closet door: first in her underwear, next wearing her dress, and finally her shoes. It seemed to work . . . a little."

This idea wasn't completely successful, but it was fun. It only worked when the caregiver's mother looked at the cut-out dolls and realized they were guides to help her get dressed. But the whole family enjoyed the exercise, including her mother. Trial and error are very important tools. Some ideas will work and others might not. You have to discover what works in your particular situation.

As mentioned earlier, people with AD often make lists and maps. Many caregivers find them in their loved one's clothing: Lists of the right ingredients to put in the cereal bowl or maps to and from the kitchen. If it works, learn from your family member, and encourage their use.

Create with your family member a list of clothing in the proper order for dressing. Tape it to the closet door or in the area where he gets dressed.

Refusing to Get Undressed

Sometimes refusing to take one's clothes off is just what it appears to be—a stand. Your family member may be fighting to maintain control over his life, and only he is going to decide when he will get undressed. After all, when one's freedom and choices are taken away, it's only normal to resist.

Is it possible that your family member is embarrassed to get undressed in front of others, perhaps the "person" in the mirror? In this case, you may want to cover the mirror, so the "stranger" will no longer be in the bathroom with your father. Could your family member be associating undressing with more frightening activities (perhaps bathing)? (Refer to the discussion of fears chapter 2.)

Create a Special Dressing Area

Setting up specific areas to assist your loved one to complete daily activities could be very helpful. Introducing subtle cues often helps suggest correct behavior (toileting in the bathroom, eating in the dining room, and dressing in the dressing area). In addition, these spaces can be specially prepared to assist and offer gentle reminders: a comfortable, stable chair to sit on and perhaps an appropriate piece of artwork of someone getting dressed. (The chair will also be a good place for friends to sit and visit.) If space is limited, the bed will do, but it isn't as good as a chair with a high back offering different levels to hold (seat, arms, and back).

Imagine how much support a grab bar or chair might offer when trying to balance on one foot, putting on a pair of pants. We often take the process of dressing for granted. For a person with AD multiple tasks performed simultaneously (balancing and putting on pants) may be impossible.

A special dressing area that is close to both the bathroom and the closet will make it more convenient to undress and enter the bathroom, as well as shorten the trip to the closet when dressing.

"Allen can't dress himself anymore, so we placed a grab bar on the wall in the bedroom. Now he holds onto it while being dressed. This provides a small, but to him significant, responsibility in dressing. It seems to make an otherwise undignified and impossible task a little more acceptable, since he can now help and contribute."

Grooming

Grooming is an important activity that you will want your loved one to continue and enjoy for as long as possible. We spend a lifetime making ourselves presentable and trying to look our very best. These lessons have deep roots in our long-term memory. As long-term memory replaces short-term memory, these values and concerns may resurface.

A caregiver's assistance, however necessary, may be seen as an intrusion or a reminder of the disease. It could result in hostility or agitation. Giving your family member a role or responsibility (however slight) in his own care may help.

Create a Pleasant Grooming Area

Create a special area in your loved one's bedroom where she can sit in front of a mirror and groom herself comfortably, at her own pace. Requiring your loved one to stand at a bathroom mirror imposes a time constraint based on how long he can remain standing comfortably and safely. Other tasks besides grooming must occur simultaneously when standing at the mirror, such as balancing or holding onto the sink's edge or a grab bar.

A table, desk, or vanity with plenty of light and a comfortable chair is a good idea. Simplicity is a repeated theme that applies here, too. A makeup table overflowing with too many

"As a young girl Mom taught me to stroke my long hair with a brush 100 times every day. Suddenly she has begun doing it, though now her hair is very short."

*"Yesterday was Irene's birthday.
We turned it into a special event.
Eileen from the beauty parlor
came over to our house before the
party to do Irene's hair. We really
didn't have a good place for this,
so we went out on the porch,
brought pans of warm water and
towels and we all had our hair
done in the sunshine. Irene
loved it!"*

brushes, combs, colors, and products may be overwhelming and self-defeating. Instead, provide only a few items.

Provide a comfortable chair. Two chairs would be better yet (the second for a caregiver, granddaughter, or friend, who might want to help, chat, or join in and groom herself).

At some point it may become too difficult to take your father to the barber or mother to the hair dresser. Yet you could create another special place in the den or on the porch (at least while weather permits) that could be used for a visiting barber or hairdresser. Imagine the pleasure of sitting in the den or on the back deck, watching the grandchildren playing in the yard, while getting a shave or your hair cut or shampooed. This could turn an otherwise difficult occasion into a unique and fun experience. Maybe other family members could get their hair done, too, making this a family affair!

Mirrors

Mirrors are important tools for dressing, grooming, and looking our best. Yet, there may be problems with mirrors related to AD. Your family member may not be living in the present and recognize himself in the mirror. His image of himself may be that of years ago, a younger man, and he may insist adamantly that the person in the mirror is just not him.

A full-length mirror allows you to see yourself from head to toe. There are advantages and disadvantages. Suspicions of strangers in the room can be triggered by a reflection in the mirror or movement seen out of the corner of the eye. Furthermore, a full-length mirror allows one to see a full-height figure, while a smaller mirror reveals only part of one's body and may be less likely result in misunderstood reflections.

Mirrors may be upsetting to your family member if she is not happy with how she looks or how she has "let herself go." Imagine the horror your mother might feel seeing herself with lipstick all over her mouth, instead of the meticulous detail she expected.

Try a smaller, table-top mirror that reveals only partial glimpses of the face, rather than the whole face. Your family member may then focus only on the details, rather than the whole image. If she doesn't get a look at her whole face, what she does see may not be so upsetting or likely to be misinterpreted.

Mirrors that present problems may have to be removed or covered. Observe your family member's reactions, making sure that fear or defensive actions don't result. (See chapter 2 for more discussion on mirrors, fears, and related problems.)

Lighting

Along with mirrors, lighting also plays an important role in grooming. Too little light or the wrong type of light bulb may result in a less-than-flattering reflection. Incandescent light bulbs, for example, generate a warmer light, higher in the warm colors of the spectrum: yellows, browns, tans, and reds. We all look better under light that reflects warm color in our skin, rather than cool fluorescent bulbs (higher in blues and greens) that make you look pale.

"We changed the lights in Mom's bathroom. Now they giver her a 'rosier' appearance."

If you are stuck with fluorescent fixtures in your bathroom, replace the bulbs with ones that say "natural light," "warm white," or "full spectrum" for a more natural display of color. These bulbs will provide more flattering light.

Too much or too little light can also be a problem. Older people need two to three times the amount of light as when they were younger. But with Alzheimer's disease, too much lighting can result in distracting and irritating glare or too much environmental stimulation. Replace clear bulbs that allow a view of the glaring filament with low wattage frosted bulbs.

Socializing

Alzheimer's, with all of its unusual behaviors, is a difficult disease for the person with AD, family, *and* friends. With this in mind:

- Make talking, listening, and socializing as easy as possible for everyone.
- Make the experience as enjoyable as possible for everyone.
- Provide activities (food for the birds in the back-

yard, crossword puzzles) and conversation pieces (photos, knickknacks) in your social area.

- Recognize, remove, and minimize triggers to possible upsets and problems that might occur and discourage future visits.

Once again, create a special place in the home where the surroundings encourage socializing. (You may fashion one special place that can serve more than one purpose.) This could be a separate room or just a corner—a quiet, remote location without distractions or background noise. Anticipating possible agitation, this special area should be safety-proofed, with soft edges, and free of dangerous items that can be picked up and thrown.

Provide conversation pieces and activities that make it possible for friends to participate. These might include music, puzzles, and religious items, as well as photos and memorabilia for your family member to recall and share his memories with family, friends, and visitors. Provide plenty of comfortable chairs for everyone.

Reminiscing

Frames, photo albums, and photo displays:

Exposures or crafts or photo supply stores.

Reminiscence Magazine, full of pictures and articles from years gone by–(800) 344-6913.

Reminiscent products:

Nasco.

As your loved one depends more upon her long-term memory, the therapeutic value and pleasure of recalling and sharing life experiences are likely to grow as well. Reminiscing and reviewing the "good ol' days" is one of the most-enjoyed sports of those with AD. Some stories get told several times a day, with very few changes, yet a lot of pleasure.

Encourage stories from the past with photos of neighborhoods where she once lived, pictures relating to skills, accomplishments, and jobs she once had. Photo albums, "memory books," cards, and mementos stimulate recognition and help to bring distant memories to the surface.

Add labels to the photos. Identify locations and people and other important facts that your family member can discuss over and over with friends. They will also help visiting caregivers who may not be familiar with your family member. Labels and photos help present your loved one as a person, rather than a patient—

someone who has made a difference, accomplished things, been places, and has interesting stories to tell.

If your family member worked on a train, go to a flea market and pick up books on trains and train memorabilia. If music is enjoyable, find old sheet music and display it on the walls or on a table. Perhaps your wife loved to sew—buy fashion and dress pattern magazines.

Display awards and trophies, no matter how insignificant (third place in the 40th Street Relay Race). Everyone's life is full of accomplishments, large and small. If you can't find the trophy he won at that high-school swim meet, go out and buy one; don't miss opportunities at local flea markets or garage sales where people may be clearing out their attics! (You can always say you found it upstairs in an old trunk.)

Frame and display meaningful newspaper articles. Create a collage of articles that your family member can boast about, take pride in, and relate stories about. If you can't find suitable articles, have a printing company create a newspaper page with an article about your loved one, written by you!

Be careful where you locate memorabilia. *Do* place them:

- where they can be seen and enjoyed privately while sitting down or lying in bed; and
- where they can be easily seen by family and visitors to stimulate interesting conversation.

Don't place them:

- where they might be dangerous distractions, such as hanging on walls going up stairs;
- where they are difficult to reach; or
- close to other objects that can be knocked over or broken.

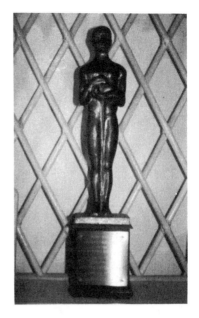

A false Oscar trophy is the source of stories and pride for someone very special to her family.

Remove photos and portraits if they become unpleasant reminders of people who have passed on. Mourning the loss of a loved one will put a damper on any social event. If your family member mourns the loss of her spouse every time she sees a photo of him or asks where he might be, remove these triggers. This may or may not be true in your case. Just as the reflection in the mirror can be a "stranger" to fear or a "friend" to talk to, photos of departed loved ones may or may not be upsetting.

Communication Difficulties

Certain environmental factors can be barriers to successful communication. They can include background noises, poor lighting (making it difficult to see facial features), and orientation of the seating.

One of the biggest obstacles to effective communication is background noise. Older ears find it harder to isolate and distinguish conversation from annoying environmental sounds. For those who are confused, this is also another form of over-stimulation, too much going on to understand. The result may be agitation.

Sources of background noise include:

ringing telephones	buzzing ceiling fans
outside traffic	family conversation
the dryer	fluorescent lights
telephone conversation	air conditioners
children playing	airplanes overhead
neighbors arguing	barking dogs
the washing machine	the dishwasher
water running	flushing toilets
the television or radio	fans

Your fluorescent lights may have ballasts that are going bad and create a buzzing sound. These sounds can be annoying and make it difficult for your loved one to hear, especially if the buzzing (which you may not notice) is amplified by a hearing aid.

"We would tell Lenny what to do. He'd say 'okay' and then go right ahead and do it his way. This happened over and over, and we would get so mad. We finally decided to have his ears checked and found out they were full of wax. Lenny couldn't hear us!"

Identify causes of background noise in your home, especially in areas where conversation typically takes place. Remove those that you can and soften the room with carpeting (on the floor and decorative pieces on the wall) to absorb excessive noise. Add soft pillows, curtains, and upholstery. All will help.

Any hearing impairment, including background noise interference, can result in failure to hear, yet appear to be an inability to understand or remember. If you suspect a medical hearing or visual impairment, consult your doctor.

Provide plenty of light where conversation typically occurs. This will make it easier to see visual cues. Physical components of conversation, such as reading lips, hand gestures, eyebrows that rise with a question, and smiles that delight with laughter are also a part of communication. Often these gestures are as important as the conversation itself, offering the cues to laugh or smile (signs of understanding and participation).

Some visual problems, such as tunnel vision, visual cliffing, and poor depth perception do seem to be related to Alzheimer's disease. Your loved one may not be able to hear, understand, or realize that he is being spoken to unless he is facing his guest directly. Both lighting and furniture arrangements will help.

Arrange the furniture to encourage eye contact and face-to-face conversation. When sofas, chairs, and benches face each other or are perpendicular to each other, you can sit facing your family member, so that he realizes when he is being spoken to and experiences all the cues that contribute to the conversation.

Large ottomans have been praised for how they can be pulled up for sitting in front of a loved one without the formality of a chair. The warmth and proximity they offer create opportunities for close and caring conversation. They offer other benefits as well, including the obvious one of providing a place to rest your feet. Make sure yours is large and easy to see and won't create an obstacle.

"I used to have trouble talking to Mom. Whenever we talked it seemed that she wasn't listening to me and sometimes she wondered where my voice was coming from. One day I noticed that if I sat right in front of her she had less difficulty. I realized that I had to be right in front of her face before she would realize I was talking to her."

It's always better to have two chairs or benches rather than just one, so there will always be a place for a friend.

Using the Telephone

To help someone with Evelyn's problem try placing labeled pictures of friends and relatives next to phone. Perhaps your loved one will be able to associate the picture with the name.

Provide a paper and pen next to the telephone for notes that your loved one may want to take during the conversation (appointments, names, telephone numbers, messages, reminders, lists, directions, etc.). Since short-term memory may be limited, this may be a helpful and much-appreciated gesture.

"Evelyn doesn't recognize me on the phone anymore. I tell her my name is Karen, but she can't place the name. I've been her best friend for 20 years."

"Uncle Dan can't dial the phone anymore. He keeps getting the wrong numbers."

Telephones with large buttons:

Easy Street, Hello Direct, HITEC, Independent Living Aids, LS & S.

Easy-to-read telephone number attachment:

Independent Living Aids, LS & S, Sammons Preston.

BackTalk number announcer:

Independent Living Aids, LS & S.

Telephones equipped with Backtalk number announcer:

HITEC.

Automatic dialing phones with pictures:

Ameriphone, Crestwood, Dynamic Living, DTE Edison America, Independent Needs Centre, Polyconcept USA, Sears Home Healthcare, The Sharper Image.

Mainstreet Messenger:

Elcombe Systems Limited, Maxi Aids.

Perhaps Uncle Dan can't remember the right telephone number to dial. Maybe he has a visual impairment and is struggling with numbers that are too small for him to see. He might have poor hand/eye coordination, trembling, or unsteadiness, making it difficult to hit the right button.

Uncle Dan might do better with a telephone with large buttons, or a large-button attachment for the phone he's using.

Your family member might have more success with a back-talk number announcer that audibly announces the numbers as he pushes them. If he wants to push 4-7-7 and accidentally pushes 4-6-6 he will hear his mistake as it happens.

Or he might be able to use an automatic telephone dialer that remembers and dials certain telephone numbers at the push of only one button. Many telephones and answering machines come with buttons that can be programmed to dial numbers automatically.

One possible problem with programmable phones is that one button is often reserved for emergency numbers (911 or HELP). For a person with Alzheimer's disease this may not be a good idea, since that button may get pushed by mistake or too often. In most communities, when 911 is dialed, rescue units must respond, even if the caller hangs up without saying a word.

You might try placing a label (and a small photo) next to each button to identify the person whose number it dials. Make sure there is plenty of light to see the labels and photos. A magnifying glass kept on the table may also help. (Magnifying glasses are available at eyeglass stores and drug stores.)

You might consider special telephones with pictures or the MainStreet Messenger, which offer convenient communication access, even when there is difficulty dialing conventional telephones.

Some automatic dialing phones with pictures provide numbered buttons large enough to insert photos of the people one wishes to call. Pre-program their telephone numbers, and all that is necessary is to push the button with the appropriate picture.

The MainStreet Messenger is a telephone and automatic dialer. In addition, your family member can wear a pendant

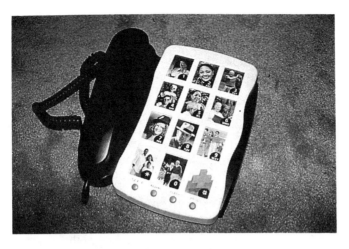

The Photo Dial Phone. Photo courtesy Polyconcept USA.

with a button. When this button is pushed (in case of a fall, for example), the telephone automatically begins calling the pre-programmed emergency numbers until it receives the proper response. The person called can then push a number on his phone (according to the taped instructions) to activate the two-

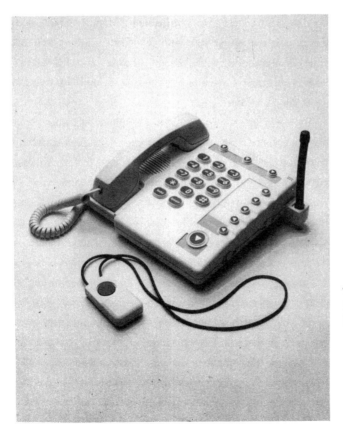

The MainStreet Messenger Phone. Photo courtesy Elcombe Systems Limited.

way speaker on your MainStreet Messenger phone (or phones, if you locate several throughout your home). Furthermore, the phone will monitor its own use and dial out for help if there is no activity (for 12, 18, or 24 hours). You can also add smoke detectors, motion detectors, or a number of other accessories. The unit will identify which one was activated and automatically dial for help.

With the MainStreet Messenger you have the option of using a 24-hour monitoring service for a monthly charge or having family members and friends respond to emergencies, thereby eliminating monthly fees.

Whenever purchasing emergency equipment that requires the use of pendant buttons, we recommend purchasing extra buttons to locate in key locations (by the bed, at the foot of stairs, next to the toilet and bathtub).

Another problem with telephones is getting to them in time when they ring, for both family member and caregiver. The cordless telephone is a marvelous invention and serves this need well. If you are giving your family member a bath, doing the laundry, or sitting with your loved one on the porch, take your cordless phone with you. No running to catch the phone, leaving your loved one alone in the tub, or fumbling with awkward telephone cords.

You could also install an additional telephone jack wherever you might need one. These could be conventional wall jacks (installed by your local telephone company) or remote jacks that work through your home's electrical system and require no new wiring.

If your loved one doesn't hear the telephone when it rings, have both her hearing and hearing aid checked. You may also want to consider telephones that are clearer and amplified, or devices that flash a light to indicate when the phone is ringing.

And, of course, there are always telephone answering machines or services to pick up calls for you. Check your local home improvement center or telephone store. Your local phone company probably offers an answering service. Contact them and discuss their charges. Among the advantages of using the telephone company's service is that there is one less piece of confusing equipment cluttering the table that can be broken.

Wireless telephone jacks:

Brookstone, Comtrad Industries, Hear More, Phonex, Radio Shack.

Amplified telephones:

Ameriphone, Hello Direct, Independent Living Aids, LS & S, Sammons Preston.

Telephone flashers and accessories:

Ameriphone, Envirotrol Company, Hear More, HITEC, Independent Living Aids, National Flashing Signal Systems.

Automatic telephone recording devices:

Canwood Products, Hello Direct, LS & S, The Safety Zone, or security equipment, telephone equipment, or electronics stores.

Install an automatic telephone recorder. These are tape recorders that automatically record all telephone conversations. They can be used to monitor calls and take messages, then you can just listen to the tape each day and follow up on the messages.

"Dad still answers the phone and has nice conversations—but never remembers to take a message or tell us who called."

Personal Emergency Response Systems (PERS)

PERS systems are devices and services that allow a person to summon help in the event of an emergency. Basically, they are made up of two components—a transmitter button (wall-mounted, set on a night table, or worn as a bracelet or necklace) and a telephone dialer. If help is needed, the button can be pressed, activating the dialer. Operators will then respond to determine if there is a real emergency and the appropriate action to take (call a family member, friend, neighbor, distant caregiver, or 911).

There are many variations among PERS systems. Some services offer options to lease or buy the equipment, additional wall-mounted buttons (for the tub or shower, next to the toilet, and at the bottom of the stairs), daily "check-ins," battery back-up, connections to pagers, fire and smoke alarms, home security systems, and medication reminders. Some systems even work if the phone is off the hook or someone else is on the line (to date none of the systems allows you to talk through the bracelet or pendant). Each company is different, with different services, options, and rates.

Discuss individual monthly service charges and system options with the company representative. PERS systems are among the many devices that allow a person to live independently longer and offer peace of mind for long-distance caregivers.

For more information on PERS systems, contact AARP and ask for their product report on PERS (stock #D12905—latest edition).

You may contact AARP at the following address:

PERS Systems:

American Medical Alert, Colonial Medical Alert Systems, Elcombe Systems Limited, Fidelity TeleAlarm, Guardian Medical Monitoring, Interim In-Touch, Lifeline Systems, Link to Life, Magnavox SecureAlert, Maxi Aids, Medic Aid Response Systems, PERSYS, Pioneer Medical Systems, ResponseLink, SecurityLink, SOS Wireless Communications, Transcience.

American Association of Retired Persons
601 E Street, NW
Washington, DC 20049
(800) 424-3410

Food Preparation

Preparing meals and feeding one's family represent primary means by which people care and show their love. With Alzheimer's disease your wife or mother will continue to be able to prepare meals for only so long. Until then, you will want to take steps to preserve this important act, making changes gradually.

Replace fragile dishware and glasses with more forgiving, non-breakable pieces. (If you have grandchildren, maybe you can say you are doing it for them.) Organize cabinets and pantries to minimize and streamline their contents, making items easier to see and find. Group ingredients, bowls, and utensils for certain recipes and meals together. This will remind your loved one of all the ingredients required and help him find them. (See also chapter 2.)

As suggested earlier, post lists that you and your family member create together. Encourage your family member to display them as she sees necessary. One of the earliest and most distressing mishaps that occur in the kitchen is when a meal or treat is prepared short of one or two ingredients. This can be a major disappointment, especially when preparing goodies for others has been a lifetime family delight. It may be upsetting for your mother or wife to give up or accept her inability to perform this.

Remember also that lists not only serve to remind your family member of all the ingredients that go into a dish, but also the steps necessary to prepare it. Even the most mundane steps that we might take for granted can be overlooked. It wouldn't be the first time someone with AD tried to remove a hot pan from the oven without protective mitts! Make sure your loved one's lists include all the important steps, especially turning off appliances.

Make it possible for older eyes to read lists and recipes. Replace burned-out bulbs. Add stronger bulbs where they might help, providing you don't exceed the allowable wattages (usually indicated on a label or tag). If budget allows, consider having additional lights installed on the underside of your cabinets.

Remove unnecessary countertop clutter. Too many items on the counter make it difficult to find specific items and make selections.

Safety-proof the kitchen, and remove appliances and products that are dangerous, require special skills, or may now be too difficult for your loved one to operate. Continue to observe your family member and remove unsafe products and appliances as the disease progresses. Eventually certain cabinets may need to be locked and remote switches installed on dangerous appliances that cannot be removed, such as the disposal and stove. (See also chapter 9.)

Try to recognize unique dangers, such as plastic freezing containers that might be put directly on stove burners or items wrapped in aluminum foil the that might go into microwave ovens (foil and all). Perhaps a list would help, suggesting all appropriate steps, including removing the burgers from their containers.

Provide a grab bar at the kitchen sink and at other locations in the kitchen to make standing easier and safer.

Create a special safety-proofed place in the kitchen where your loved one can sit and prepare dishes, read recipes, talk with you while you prepare a meal, or help with stirring, etc.

Remember, far more goes on in a kitchen than just cooking. You will want to make sure that everyone is comfortable when the family gathers to talk, read the paper, do puzzles at the kitchen table, or just admire the pie you and your mother made.

Your kitchen should also be wheelchair accessible, making it easy and convenient to use when your family member requires a wheelchair. Provide room for her to sit and "help" you, in her wheelchair. (See chapter 8.)

"Dad used to cook dinner himself. He'd take the hamburgers out of the freezer and put them on the stove. But sometimes he would forget to take them out of the containers! The burgers and plastic all melted together, they looked like blue cheesburgers."

Eating and Dining

Meals, too, are a family affair. In addition to eating, other activities also occur at the table—family conversation, updates on what happened that day, and enjoying the family all at one place, at one time. You will want to create an atmosphere that makes mealtime as pleasant and enjoyable as possible for everyone. (See also the discussion on the dining room in chapter 1.)

Create a Special Place at the Table

Create an environment that allows your family member to contribute to family responsibilities. Locate her place at the table, not only to eat, but also to direct or help. Your loved one can continue to make important contributions long into the disease, whether it is wiping down the table, setting the table, carrying safe items into the dining room, saying the prayer before the meal, or just folding napkins.

Your loved one's place at the table should be clearly defined and distinctive. Provide him with a chair that is comfortable and stable. Using a chair different from the others further defines his place at the table.

Do not isolate your family member at one end of the table. One of the greatest pleasures derived by families is sharing stories at the dinner table. Eating is not the only activity that occurs there. Placing your loved one near the middle of the table will help her hear everything and for all to hear her. Remember, speaking, organizing thoughts, and finding the right words may be difficult for her. There is no need to complicate matters by stranding her at the end of the table.

A simple place setting with minimal items results in fewer choices and less confusion. Replace clear glasses and containers with larger, more stable, colored versions, which are easier to see and handle and are less likely to be knocked over and spilled. Using plates and table accessories with colors that contrast with the table makes them easier to see and defines your loved one's place at the table.

Look through catalogues offering gadgets and utensils especially designed for people having difficulties. There are utensils that are easy to hold, distinctively colored plates with lips, and table mats that can differentiate your family member's space from others. Using table cloths and place mats that contrast to the dishware, for example, might help with some visual impairments common with AD.

You may need to place items that can be grabbed out of

"Mom spends almost the entire meal telling the family and her friends about her earlier days selling fruit in the open market. I must have heard the same story a hundred times, but she enjoys telling it and we just listen."

Home utensils and gadgets:

Accent on Living, AdaptAbility, Aids for Arthritis, Easy Living Specialties, Enrichments, ETAC-USA, Improvements, Independent Living Aids, J.C. Penney "Special Needs Catalogue," Lifestyle Catalogue, Maddak, Maxi Aids, Rifton, Sammons Preston, and Shamrock Medical.

reach, such as silverware or someone else's food. People with AD often invade other people's space, try to take their utensils, or eat their food. You can define his space with color, which can also define a reassuring buffer space around what is his.

People with Alzheimer's may find inappropriate uses for certain foods and utensils, so it might be best to keep them out of reach. Pepper may be added in excess, salt shakers thrown in outbursts of rage, olives may be grasped and put in one's mouth, but not chewed or swallowed, resulting in choking. Metal forks are pointed and eventually should be replaced with spoons. Avoid plastic forks, as their tips can be bitten and eaten by mistake, as your loved one is no longer able to make the distinction between them and real food.

Make room for a wheelchair or walker, even if you don't need one yet. Although this may require a little furniture re-arranging, you will want to make sure that your loved one can still come to the table. Provide extra room for an assisting caregiver, as well. Since change is confusing for people with AD, you will want to maintain the same place at the table throughout the entire course of the illness, rather than change later when more space is needed.

Create space that allows:

- access by a wheelchair without blocking travel paths;
- convenient storage space for a walker or wheel-chair; and
- space for a caregiver to sit and assist when necessary.

Use subtle cues to stimulate your loved one's appetite. Your family member may no longer remember or be able to make the appropriate connection between food and what to do with it. Hang pictures of food and people eating on the wall in front or to the side of your family member's place at the table.

Accidents Happen

Messes are a part of life, they just happen—so be prepared for accidents and spills. Dycem is a slip-resistant, plastic material that creates more friction and minimizes the possibility of plates

Slip-resistant (Dycem) place mats:
AdaptAbility, Maddak, Maxi Aids, North Coast Medical, Sammons Preston, Smith & Nephew.

sliding or glasses being knocked over. Several companies offer Dycem place mats in decorator colors so that you can choose one that contrasts to the color of your table and dishes, making them easier to see.

Store towels and wash cloths nearby to clean hands. Utensils may be difficult or impossible to use and fingers may replace them. Handling and playing with food at meal time is not unusual for people with AD. The more convenient these towels and wash cloths, the easier cleanup will be, and the less likely you will have to get up and leave your loved one to get them.

Unfortunately, dinner and sundowning often occur at the same time. Be prepared for upsets and emotional reactions. You may need to remove throwable, dangerous items from reach and create a soft and more forgiving dining room. (See chapter 9.)

Wireless telephone jacks:

Brookstone, Comtrad Industries, Hear More, Phonex, Radio Shack.

Finally, provide a comfortable chair for the caregiver. Meals involving people with AD can take several hours to complete. Install a telephone nearby so you don't have to get up from the table to answer the phone in another room.

Housekeeping

Great pride is taken in keeping the home clean and presentable for family and guests. As the disease progresses, your loved one may not notice her diminishing abilities or the decline in her home's cleanliness, though continuing to go through the motions of keeping house. To make housekeeping safer, take certain precautions and be aware of several concerns.

"Hal takes his mother, Gail, out for afternoon excursions while a cleaning lady comes in and straightens the house. The family raves about how clean their mother keeps the house, and she glows with pride."

At the same time make it possible for your loved one to continue to keep house. Just as was true for preparing meals, there are plenty of safe ways that your loved one can continue to contribute: dusting with a feather duster, straightening shelves and table decorations, sweeping, watering indoor plants, etc.

Because hallucinations are common with Alzheimer's disease, housekeeping concerns may arise from imagined dirt or lint. Carpeting with white spots may suggest fuzz, certain patterns may be seen as spots and hours may be spent obsessively trying to remove them. Your loved one may be hallucinating or seeking the pride she once felt in a job well done, taking care of the home (despite the handicaps of her disease). Providing simple, completable tasks may provide the satisfaction and sense of accomplishment she needs. Provide the opportunities and then the praise.

As your family member travels through the house "cleaning," it is important to recognize and minimize opportunities for accidents and upsets. Safety-proof the home. Look out for common and obvious dangers, as well as problems that are specifically related to dementia. (See chapter 9.)

If your family member has trouble with equilibrium, remove the vacuum cleaner so she won't push it while using it for support. Many people rely on equipment with wheels as rolling walkers, and it's definitely not safe to use a vacuum cleaner this way.

Make your home easier to move about in and clean. A less cluttered room is easier to maintain, especially for people who are confused. Even if your loved one can no longer really clean, just "making the rounds" or checking your work may be important to her.

Open furniture arrangements and spread furniture apart to create wider lanes. Remove tables and pieces of furniture from in front of windows. Windows often "need to be cleaned." Furniture blocking the way creates problems and hazards.

Laundry

Doing the laundry is another way of caring for one's family. If doing the laundry is no longer possible, your loved one may feel useless. (See also chapter 1.)

To help your mother continue to do the laundry here are a few helpful hints:

- safety-proof the laundry room (See chapter 9);
- leave only those supplies that are safe and necessary for doing the laundry in view, on open shelving;
- provide plenty of clothes that "need cleaning" and can afford to be ruined (old clothes you would have otherwise thrown out, etc.);
- purchase pre-measured boxes of detergents;

"Mom insists on ironing my shirts. Last time she left to pet the dog and forgot about the iron. My shirt was ruined, but fortunately that's all that was damaged."

Combination washer/dryer that requires no venting:

Bendix, Equator Corp. Many appliance dealers also offer small, compact washer/dryers for apartments.

- provide a chair and table for sitting and folding the laundry.

Consider installing a compact washer/dryer upstairs near the bathroom or bedroom to:

- allow your family member to do laundry without having to go downstairs or to the basement;
- satisfy his need to make a contribution to the family or to his own care;
- provide laundry facilities closer to the source of most laundry (the bedroom and bathroom);
- make incontinence easier to deal with by minimizing the distance wet towels and sheets have to be carried for laundering.

Talk to a local contractor or architect to find out what would be necessary to install a compact washer/dryer upstairs in your home.

Consider your loved one's history. When she was younger, clothes dryers may not have been available—she may have used clothes lines. Take advantage of this. Clothes lines are not only safer to use, but also offer the opportunity for a pleasurable family activity that you and your loved one can enjoy together. (Be careful to locate it and keep it high enough so that no one will walk into it when wandering in the back yard.)

Locate the line where your loved one is able to see it from her favorite chair and bed. Eventually she is likely to become bed-bound, and every little bit of entertainment (especially involving the family) will be a treat and cause for a smile.

Appliances that shut off automatically:

Black & Decker. Also check with appliance dealers.

As the disease progresses, certain appliances and products will become dangerous for your family member. The iron can be dropped or left on a piece of clothing too long. Eventually, activities such as ironing will have to be supervised, then discontinued. Until that time, use irons and other appliances that are lightweight and turn off automatically. You will also have to keep your eyes open for toxic or caustic laundry products, such as bleach, that if improperly used or mishandled could be harmful. (See chapter 9 for more suggestions.)

When it is no longer safe for your loved one to perform basic laundry chores, hide the laundry and use closed hampers. This way she won't see the dirty clothes piling up and may not feel the need to do the laundry. Store laundry supplies only in the laundry room. Place a secure lock on the door. (See chapter 6.)

Medication Administration

Eventually all medications will need to be locked in a secure cabinet to prevent overmedication, but until then, here are a few suggestions that might help.

The home environment can't ensure that your loved one takes his medications on time. But it can help contribute to your family member taking the *correct medications* and making it possible for him to know the *correct time,* which together might help accomplish the original goal.

Provide a large-faced or talking clock to help your loved one know the correct time, in both the bedroom and the kitchen. A push of the button and a voice will accurately tell him the time. There are also talking wrist watches.

Some older people often have difficulty seeing and identifying medications by reading the label on the bottle. (Given the size of the writing on most prescription bottles, this should come as no surprise.) Most identify their medications by the pills' size, shape, or color, or of the bottles containing them. So it is important to ensure that your family member can clearly see his pills.

Provide sufficient lighting in the bathroom. Lighting can make all the difference in the world, especially when trying to distinguish the pink pills from the violet ones, or the light blue ones from the light green ones. Furthermore, if small items like pills get dropped on the floor, proper lighting in the bathroom will go a long way to making them easier to find.

Keep a magnifying glass close by, so your family member (or caregiver) can read the instructions on the prescription bottle—the expiration date, the name of the medicine, the name of the patient, incompatible medications or foods, when to take the pills,

"Dad made a list so he would know what pills to take and when to take them. The problem is that he can't tell what time it is and he is always calling me or the operator to find out."

Large-faced and talking clocks:

Bossert, Easy Street, J. C. Penney Special Needs Catalogue, Lighthouse Enterprises, Lighthouse of Houston, LS & S, Maxi Aids, McKesson, National Federation for the Blind, TFI Engineering.

Talking watches:

Bossert, Easy Street, Independent Living Aids, Lighthouse Enterprises, LS & S, Maxi Aids, McKesson, TFI Engineering.

Free-standing countertop magnifier:

Graham Field, Independent Living Aids, LS & S, Science Products.

Automatic medication dispenser (with or without a recorded reminder message):

Home Remedies.

etc. Magnified reading glasses or a countertop magnifying glass may not only prevent a mistake, but save a life.

For those having difficulty remembering to take their medications, or which pills to take, or whether they already took their medication, consider an automatic medication dispenser.

Consider your loved one's history. A lot of older people lived through the Depression, when times were hard and every penny counted. For those with AD, long-term memory and values instilled in the distant past often remain very much intact. Dropping a single "expensive" pill on the floor and not being able to find it might provoke considerable concern.

Bathrooms are no place for Oriental rugs or other multi-patterned rugs or carpets. As beautiful as they might be, they are nightmares when small pills are dropped on them. A small pill can blend into the patterns perfectly and be impossible to find—a potential upset for your family member striving to maintain independence or care for another.

Recognize that medications are kept and administered not only in the bathroom, but in the kitchen as well. Some medications are stored in the refrigerator, not the medicine cabinet. Any consideration that is applicable for medicines in the bathroom is equally applicable in the kitchen.

"Going to the Office"

"Dad gets up in the middle of the night, puts on his clothes, and says he's going to the office."

For many, another essential daily activity and means by which one cares for the family is working, or going to the office. Your loved one may not want to face the reality that he can no longer provide for his family or perhaps it is a habit hard to give up.

Dad may also be retreating into his long-term memory, to a time when habits and daily activities included getting up each day and going to the office.

Create an "office" at home, where your loved one can maintain his self-esteem, yet not endanger himself by trying to leave home. Set up a table or desk complete with telephone, adding machine, paper, and a file cabinet. Provide plenty of "mail" and "important" papers that will need filing, sorting (maybe now by color, rather than name), and attention.

Windows and People Watching

Staring out the window or watching people from the porch are wonderful activities that can entertain for hours, harmlessly and inexpensively. Any action can be pleasurable and worth watching:

people walking their dogs   traffic
birds, butterflies, and wildlife   children playing
family pets playing in the   grandchildren visiting
  backyard.   and playing
family members tending a garden

Any view and any backyard can be made more interesting. (See chapter 1.)

Religious Activities

Don't overlook the importance and benefits of continued or renewed religious involvement and your family member's commitment to his religion, church, and congregation.

Place a radio near your loved one's chair or bed. Although she can't get to church or temple, there may be religious services she can still listen to on the radio. Make listening comfortable and as easy as possible. Minimize background noises. Make sure there is a convenient and accessible electrical outlet nearby.

Provide religious items, pictures, framed scriptures, etc. near his favorite chair and bed.

Request home visits by a local religious leader. Make sure there are comfortable seats for all, free of distractions and background noises, to ensure that your loved one can enjoy and benefit from the visit. (See chapter 1 for ideas on making it easy for visitors to find your home.)

Hobbies

Activities of daily living should also include the little things in life that give pleasure. These activities may include gardening, cooking, making little toys for friends and family, whatever.

"In college, as part of a class proj-ect, I visited a nursing home. The group got ahead of me and I found myself walking down a cor-ridor by myself. I passed one room, and the lady inside tried to sell me tickets to an imaginary circus. At the next door, a lady was using a thermometer to take the temperature of all the plants in her room. She carefully mea-sured each plant's temperature in three places—the surface, the mid-dle of the pot, and the bottom—carefully recording the numbers. She began to explain to me the importance of this, which frankly I didn't get. However, her room was exploding with color radiat-ing from the blooms each plant provided. As it turned out, she was an expert in raising and de-veloping African violets. Taking their temperature wasn't the re-sult of her dementia, but rather necessary for growing African vio-lets so well and for her to con-tinue activities that were so im-portant to her."

Make it possible for your family member to continue hobbies in some way, or surround him with examples of his accom-plishments, skills, and special knowledge.

Gardening can be a wonderful activity for your family mem-ber and the whole family, as well. Alzheimer's care facilities across the country offer waist-high planters and gardens that their residents maintain and enjoy. You can do this, too. Create family projects that your loved one can supervise and direct, with or without getting her hands dirty. Weeding, planting, trimming, and picking fruit can happen in even the smallest of patios or planters. (Continued pleasure can be gained from cut flowers purchased at a store, yet claimed to come from the garden.)

For those less able to continue more complicated tasks, search your loved one's past for what once gave her pleasure and skills that she once had:

- For the mechanic: a box of large nuts and bolts to put together and take apart;
- For the carpenter: blocks of wood that need sanding;
- For the homemaker: napkins that need folding, a feather duster to be put to use around the house, colored socks that need sorting, ingredients that need mixing;
- For the gardener: watering the garden or picking weeds, raking leaves, potting plants;
- For the handyman: PVC plumbing fittings that can be put together and taken apart (straight sections, angles and end caps), available at your local home improvement center or hardware store.

Use your imagination and recognize that even the sim-plest tasks may represent a significant contribution that your loved one is still able to make. What may appear small to you or me may signify tremendous sources of pride and accom-plishment to him.

Exercise

People with Alzheimer's disease are not limited to only seden-tary activities. Exercise may have been a major part of your

wish to continue
nich demonstrates

: can use for exer-
ly in the nursing
report, telling me
down his favorite
re also companies
r adults. (See also
s.)

m just those tasks
loved one's abili-
d in this chapter.
es will emerge that
, this chapter has
steps to take and
your loved one to
ks become too dif-
tivities that he can

he transition from
ance, dependence)
one learns to deal
ner's disease.

Activity products and exercise equipment for older adults:

AdaptAbility, American Health Care Supply, Bailey, Carex, Easy Street, Enrichments, Hammatt Senior Products, Independent Living Aids, McKesson, Nasco, North Coast Medical, Sammons Preston, Sears Home HealthCare Catalogue, Senior Products, St. Louis Medical Supply.

5

Wandering

Wandering is the repetitive, sometimes incessant, behavior of roaming, pacing, or attempting to leave home. It is a major concern for those caring for someone with Alzheimer's disease.

Persons with AD wander for a variety of possible reasons. They may be industrious, with a specific purpose in mind: in search of a specific person or destination, attempting to escape a discomfort or condition (imaginary or real); or they may just be meandering aimlessly.

"My father has Alzheimer's disease and has moved in with us. He started walking off and he can't find his way home."

Some caregivers whose loved ones wander at night have to sleep with one eye open, fearing that at any time their loved one may wake up and wander into the kitchen or out of the home. They worry about their family member falling, eating something dangerous, or starting a fire while everyone else is asleep. At night especially, when the family member can go unobserved, the concern is not only for his or her well-being, but also for that of the whole family (and others living in the building).

"Gramma gets up at night, goes into the kitchen, and turns on the stove. Then she puts a napkin on each burner and goes back to sleep."

In the early stages of Alzheimer's your loved one may struggle to remain independent. She may be capable of handling most situations, able to hide her condition, get away with minor episodes of forgetfulness, and navigate from one place to another without incident. At some point, your family member's memory and image of the once-familiar home may disappear, leaving her stranded and unable to recognize her own home, though she may be standing right in front of the door. A trip to the mailbox can result in your loved one turning around and not recognizing the right building, or a trip down the hall can result in an endless attempt to find the right apartment. As the disease continues its course, trips within the home, from one room to another, in search of specific rooms, and even within a single room can result in your loved one becoming lost. Eventually, such episodes may become more frequent, more terrifying and more dangerous. This chapter is intended to help you and your loved one avoid such experiences for as long as possible.

Wandering Basics

Wandering is not always bad or undesirable. Controlled wandering in a safe environment can be a stimulating and therapeutic source of healthy, pleasurable activity, exercise, and entertainment, occupying your family member for hours at a time and providing much-needed relief and relaxation for the caregiver. It gives your loved one exercise that can contribute to a better night's sleep, afternoon naps, better health, and respite for the caregiver. Daytime wandering may also deter less desirable activities, such as sundowning and nocturnal wandering. But most importantly, wandering can allow your loved one a degree of independence within the limits of his capacity, in a safe, controlled environment.

Whether wandering should be discouraged or limited depends on your situation. Your loved one may not know when to stop and may become so tired that she loses her balance and falls down. She may not realize how exhausted she is, why she feels the way she does, or be able to find a place to sit down.

Be on the lookout for signs of exhaustion or silent injury (swollen ankles, for example). Provide plenty of places to sit down and rest in convenient locations. Create a soft, safe environment, just in case a fall does occur. Install railings for added help and guidance where your loved one may need it.

Wandering can also be life-threatening. Fearing that a loved one may leave the house and be unable to return home is a realistic concern. (The book *Gone . . . Without a Trace* by Marianne Dickerman Caldwell (Elder Books, 1995) is a testimony to this problem.) Your loved one might leave home without warm clothing in the middle of winter, walk in traffic, or fall victim to abuse. (Refer to the section at the end of this chapter entitled "Just in Case.")

Unexpected dangers could lurk close to your own front door, such as:

a busy road or highway	a crowded downtown area
a construction site	railroad tracks
a bridge	wild, open country
a cliff or steep incline	a cave or mine
dense woods	a river, canal, pond, lake

On the other hand, some people with dementia never wander at all.

Freedom to Wander

Safe and beneficial wandering or pacing can be encouraged by providing well-lit, hazard-free pathways. Calm, quiet, understandable environments, free of agitating factors, can make wandering a pleasant, rewarding, and enjoyable experience—and less of a concern for the caregiver. Wandering paths offer the benefit of repeated trips along the same path, limiting the area that needs to be carefully safety-proofed and constantly supervised.

In addition to creating safe areas to wander, you can minimize the "bad" areas through:

- "Access denial"—denying entry to dangerous areas (Danger Zones) and availability of hazardous products, chemicals, tools, and appliances. It also restricts entrance to inappropriate areas, including the Respite Zone. The result of access denial is that your family member is limited to only those areas that are safe and properly prepared for him to wander. These areas may be different during the day from those at night and change according to the various stages of the disease. (Refer to the section entitled "Identify the Zones of Your Home" in chapter 1.)

- "Activity notification"—alerting the caregiver to wandering, doors opening to the outside, or to locked areas storing dangerous and valuable items. This can be accomplished with alarms, motion detectors, remote signalers, etc.

- "Wandering prevention"—strategies and equipment specifically designed to discourage and prevent "elopement" (wandering away from home). (Refer to the section entitled "Devices and Equipment" later in this chapter for more discussion on alarms and equipment.)

- Creating "perimeters"—defining areas within your home where your loved one can wander and that are appropriate for his particular abilities, condition, and risk of becoming hurt. (Refer to the section later in this chapter on perimeters.)

Causes of Wandering

Very little is known about the causes of wandering. Some theories suggest that people wander as a result of restlessness, searching, disorientation, to avoid feelings of confinement, or as random behavior. Today's reason may not be the same as tomorrow's, this afternoon's, or tonight's. Everyone is different, and your loved one may have her own unique reasons for wandering.

Wandering in Search of . . .

Wandering may be a desperate quest to find something familiar. What once was familiar may no longer be recognizable. She may be searching for something (anything) that will make sense in her world of confusion.

Alzheimer's disease erases memories, first those of only moments ago, then those of years ago. Remember our theory of "last in, first out." Your loved one might be wandering in search of an earlier time when things and places were different.

Your family member's current home may no longer be a place she relates to. She may be searching for what she recalls as "home"—her childhood home, along with the warmth, nurturing, and comfort of a time and place where she wasn't burdened by the terrible effects of this disease. (See chapter 2.)

"I want to go home. Take me home."

Your loved one may be looking for a specific destination, exit, entrance, item, or person. Wandering may be an attempt to find the bathroom, bedroom, a lost spouse, or the caregiver. She may be lost within her own home, looking for some clue that will help orient her. She may be looking for something she doesn't remember hiding, but realizes is missing. She might even be looking for something that was once in her room, but removed long ago.

"Mom walked in our room tonight at 3 A.M., crying. She just sobbed that she couldn't find the bathroom and had been looking for it for hours."

Every room in your home is different. Each has its own set of cues that help identify it. Alzheimer's disease makes some of those cues invalid. It destroys the information paths within the brain, making it difficult to apply the proper meaning to the information received. Though the toilet is completely visible, there is no reason to assume that the room containing it is the bathroom. However, maybe if you provide additional cues, as many as possible, perhaps one will find a pathway still intact and make the complete journey, allowing your loved one to once again recognize the bathroom, dining room, bedroom, etc. (See chapters 2 and 8 for more ideas and more discussion on this important topic.)

Change (moving to a new apartment or in with a family member, for example) is often blamed for confusion, leading to wandering. Suddenly, the surroundings are not familiar. The recent change, now gone with the short-term memory, is no longer recalled. Your family member seeks something familiar, that was there yesterday, but gone today.

Your loved one may be looking for a place to hide something or rummage. Rummaging and hiding are often intended to be secret activities. Your loved one may be disguising his intentions. His wandering may just appear to be random meandering, when in fact he may be secretly hiding something, collecting, or looking for something. Your family member may be looking for the "stranger" he saw in the mirror or the culprit responsible for all of those "missing" items.

Wandering to Escape

Your family member may be trying to escape from a threat or from something that annoys, irritates, or disturbs him. This could be a television show, a voice on the radio, disturbing music, or an imagined "stranger." He may be seeking refuge from a situation he does not understand, perhaps a room with too many decorations or features for him to comprehend, or a task he is unable to perform.

Delusions are common with Alzheimer's disease. Your loved one may feel that people are out to get him, conspiring against him, or that he has been abused. Wandering may be an attempt to escape this perceived mistreatment.

Your family member may be wandering to get out of doing something—a bath, for example, or a task that is too challenging. Alzheimer's may be active in some people for as long as ten years before it is recognized or diagnosed, giving them years to learn how to cloak and hide the disease and get out of tasks that they find threatening.

Wandering with a Purpose

"Arlene walks around day after day, holding and caring for her 'baby doll.'"

Your family member's wandering may be an attempt to satisfy and fulfill family responsibilities: cooking, house cleaning, caring for her children, etc.

Your loved one may be attempting to maintain a previously active lifestyle. Many older people are aware of the benefits of exercise. Walking for exercise may have been a part of their lifestyle for years. Your family member may be recalling this habit and performing what she considers healthy activity.

"It seems that every time I talk on the phone Mother begins pacing back and forth in front of me. This has to be more than just a coincidence!"

Wandering may be related to "shadowing," following the caregiver or imaginary people around the house. This may be due to a fear of being left alone or abandoned, a desire to be involved in home activities, or contribute to taking care of the home.

Wandering or pacing close to you may be a request for attention.

Aimless Meandering

Most wandering has purpose and meaning. However, it takes careful observation to discover the underlying reasons and significance. They may be only logical or apparent to the person doing the wandering. Yet, admittedly, some people may wander aimlessly, in confusion.

Your family member's wandering may be stress-related. Alzheimer's disease is one disappointment and frustration after another. Your family member wants to understand, but can't. He is living in a world with rules he can neither remember nor understand. He has no control over his life or surroundings. Wouldn't you be frustrated?

Wandering may be all your loved one can do that is safe and entertaining! A common explanation for wandering, from the people with AD themselves, is that they simply don't have anything else to do—they are bored. Look for opportunities to create meaningful and entertaining activities for your loved one, including a safe and interesting wandering path.

Your loved one may be unable to sleep, and wandering may be the only activity available.

Sleep disturbances are common among Alzheimer's sufferers. Daily exercise, soothing music, clean bedding, a nightlight, and proper temperature settings can help contribute to a good night's sleep.

Wandering may be a coping reaction to a situation your loved one can do nothing else about. For example, pain may be keeping your loved one awake: arthritis, osteoporosis, an injury, or some other condition that she doesn't understand or can't explain. Getting up and wandering or pacing may be her only way of coping with the discomfort.

Wandering may be an emotional reaction to a loss that he is just unable to deal with or understand. Constant reminders of a loved one who is now gone may cause your family member to mourn over and over as the memory is recalled or her presence is missed. Your family member may wander (or pace) out of grief or in search of the departed loved one, a common reaction for even those not suffering from dementia.

Nothing that you can do to your home can eliminate the

pain of losing someone close to you. But you can survey your home and eliminate reminders of her loss: photographs, possessions of the departed loved one, even sculpture in the garden that may resemble a cemetery stone. Be extra sensitive to invisible memories lurking in the home that only your family member may recognize: the table they built together, the pillow they both spent all night looking for, etc.

Recognize that people become integral parts of the home and one's life. The absence of a familiar figure, one who has been around for many years, may make the home seem different, empty, and unrecognizable. Your loved one may wander in search of familiarity, something else to tell her where she is or that this is in fact "home." Your loved one may be seeking something that will offer the comfort and warmth that went when the loved one passed away.

Your family member may be wandering out of fear that if he sits down he won't be able to get up. Or his chair may be uncomfortable. Providing an elevated chair, with strong arms and room underneath to place one's feet for leverage, may help dispel this fear. (See also chapter 8.)

Wandering may be the result of medication side effects. Medication can cause or increase anxiety, sleeplessness, and other symptomatic behavior.

Finally, wandering may have no logical explanation beyond whatever may be going on in the mind of your family member.

Types of Wandering

We identify four general categories of wandering:

- indoor wandering
- outdoor wandering
- nocturnal wandering
- wandering away from home (elopement).

Indoor Wandering

Though sometimes very trying for the caregiver, indoor wandering is the least serious and dangerous of the four types. It is often characterized by pacing, cyclical patterns, or following the caregiver around the house.

As your loved one's mobility and abilities decline, it may only be safe for her to wander in certain parts of the home that have been properly prepared. As the days become shorter and colder in winter, it may be best that she not go outside without supervision. Indoors may become all that remains of her world. If wandering indoors is an activity that your family member can still enjoy and it does no harm, who are we to argue?

Create a Safe Home

Wandering may eventually put your loved one at risk due to frailty; difficulties with stability, vision, or equilibrium; or a desire to leave home. But wandering indoors occurs *within the home,* in a limited and controlled environment, close to help and supervision. This provides the caregiver with better control and proximity when accidents or upsets do occur, allowing for quick corrective action.

Making the home as safe as possible is the first step in creating a home conducive to wandering, making it a healthy activity, rather than one that is dangerous or that can result in upsets and frustration. Limit the area accessible to the wanderer to only that portion of your home that is safe, with no hidden dangers that your loved one can get into. Go beyond normal safety standards, taking into consideration the unique kinds of trouble your loved one can now get into and the difficulties that he seems to be having.

Create a Simple Home

Simplify the home environment. Choose a few large pieces of furniture, in solid colors rather than confusing patterns. A room with large, simple shapes will be a lot easier to understand and navigate than one with a lot of smaller ones. Create clear and straight pathways. Your loved one should never have to walk around a piece of furniture to get where he wants to go. Even a simple detour may be confusing, when a more direct route might be within his abilities to understand.

Clear the pathways that develop into wandering paths.

- Remove clutter. Many older people move from larger homes to smaller apartments or condominiums, bringing every piece of furniture they can. Hallways become popular locations for extra tables and chairs. Extra furniture is often fit in instead of given up.
- Survey the home frequently, removing items that accumulate and modifying areas that pose difficulty. Don't overlook changes that your family member may have made himself.
- Remove obstacles that may be outside your family member's field of vision. Check right, left, at floor level, and at eye level for furniture, decorations, and wall-mounted objects that he might walk into.
- Remove hard-to-see glass items along the way. For people with dementia, clear objects may be almost invisible. Your loved one may try to reach right through a glass door of a china cabinet or walk into the glass shelving or sliding glass doors. Better to remove them than risk an accident.

Check lighting along frequented pathways and make sure there are no poorly lit, dead-end corridors or areas with shadows that might be misinterpreted.

Increase lighting to help your family member see and avoid "trippers." Remember, unless the objects are blatantly obvious they may not be seen. Look for areas within your home that are dark or create shadows, where "trippers" may be difficult to see.

Use lighting to help your loved one discover the correct routes and see their destinations. Use signage, maps, and cues to direct and guide your loved one. Take advantage of color, landmarks, and lighting to highlight important doors and destinations, making them more recognizable and easy to find. (See chapter 8 for more discussion on cues and landmarks.)

Make your home and rooms within it as easy to navigate as possible, so that routes are clear and defined. Given that people with AD seek the paths of least resistance, make routes direct and failure impossible. Make sure that as long as your family member keeps moving he will inevitably find his way.

Wherever possible, take advantage of the "reverse funnel" effect. Widen the mouths of pathways to make their exits and entrances impossible to miss. Moving furniture just a little may help the lone traveler when she finds herself unsure of where she was going or how to get there. Visualize the wandering path as a series of trips, from one landmark to the next, rather than a long one. Subtly cue your loved one to each destination: to the chair, to the living room, to the window, to the doorway, etc.

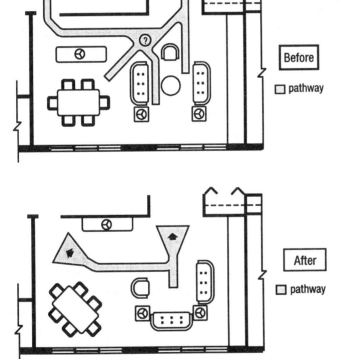

Before

☐ pathway

These pathways are not direct and clear. A person with AD might have to walk around something to get where he wants to go, which creates confusion.

After

☐ pathway

Furniture has been moved to help direct traffic and widen pathways at room exits. This open arrangement allows a clear view of all exits from each chair and sofa. Note also how the angle of the dining room table offers a gentle directional cue. (Be careful, however, not to make too many changes which might confuse a person with AD.)

Visibility

Take steps to make your loved one more visible to you in case she becomes disoriented, frustrated, or lost. Make it possible to discover problems as soon as they occur, minimizing the opportunity for them to develop into something more serious and upsetting.

Make it easier for your family member to see you as she roams through the home and as you go about your daily activities. Open up views and lines of vision within your home. Remove or relocate furniture in awkward locations that block important lines of sight. Keep in mind that not being able to see you for only a second may seem like an eternity to a person with AD and trigger thoughts of being abandoned.

Create a "Wandering Path" in Your Home

A wandering path can be a continuous looping route or meandering within an open area that allows multiple directions and routes. More than likely, if your loved one is prone to wander, he will discover his own path. So identify paths where wandering has already begun. Emphasize the primary route and remove diversions that might lead him astray, perhaps down "side streets" or into potentially confusing rooms along the way.

Wandering paths should be simple and obvious, allowing for few (if any) decisions about which way to go. Routes that your loved seeks will be those that have a proven history of success and offer no possibility for failure.

Circular or looping pathways are best, since no matter which way you go or what decision you make, you always end up back at the beginning. Linear paths can result in your loved one wandering to one end of the house, where suddenly nothing may be familiar. Also pathways that lead to dead ends should be avoided. Your loved one may walk down a corridor, come to the end, and not know how to turn around or find his way back.

Closing off and locking certain doors can create simple loops, directing your family member along pathways that are safe and provide a continuous, returning route. Sometimes rearranging or removing a single piece of furniture will eliminate an obstacle and allow your family member to continue on her way. In larger, more open rooms, placing something in the middle (to walk around) will suddenly create a looping path.

Railings

Add railings where they might be useful. Pathways with railings are safer, better defined, easier to use, and therefore more likely to be used. They offer a sense of security.

Railings make great directional cues. Continuing them around corners leads the follower in a steady, pre-planned direction. Hallways with railings on *both* sides may become routes for both coming and going along the same wandering path.

Use railings to redirect your family member where necessary. A continuous railing that wraps around a dead-end corridor (allowing your loved one to follow it around the wall) can lead him on a continuous path in the right direction. Without it, he may find himself hopelessly lost at the end of a corridor with nowhere else to go.

Make the Wandering Path Interesting

Make pathways entertaining and stimulating, create a sense of journey. Add things to look at, do, and observe along the way—pictures on the wall, drawings by grandchildren, plants, tables to straighten, a "safe" trunk to rummage through, a stack of interesting magazines, a bird cage, etc.

Also consider some of the causes for wandering mentioned earlier. How might you incorporate this knowledge into your wandering paths? Is your family member wandering to escape something? To find something? Or does he have a purpose that can be emphasized to help give meaning to his journey? Can things be added to the path recognizing these motives? Are there activities that can be encouraged along the way: dusting, looking in drawers, etc.? Can you divert his attention from thoughts that may be upsetting to more pleasant thoughts and fascinations? Once the wandering path has been established, add to it, make it a real journey, turn it into an activity instead of a mundane, repetitive task.

Incorporate landmarks to guide your family member. Your dad's favorite chair in the den may be a recognizable landmark and a popular destination, plus a great place to sit down and rest when wandering becomes a little tiring.

Provide places to sit, rest, or observe something happening along the way. If the path goes by a window, for example, place a chair there to watch outdoor activity. Where the path seems a bit long, look for a place for a bench or a chair. Be careful not to locate these seats where they can be tripped

Residential railings:

IPC, Tepromark International, or have a local contractor provide and install them for you.

over or walked into. And finally, be careful there are no distractions or items of interest too close to hazards (such as steps), distracting your loved one from seeing dangers he needs to avoid.

Outdoor Wandering

"Myrtle loves to walk in the backyard. She walks around the path for hours, talking to herself and the birds."

Both the home's interior and the backyard should be made safe and available to the wanderer. The outdoors has all kinds of magnificent benefits and therapeutic values: stimulation, diversity, sunshine, fresh air, plants and animals, watching neighborhood activity or children playing from the porch, and so on.

Free and independent movement is a natural and pleasurable activity that, if denied, is usually missed. When a person begins to wander, the caregiver's natural reaction is to limit her range of movement for safety and ease of supervision. Safe, fenced backyards (with locked gates) are ideal for enjoying all the outdoors has to offer. Another benefit for the caregiver may be valuable rest and relaxation (sitting and watching from a distance).

Outdoor Wandering Paths

Everything that applies to an indoor path also applies to an outdoor path. It needs to be safe, interesting, and complete with opportunities to sit down and rest. In addition, an outdoor path needs to direct your loved one back to the door leading inside. Becoming stranded outside, with no idea how to get back, has more serious implications than just becoming lost within a room indoors, especially during inclement weather.

Create a safe and well-planned wandering path, however long or short. Consider appropriate precautions for someone in your family member's condition, and for her particular habits and behaviors.

Wandering paths should be:

- a minimum of four feet wide, so two people can walk side by side, one assisting the other;
- circular or looped so that your family member is always led back to the beginning;

- simple and continuous, with no side paths leading away from the main path;
- full of interest and activity—with bird houses, gardens, flowering trees and bushes, wind chimes, mobiles, bird baths and feeders;
- most of all, *safe*. (See also chapters 1 and 9.)

A wandering path needn't be long to be beneficial. Even a small patio offers opportunities to meander, pace, walk, and enjoy the outdoors. Simply placing a planter in the middle of an open area will suddenly create a circular path, something to walk around. Adding a continuous bench surrounding the planter gives your loved one a place to rest, anywhere along the path.

"We put a clay squirrel in the bushes in the back yard. Every time Annie sees it she tells us to be quiet and carefully tiptoes so as not to scare it."

Create a sense of journey along the path, with fascinating items for your loved one to discover right and left, above and below. Each trip will be different. Going down the same path, time after time, will allow your loved one to discover new things that weren't noticed before—different flowers, animals, scents, wind making chimes sing or mobiles move, etc. Provide plants that attract butterflies, birds, chipmunks, and squirrels. For those times of the year when flowers don't normally bloom or animals have gone away for the winter, consider a few artificial plants and animals.

Place various objects along an outdoor wandering path to create a sense of journey.

The sense of journey and discovery can be even greater for

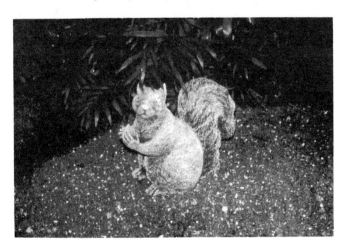

Place various objects, like this ceramic squirrel, along an outdoor wandering path to create a sense of journey. Remember to avoid objects that could cause your loved one anxiety.

people with Alzheimer's disease, who have the advantage of not remembering previous experiences. They can relive and enjoy the excitement, spontaneity, and pleasure of discovery each time they travel their wandering path—one of the few benefits of the disease.

Backyards and wandering paths can be made interesting and ever-changing for all the senses. Use color, fragrance, sight, and sound. Flowers bloom at different times of the year, changing your loved one's experience from month to month and season to season. Birds and squirrels create noises and movements that contribute immensely to the experience. Certain plants are aromatic at certain times of the year. Discuss with your local nursery how you might create different experiences along your wandering path for different times of the year.

Be careful not to place distractions too close to steps or other hazards along the pathway. You wouldn't want your loved one to trip and fall because he was looking at the ceramic squirrel or a beautiful red geranium rather than the dangerous step (rock, root, sprinkler head, etc.) next to it.

Create family projects along the wandering path. Imagine walking in the backyard and looking forward to visiting the family garden that you and your grandchildren planted. Have the flowers bloomed? Are the peas ready to be picked? Are there any hummingbirds or butterflies attracted to the flowers? What stories can your loved one come back with and share?

Finally, join your loved one frequently and share her pleasure. Point out the missed or less obvious points of interest that you have included for her delight and entertainment—wind chimes, artificial animals, newly blooming flowers, garden vegetables ripening, etc.

Make Sure Your Yard Is Safe

Survey the wandering path. Walk it yourself, not once, but often. Things change! Look out for:

- items that can be tripped over, such as hoses, children's toys, sprinkler heads, holes, tree roots, etc.;

- sidewalks that have been pushed up by roots or ice;
- irregular surfaces, uneven pavers, gravel from nearby planters, fallen branches;
- ice patches;
- fruit or nut trees that drop their bounty on pathways;
- planters or pots in the paths of travel;
- thorny bushes and shrubs, foliage that can cause irritation, or plants that may be toxic if eaten;
- movable furniture that can be carried to a fence and used as a ladder.

Wandering is often an incessant behavior, performed over and over, continuously. Create opportunities to stop, sit down, and rest, however devious, even if it means placing a chair in front of the plastic bird at the feeder. Not realizing how exhausted she is, your loved one may just sit down to watch. The feeling of exhaustion or pain from swollen ankles, not understood by your family member, may now (having rested), just as inexplicably, go away.

Place sturdy chairs or benches in the back yard where your loved one can sit and rest.

- Two benches or a bench and a chair will encourage friends to join your family member, to talk and visit. If there's room for only one, only one person will sit there!
- Locate seating areas where your loved one can be seen and supervised from key locations inside the home.
- Select an interesting spot with a view of activity— children playing outside, people walking their dogs, traffic, people parking their cars and walking into stores, etc.
- Make sure chair or bench locations allow your loved one to feel safe, secure, and comfortable. Locate them where she can observe but not feel violated or threatened by passers by, neighborhood children, wandering pets, workers, etc. Use subtle

"My sister wanders all day long, going in the same circle, nonstop. I'm afraid she is going to get exhausted or fall."

Outdoor benches:

American Health Care Supply, Brookstone, Plow & Hearth, Smith & Hawken, or home improvement centers.

barriers and lines of demarcation that allow your
loved one to watch, yet not feel threatened.

- Sitting areas should be protected from sun, wind,
  and weather (especially if your loved one exhibits
  fear of water, storms, or rain) and not too far from
  the house or shelter, in case of a problem or if the
  weather changes suddenly. Take advantage of
  shade trees or use a table with an umbrella.

A gazebo might make the backyard a special place for your
loved one, creating a safe place to sit and enjoy the outdoors
protected from weather and sun, a recognizable feature to walk
to, and a great spot to rest. (Check in your telephone book
under "sheds.")

Walking surfaces and pathways should be level, smooth,
solid, and firm (especially for use with a wheelchair, walker, or
cane). Mulch, gravel, stepping stones, pavers, cobblestones,
dirt, and sand are poor choices for wandering paths. Soft, gran-
ular materials are not stable and require skill, balance, and
strength to walk safely. Dirt can become wet and slippery mud
after just a little rain. Consider the future when designing pathways: assistive walking devices may enter the picture, and firm
footing is always important.

Remove or repair "trippers," including uneven, cracked sidewalks, roots protruding from the ground in pathways, and uneven pavers. Fix what needs to be fixed—nails protruding from
wood decks or stairs, worn steps and wobbly railings, splinters
in railings, warped planks in your deck or patio.

Call attention to "trippers" that can't be removed, like ramps
and steps, with color and railings. To make dangers really obvious, use bright fluorescent paint (available from any paint
store, hardware store, or home improvement center). A convenient railing provides something to hold on to. Your loved one
may or may not recognize the danger, but when there is a
railing present it is often grasped.

Even a safety-proofed backyard may not be safe all year
long. Your loved one may wander outside in the middle of
winter underdressed. There are seasonal dangers as well: icy

patches, exposure to the hot sun, etc. You may want to place locks or alarms on doors leading to the backyard to notify you and help you control when your loved one can go there.

(See also chapters 1 and 9 for more thoughts on eliminating special dangers that might lurk in your backyard, such as toxic plants.)

Fences

A wandering path is not safe if your loved one can walk out of the yard. The last thing you want to see is an empty backyard when you know your loved one was there a moment ago. A fence around the yard can safely and sufficiently restrict the area available for your loved one to wander.

Make sure all gates in the fence have locks to prevent leaving the yard and keeping strangers from entering "territorial" spaces. If you use latches rather than a lock, install multiple latches, since opening more than one simultaneously requires skills your loved one may no longer have. Locate them in obscure locations (high and low) to make the task a little more difficult and the devices less obvious.

Consider a waterproof, weather-resistant gate alarm. (If it is battery operated, be sure to check it frequently to make sure the batteries are still working and the alarm is operative.) (See chapter 6 for more ideas.)

Your fence needs to be high enough to ensure that your family member cannot climb over it. We recommend a minimum of six feet. (Check your local zoning and development rules.) There have been cases of older people with AD trying to, succeeding at, or getting hurt attempting to, climb their backyard fences. Delusions can result in very convincing stories in one's mind—stories that to your family member may justify extraordinary means to avoid perceived threats.

Make sure lawn furniture cannot be carried or pushed to a fence and used as an aid to get to the other side. Anchor or bolt chairs, tables, and lounges to the patio deck or chain them to something secure nearby to ensure that they cannot be moved. This precaution offers the added advantage of

Chair and bench anchors:

Smith & Hawken (brass anchors); or check your local hardware store for metal angles that will serve the same purpose.

fixing the furniture exactly where you've located it to maximize your view of your family member.

Remove incentives. Fences that you cannot see through provide less attraction to get to the other side.

Wrought iron fencing may resemble prison bars. People with delusions of being confined or who flash back to times when they actually were in jail may take exceptional steps to escape. Such a reminder of traumatic times in the past may also upset them. (See chapter 1.)

Wayfinding for Outdoor Wanderers

Make it easy for your loved one to realize where he is, where he has been, and where he is going. Trim shrubbery and remove obstacles that hinder views. It's a lot safer and easier to travel a path if you can see what is ahead of you. Realize also that just because one can see her destination doesn't mean she can get to it. Paths need to be clear and obvious. There should never be a need to search for the path, go around something in the way, or make a decision. As long as your loved one keeps moving, she can always be led to the next stage of her journey and eventually to the way back inside.

"Mom, your chair is right there, under the big umbrella, next to the red planter."

Place landmarks along the path in key locations to help your loved one find her way and orient herself, much like a ship uses a lighthouse for guidance. Landmarks can be benches, planters, sculpture, birdhouses, bird feeders, lamp posts, wind chimes, a garden, signs—anything that is distinctive, stands out, and catches your attention. Check local nurseries, home improvement centers, and gardening magazines for beautiful and useful backyard items.

Magazines such as *Fine Gardening* feature advertising in the back for outdoor sculpture and garden pieces. Check your local book/magazine store or call (800) 888-8286 or (800) 477-8727 for a subscription or sample copy.

Create a wandering path that is a series of journeys—maybe from the door to the bird feeder, then to the garden, next to the bright blue bench, etc., until your loved one has returned safely to the door leading into the house. Divide the wayfinding process into manageable, simple pieces by breaking up the path with appealing items of interest and interim destinations.

Make it easy to find the door leading back into the house. People who have lived in the same house for thirty years can still find themselves lost in the backyard. Call attention to the door in every way possible, with color, flowers, and maybe an awning. Provide a clear path leading directly to the door. Add signs pointing the way and identifying the door. Attract attention with the motion of a mobile and the sounds of wind chimes. Place a favorite chair next to the door, turning it so that it doesn't face away from the door, but at an angle. Many a lost and weary soul has sought a place to sit down and, upon getting up, discovered he was right next to the door all the time.

For those spots where your loved one hesitates, gets lost, or loses orientation:

- Use a railing as a guide. Your family member may hold onto it and continue in the direction that it takes him, whether he needs the support or not.
- Attract your family member's attention to the correct direction or destination. Use all the senses: colorful and interesting landmarks, musical chimes, and moving mobiles, to name just a few.
- Make routes clear and obvious rather than just depending on worn paths in the grass. People with dementia tend to follow the path of least resistance. If they become lost, a clear highlighted pathway on the ground might lead them to something familiar. (One way of doing this is marking the path with fluorescent spray paint along the ground.)
- Install barriers to discourage wandering in the wrong direction, such as toward a gate or farther away from the house.
- Add arrows, labels, and signs to guide your loved one and keep her moving.

Wandering paths are beneficial, and even the smallest yards can accommodate one. Oddly enough, if you find yourself at a loss, you may seek the advice of your confused family member. If a wandering path is something that he needs and wants, he may create his own, or provide you with the clues you need to construct one.

Nocturnal Wandering

Quite often people with Alzheimer's have difficulty sleeping at night and are prone to nocturnal wandering or activity. This is especially disheartening to caregivers, torn between their need for sleep and the terrifying thought of a family member wandering throughout the home unsupervised. Yet no one can be on duty 24 hours a day.

Identify your fears. What are your biggest and most real concerns? Are you worried that your loved one might:

- hide important items or rummage in places she shouldn't;
- become lost or disoriented;
- fall or have an accident;
- eat something inappropriate;
- start a fire—smoking a cigarette and leaving it somewhere, still lit; misusing the stove;
- try to leave home?

Once you identify your concerns you can take appropriate actions to eliminate or minimize the likelihood of the problems. You can then rest a little easier knowing that your fears have been addressed and are less likely to come to fruition.

Some questions that you might ask yourself are:

- What trouble can she get into?
- What does she typically do at night? What is there for her to do?
- What behaviors do you observe during the day that might be clues to what she might do at night, when she feels she is unobserved and unrestricted?
- Does your family member experience delusions? What are some of his stories? What might they lead him to do?
- Will more exercise during the day help him sleep better at night?

Have a well thought-out plan for nocturnal wandering.

Make your home as safe as possible. This will minimize the dangers that your loved one is apt to encounter. Secondly, limit the portion of the home that is accessible at night. (See chapter 6 for suggestions.)

Create things to do and places to go. Consider favorite activities, no matter how little sense they may make to you. If your loved one enjoys arranging things, create areas for items that "need" arranging, sorting, or putting away. Create places where things can go (drawers or a chest) that are okay for rummaging. Place a comfortable easy chair in the bedroom, not only to sit in and rest, but also for stability and holding onto while walking to the bathroom or leaving the room. If your mother once again shows maternal interest in taking care of a doll, maybe you can create an area in her room for that "infant" that she can fuss over, much the same way she did for you when you were a small child.

Most importantly, make it easy for your family member to find her room. (See chapter 8 for suggestions.) Next, make it possible for your loved one to find you or notify you when she has a problem. You may post a sign outside your bedroom door identifying it as your room, add another sign in the hallway that points to your room, install a monitor or intercom system or provide a call button in the bathroom and by her bed. (See the discussion on wander-alerting equipment later in this chapter.)

Make it easy for your loved one to see and move around safely at night. Dimly lit homes may be especially difficult for people with AD, not only because it's hard to see, but also because it complicates understanding the environment they are trying to navigate. If they are unable to see their surroundings clearly at night, they are more likely to become confused, lost, or frightened.

Install night lights. Locate them to light the way and guide your family member to rooms where he might need to go at night, such as the bathroom. Add new lights where they may be needed. Leave the light on in rooms and areas that are especially important destinations, such as the hallway.

Your loved one might not remember to turn on the hall light, how to turn it on, or where the switch is located. Install automatic night lights with photo cells or motion detectors,

Motion detector night lights:

BRK Brands, HITEC, Improvements, The Safety Zone.

Motion-detecting wall switch:

BRK Brands, Improvements, home improvement centers, hardware stores.

Combination motion detector/light adapter:

Alsto's Handy Helpers, BRK Brands, home improvement centers, hardware stores.

Motion detector with detached lamp adapter:

Improvements.

Motion detector with remote plug adapter (you can plug a lamp into it):

Steinel America (photo page 238).

Compact fluorescent, screw-in light bulbs:

Philips Light Company, home improvement centers, hardware stores, and some grocery stores.

motion-detecting switches, or motion-detecting adapters in hallway lights and along routes frequented at night. Motion-detecting switches can replace your existing light switch and turn on the light when your loved one approaches. Motion-detector adapters screw into a lamp between the socket and bulb. When your family member walks within their range, the light goes on. Lights with motion detectors will not only brighten the hallway as she approaches, but also signal the caregiver to her location.

Remember that older eyes need more light. Pay particular attention to the availability of light at night so your family member can see where he is going, to make the home safer and easier to navigate, and to minimize shadows that might appear to be something else. At the same time, older eyes do not adjust quickly to sudden changes in light. Automatic motion-detectors, for example, should only control lamps with low wattage bulbs, rather than suddenly lighting up the room with blinding lights. Use compact fluorescent bulbs, which turn on a little slower, allowing older eyes to adjust.

Consider asking your electric utility company to install an outdoor security light near your house. (Be sure to inquire about the likely cost of electricity for the light and installation.) If your utility company does not offer this service, contact a handyman or electrician. The light outside will shine through windows to illuminate your home's interior as well, all night long, making your home much safer to walk around in at night. Check with your neighbors first to make sure the light won't keep them up at night. If they like the idea of the light's added security, maybe it can go between your houses and you can share the expenses.

Survey your home with nocturnal wandering in mind, from every point of view. Safety-proof it to eliminate dangers and minimize injury in case accidents do occur. Pretend you have an adult-sized two-year-old child who can get into everything. Then ask yourself how *you* could outsmart your own safety strategies:

- Are the locks you've installed strong enough?
- Should you have two locks or latches on certain

doors, cabinets, or drawers, requiring multiple tasks to be performed to outwit them?

- Will your gates really block the stairs and door openings? Can they be climbed over? Is there a nearby chair that can be moved and used as a ladder?
- Do you have alarms on the important off-limits doors that will sound if your family member outsmarts the lock or finds the key?

As the disease progresses, you may need to limit nighttime activity to specific areas of your home that are safe, have been prepared for nighttime wandering, and are not too distant from your family member's room (in case he finds himself lost, unable to get back, or in trouble). Define a perimeter that allows access to a limited, but satisfying portion of the home. (Refer to the section later in this chapter on perimeters.) Consider using a gate, Dutch door, or screen door in select locations, which will allow him to wander only in certain areas (perhaps his bedroom) yet still see what is going on beyond the door.

A Dutch door has three combinations:

- both sections (top and bottom) left open to allow free access,
- the top half only opened to allow your family member to see and hear what's going on beyond the door, but not to leave the room, or
- both sections closed to completely hide and prevent access.

Make sure that your loved one cannot climb over the Dutch door or gate. Making the barrier high enough and not locating anything nearby that can be used as a step ladder are two important steps, but not guarantees. Remove any portable furniture (low tables, hallway chairs, or floor decorations) near the barrier that can be used to help your loved one climb over it.

Please be very careful when denying access or freedom. Even those who are older and seem weak have been known to climb over gates and Dutch doors, and even out of windows

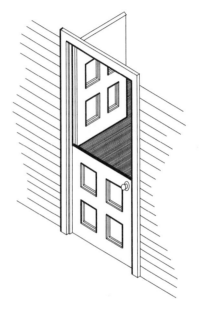

A Dutch door is a creative and less upsetting way to limit wandering. When the bottom half is closed and the top is open, your family member can still see and hear everything going on outside his room.

(sometimes on upper floors) to "escape," to regain their freedom or access areas denied to them. Whenever confining someone, even as humanely as with a Dutch door, it is wise to carefully monitor reactions. Refer to the suggestions in chapter 8 and take advantage of various devices to help you supervise your loved one's reactions.

Each stage of AD will require its appropriate perimeter. (See the discussion on perimeters later in this chapter.)

Finally, take advantage of local daycare programs to provide you with opportunities to catch up on much-needed sleep.

Wandering Away from Home

"Aunt Ethel walks very slowly and carefully. Yet all we have to do is turn our backs for just one second and she can be out the door and down the street in the blink of an eye!"

Probably nothing is more terrifying than the thought of your loved one wandering away from home, unable to find her way back or tell anyone where she lives. Wandering away from home (or elopement) is a major concern for families and caregivers. The world is not always a friendly place. There are people who prey on the weak and take pleasure in harassing or hurting them, as well as numerous dangers for confused people lost in crowded stores, in traffic, or maybe their own neighborhood.

- Take steps to alert you to attempts to wander away from home.
- Take steps to prevent leaving home.
- Be prepared if wandering away from home happens—just in case. (Refer to the discussion on this at the end of this chapter.)

In addition to installing alarms, try to identify the causes and triggers of elopement to minimize their occurrences. Remove cues and reminders that suggest leaving the house, traveling, or destinations. These might include shoes, boots, hats, or coats by the door, suitcases, keys, views of the bus stop, or even road maps lying on the table. Move hats to inside the coat closet, so they're not in plain sight and a constant reminder to your family member of trips he cannot take. Find a better place to leave your shoes than by the door.

Eliminate access to vehicles. Remove the car keys and lock the door leading to the garage, shed, or carport. Don't overlook the lawnmower, motorcycles, bicycles, etc. These too have been used for transportation. If your loved one drives away, she may get lost, forget to stop at a stop sign, drive off the road, forget how to operate the vehicle, or forget an important step in a safety sequence, such as checking for oncoming traffic before proceeding through an intersection.

Don't forget to put away the garage door remote control and disengage the wall-mounted button that opens the garage door. Your family member may recognize it as a way to open the garage door and go for a "walk."

No one can see and hear everything that is going on everywhere in the house, all the time. You may need to use several strategies, devices, and systems to alert you to attempts to wander away from home. Among the best strategies to deal with wandering is to establish perimeters in your home.

Perimeters

Perimeters are outlines defining the safe areas of your home. They allow your loved one to wander only within areas that have been safety-proofed and child-proofed for his protection. Perimeters also alert the caregiver of attempted violations (opening of doors or windows leading to danger) and they notify the caregiver of activity and its location.

Perimeters change, depending on your loved one's risk of elopement, getting into trouble, or falling. As time goes on and your loved one's mobility and cognitive abilities decline, so do the areas within the home that remain safe. We identify three perimeters:

- Stage One Perimeter—prevents elopement and access to areas of danger;
- Stage Two Perimeter—allows limited wandering in only certain areas of the home;
- Stage Three Perimeter—prevents falls, notifies the caregiver of attempts to get out of bed or up from a chair.

Pool guard alarms:

Improvements, Perfectly Safe, pool supply and home improvement stores.

Pool alarm with remote alarm:

Improvements.

Stage One Perimeters

Stage one perimeters are useful when independence is still encouraged. Yet you want to feel secure in knowing that your loved one cannot wander away from home or into areas that may be dangerous, such as the pool, balcony, attic, basement, garage, or a closet where items are being stored for safety. It is time to consider stage one perimeters as soon as your loved

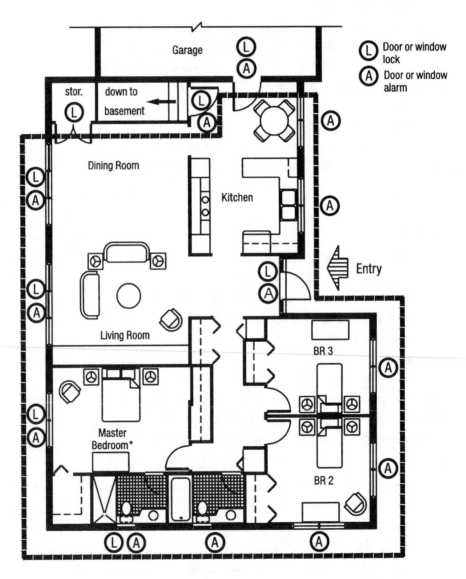

A sample stage one perimeter. The goals are to discourage wandering into dangerous areas of the home and out of the home. *The person with AD uses the master bedroom.

one leaves home and is unable to find his way back, or when there are attempts to elope, perhaps in search of "home." (See chapter 2.)

To help define this perimeter you will need a sketch or drawing of your home. Draw an outline around the safe areas, paying particular attention to doors and windows along that border. These doors and windows will need to be locked and/or alarmed. If your yard is safe you may want to have two stage one perimeters: One allowing access to the yard during certain times of the year and the other not. The outdoor perimeter includes your fence and gates leading out of the yard.

Openings in your perimeter need to be protected by locks *and* alarms (on windows, doors, and gates) to notify you that your loved one has defeated a lock and either opened the door or window, or attempted to leave. There are plenty of alarms and devices that might help you. They offer a multitude of options, depending on the degree of security that you need.

Don't overlook windows and doors leading to balconies. Your loved one may not realize that he lives on an upper floor or the danger of climbing out a window or over a balcony wall. This is especially true if your loved one experiences delusions that people are out to get him or if he has strong urges to go "home."

Add window alarms and locks to limit how far windows can open, allowing fresh air in, but not your family member out. Don't rely solely on alarms, as you might not get there in time. Even your garage door is a possible exit. It too should be kept locked and alarmed.

Use multiple window-locking devices (pins, dowels, or flip-down devices), not just one. (See the drawing on page 262.) Your loved one may figure out one lock, or the lock may break or fail. Have a backup alarm, and check regularly to make sure it works. If batteries or electricity fail, electrical devices may not work. Or one well-intentioned alarm may break and your second, back-up alarm could save the day, even if it's only a cowbell mounted on the face of the door.

Use additional strategies in conjunction with locks and alarms. Child-proof gates or Dutch doors may avert the need

Remember:

When both a lock and an alarm are installed on a window or door, the alarm will only sound if the locked lock is defeated.

Door monitor chime alarm:

Perfectly Safe.

Sliding window and door alarms:

Alsto's Handy Helpers, DAC Technologies, J. C. Penney Special Needs Catalogue, Perfectly Safe, or home improvement centers.

Garage door alarm—two part with remote receiver indoors:

DTE Edison America,
The Safety Zone.

Window-locking devices:

hardware stores and home improvement centers.

to wander by allowing visual connections to the rest of the house and avoid the feeling of being caged or confined. Hiding a gate in the backyard with a sheet may foil your loved one's attempts to find a way out. Diversions (the cat lying on her bed or a hanging bird cage) can direct your loved one away from doors leading outside or to dangerous storage areas. These may be enough of a distraction to allow him to forget his interest in leaving or what's behind that door. (See chapter 6 for more ideas.)

Stage Two Perimeters

Stage two begins when your loved one demonstrates behavior that threatens her safety or the safety of others living in her home or building. Wandering must now be limited even more. For example, you wouldn't need to be notified every time your family member got up to go to the bathroom, but if she ventures into the kitchen or near the stairs you may need to be alerted. Stage two perimeters are especially helpful in notifying the caregiver of nocturnal activity and wandering.

"Granpa just won't give up smoking. Last night he found a cigarette and went into the kitchen to use the stove to light it. He burned his sleeve and almost started a fire."

First define the area of your stage two perimeter. Again, look at your home's floor plan. Make sure the perimeter you designate allows free roaming in safe areas, such as from the bed to the bathroom. Perimeter two will be smaller than perimeter one, since the area where your loved one can wander safely is now more limited. In some cases it may include only the bedroom and the bathroom. In other homes, you may be able to include the den or the living room—but not the kitchen, laundry room, etc.

Is your family member's bathroom directly connected to his room, rather than down the hall? If so, your solution might be to alarm only the bedroom door, allowing your family member free rein in his room and bathroom, but not the hallway.

Your stage two perimeter is not a substitute for your stage one perimeter, but rather an addition. Your first perimeter remains intact. Stage two perimeters may be needed only at night. The first perimeter will still be helpful during the day and night, protecting your home's exterior windows and doors.

Areas that seem endless can always be contained by a gate,

lock, and an alarm. In a hallway that leads to the bathroom, for example, add a child-proof gate with a lock and alarm just beyond the bathroom to prevent access to the rest of the house. Often to create a stage two perimeter all that is necessary is a gate that limits travel and a motion detector chime or alarm that alerts the caregiver in case your loved one gets past it.

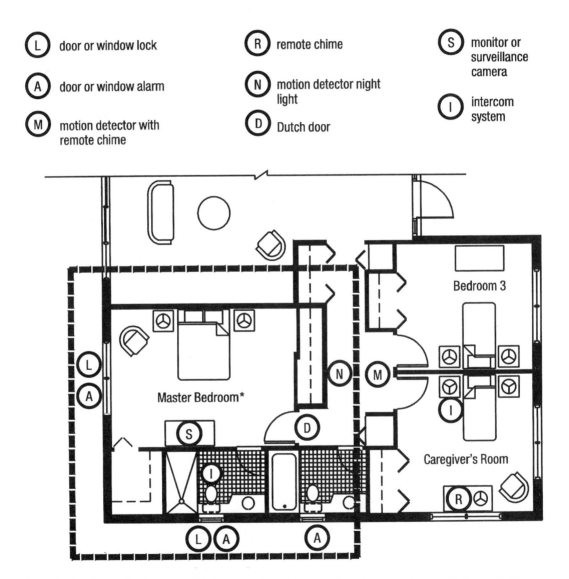

A sample stage two perimeter. The goal is to limit and notify the caregiver of unsupervised wandering within the home yet at the same time allow freedom to move about permissible areas, for example, to and from the bathroom. Setting up a stage two perimeter does not warrant or suggest removing the elements of your stage one perimeter; it is in addition to it. *The person with AD uses the master bedroom.

Stage two perimeters can also be a little more complicated. If your family member's room is next to the caregiver's room, consider installing a new door between the bedrooms and locking or blocking the original door. This way your loved one will have to go through the caregiver's room. Requiring your loved one to go through your room to get out adds alarms that won't require any electricity, providing you are a light sleeper.

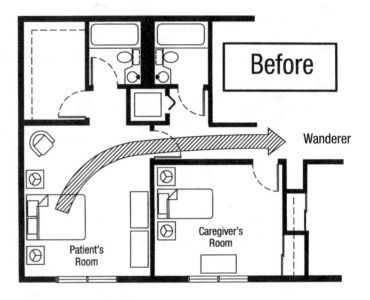

A new door redirects the wandering person through the caregiver's room to leave the area. An alarm on the door or motion-detecting chime alerts the caregiver to attempts to wander beyond that point.

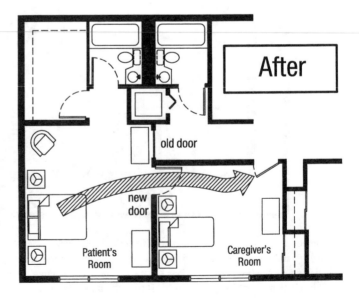

You can also add a motion detector to alert you to wandering in a certain area of your home, such as the hallway, the kitchen, or your office. (See the section later in this chapter on motion detectors.) There are also distance-monitoring devices that will notify you if your loved one strays beyond a designated distance from his bed. (See the section later in this chapter on distance-monitoring devices.)

Perimeter one or two can also be created by installing a wireless security system in your home. Contacts can be installed on certain doors and windows and motion detectors placed in key locations. If your loved one goes beyond the allowed area, you will be notified immediately. Ask your alarm company representative if there are gentler alarms that won't scare you or your loved one when they go off.

Wireless security system:
Radio Shack, Honeywell Home Security Systems, or home improvement centers.

For those noises that you hear at night and wonder what is happening, baby monitoring devices and surveillance cameras can be helpful. Monitors will allow you to hear activity when it occurs, as well as cries for help. A camera will let you actually see what is happening. This way you can feel better knowing that the noises you hear are harmless and no one is getting into trouble . . . without having to get out of bed. (See the section later in this chapter on monitoring equipment.)

Stage Three Perimeters

Perimeter three is even more confined. As your loved one's mobility becomes more impaired, with a greater risk for falls and injury, the safe area becomes smaller.

Is your loved one on medications that may make him drowsy at night? Does she have osteoporosis, which puts her at greater risk in the event of a fall? Has she already had a few falls? Is he too unstable or weak to get out of bed by himself? Is the bathroom too far away?

A stage three perimeter is intended to alert the caregiver of any attempt on the part of the loved one to get out of his bed, easy chair, or wheelchair before a fall occurs. Perimeter three is necessary when your loved one risks falling or hurting himself with any unassisted movement.

"Daddy gets up several times during the night. In the last few weeks he has fallen four times trying to get out of bed."

The primary means of creating the third level of protection are "fall prevention devices." They alert the caregiver as soon as a family member attempts to get out of his bed, wheelchair, or easy chair. There are several types of fall prevention devices. (See the section dedicated to fall prevention devices later in this chapter.)

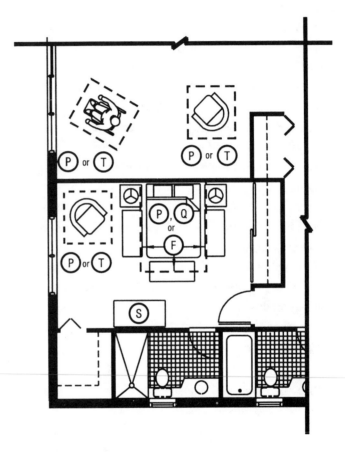

(T) pull-tab alarm	(P) pressure-release chair or bed mat and alarm
(F) pressure-sensitive floor mat with alarm	
(S) monitor or surveillance camera	(Q) distance-monitoring device and alarm

A sample stage three perimeter. The goal is to notify the caregiver of any attempt to stand or get out of a bed, chair, or wheelchair. This is especially important when such attempts risk a fall.

Devices and Equipment

For each stage of the disease and each perimeter there are devices and equipment that can help. You've got plenty to choose from with a variety of options. This section will describe your choices and where you can get them. All have appropriate uses, and you will need to determine which best meets your needs.

	Perimeter One	Perimeter Two	Perimeter Three
Wander-Alerting Systems	✔		
Alarms	✔	✔	
Simple Bells, Chimes & Buzzers	✔	✔	✔
Motion Detectors		✔	
Notification, Signaling, and Alerting Devices	✔	✔	
Monitoring Equipment		✔	✔
Distance Monitoring Equipment	✔	✔	✔
Fall Prevention Devices			✔

Wander-Alerting Systems

Wander-alerting systems are alarms or systems specially designed to prevent elopement or to notify you if your loved one leaves or attempts to leave home. This equipment ranges from devices that automatically lock doors when your family member approaches to alarms that signal when your loved one has exceeded a specified distance from the device. Some wander-prevention equipment will also help you track and find your loved one once she has left home.

Some wander-alerting systems sound an alarm only if your loved one opens certain doors. These systems consist of a base unit and a small bracelet or anklet that is actually a transmitter. If the wearer opens a door fitted with a special sensor, an alarm sounds. For those not wearing a transmitter the door works normally, without sounding any alarm. To open the door and take your loved one along with you, all you have to do is enter a special code in a keypad that temporarily disables the door alarm.

Wander alerting/prevention systems:

Alert Care, Guardian Electronics, R. F. Technologies, Secure Care Products, WanderGuard, Wander Watch.

Alerting systems that include tracking equipment:

Care Electronics.

Electric sensor locks:

Secure Care Products,
WanderGuard.

"Mom follows me everywhere I go, even outside when I get the mail. I sometimes don't even realize she is behind me. I'm afraid one day she will turn and start walking down the street and I won't even know."

Anti-tailgate feature:

Secure Care Products.

Other devices automatically lock the door when your loved one (wearing a special bracelet) gets too close. When he retreats, the door unlocks. The lock can be overridden by entering a special code in a keypad or applying pressure to the door for several seconds. Each system is different. (If you purchase this type of system, make sure that you can override the system with a button or keypad from the *outside* as well. Imagine going outside to get the mail or the paper and when you tried to get back inside you couldn't, because your loved one is standing at the door waving to you and, in doing so, locking the door!)

Quite often family members will follow you right out the door. Anti-wandering door alarms, once disabled by entering a code, allow a certain amount of time before re-alarming. An "anti-tailgate" feature re-alarms the door immediately upon closing, so your loved one can't follow you.

Hard Alarms

There are "hard" and "soft" alarms. Hard alarms are those that sound loud, frightening noises that ensure they can be heard from remote locations. This type of alarm has been controversial among caregivers because of the distress and trauma that can be caused by loud noises. However, we feel that certain dangers, such as doors leading out of the home, to a pool, to a balcony, or a stairway, justify a loud alarm. Furthermore, the startling effect of an alarm may not only alert you, but also stop or delay your loved one, giving you additional time to get to the scene and take appropriate action.

Use hard alarms with caution. They are only warranted at the most dangerous locations. Loud, scary alarms can cause stress and anxiety that your loved one will not understand. If you use locks in conjunction with the alarms, the loud warning will only sound if the lock is defeated and the door is opened.

Alarms don't have to be expensive. There are simple, inexpensive alarms that may work perfectly well for you. Do keep in mind, however, that they may have been designed for a different purpose—and you may get what you pay for in dependability and quality.

Travel alarms are intended to hang on the doorknob of a hotel room and are activated by the slightest movement. You can use one for a door alarm at home. When the doorknob is turned to open the door, the alarm will sound, alerting the caregiver. Keep in mind, however, that these devices may be very loud.

Personal security devices (those pendants that you carry or hang around your neck when walking or jogging that sound an alarm if you pull a string to release a pin) can also be attached next to a door, with the string attached to a hook on the door. When the door is opened, the string will be pulled and the alarm will go off. To reset them, all you have to do is re-insert the pin. These devices also are hard alarms, often very loud, intended to attract attention to a mugging or personal emergency.

Don't overlook windows as appropriate places for alarms. It is not unusual to hear a story of someone suffering from delusions or desperately wanting to go "home" trying to escape out a window. Refer to our discussion of perimeter one and decide how appropriate window alarms may be in your situation. Check your local home improvement center for inexpensive window alarms that alert you if certain windows are opened.

Soft Alarms

Simple bells, buzzers and chimes are referred to as "soft" alarms. Soft alarms are gentle. They might be a simple jingle bell or cowbell attached to the door. When the door is opened, it pleasantly alerts the caregiver. Another example is a visitor chime triggered by a motion detector, which could be used to alert you that your loved one is walking in the hallway. (See the following section on motion detectors.) There are a lot of available products that may serve your purposes. Check your local hardware store or home improvement center.

Remember that battery-operated devices depend on the strength and freshness of their batteries—and batteries wear out! Check and replace your batteries on a regular schedule.

Finally, there are devices that don't sound an alarm at all, but activate a recorded message. (See the section on fall-prevention devices later in this chapter.)

Door or doorknob alarms:

Alert Care, Crest, DAC Technologies, Enrichments, J. C. Penney Special Needs Catalogue, LS & S, Perfectly Safe, Radio Shack, The Safety Zone, WanderGuard, or stores specializing in travel products.

"Dad kept saying people were after him. Finally one night he climbed out of the bedroom window and we found him three miles away hiding in some bushes."

Sliding window and door alarms:

Alsto's Handy Helpers, DAC Technologies, J. C. Penney Special Needs Catalogue, Perfectly Safe, or home improvement centers.

Motion Detectors

Motion detectors seem to be a well-kept secret. Regardless, in the course of my research for this book I encountered several models with some unique features and applications.

Place a motion-detecting bell or buzzer in important doorways or openings to alert you when your loved one walks past. When the light beam is interrupted or the motion detector is activated, a chime or buzzer will sound. These are called "visitor chimes"; retailers use them to signal when customers enter their stores. You can use visitor chimes to alert you of activity in certain areas of your home.

Visitor Chimes:

Independent Living Aids, Telko.

Light beam alarm/monitor:

Radio Shack.

Battery-operated motion-detector alarm:

LS & S, Telko.

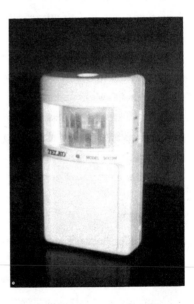

A motion-detecting visitor's chime can gently alert you to nocturnal wandering without frightening your loved one.

Wireless motion detector that sends a signal to a remote chime or alarm that plugs into any outlet up to 100 feet away:

American Health Care Supply, Steinel America.

Motion detector with detached wired alarm:

Snyder Electronics.

Motion detector with plug adapter (you can plug a lamp or radio into it):

Steinel America (photo page 238).

Some motion detectors activate remote chimes or adapters that plug into electrical outlets, which can be located in your bedroom to activate a light, radio, etc. Motion detectors with remote receivers can also be located in specific rooms to alert you to activity in them, the kitchen or your office, for example.

Your home improvement center probably sells motion-detecting adapters that screw into your lamp (between the bulb and socket). When the device senses movement, it turns on the table lamp, as simple as that! After a few moments the light will go off, only to be turned on again when your loved one returns.

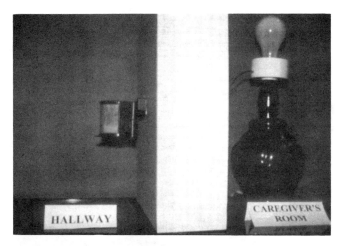

The motion detector senses movement in the hallway and turns on a lamp in the caregiver's room. (A clip-on lampshade may be necessary if the adapter is too large for the arms that attach the shade.) The detector could also be modified to turn on a radio.

Be aware that pets can set off motion detectors at night, notifying you that they are on the prowl, not your family member! Some motion detectors can be aimed, focused, or limited to exclude low areas where pets walk, thus avoiding false alarms.

Wall switches with motion detectors can be used to signal the caregiver, illuminate the hallway (for the wanderer), or turn on a light to let the caregiver know where in the house the loved one may be wandering.

Motion-detecting wall switch:

BRK Brands, Improvements, or home improvement centers.

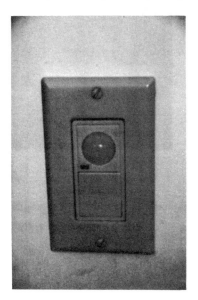

Your regular light switch can be replaced by one that has an option allowing it to go on when it senses motion in the general area.

This motion detector (top) is battery-operated and sends a wireless signal to a remote alarm (center) or to an outlet adapter (bottom) to turn on a lamp or radio. Photos courtesy Steinel America.

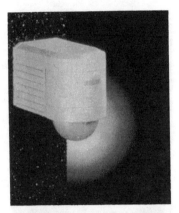

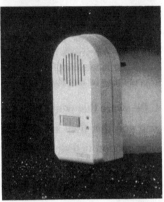

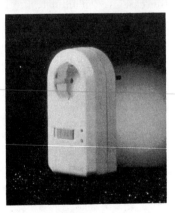

Notification Systems

Notification systems were originally designed to warn people who may be hard of hearing of different happenings within the home.

Notification/alerting systems:

Deaf Products, Harris Communications, Hear More, HITEC, Maxi Aids, The Safety Zone.

For our purposes, these range from devices to notify the caregiver of various types of activity within the home to pagers intentionally activated by your family member. For example, they can let you know that your loved one is calling you or she is stuck on the toilet or in the bathtub. They can also alert you to the motion of nocturnal wandering or that a certain door has been opened. Some can even tell you that a smoke alarm has gone off in the house.

Notification systems employ several techniques to warn you. They can:

- flash a lamp (any lamp plugged into a special adapter);
- signal a pocket or wrist-worn vibrator;
- signal a flashing strobe light;
- sound a remote horn; or
- set off a pillow or mattress vibrator that can wake even the heaviest of sleepers.

Not all notification systems offer motion detectors. This may be important to you if you intend to use the notification system to alert you to nocturnal wandering or if your family member strays beyond a check point. If you have a hearing impairment, a bed vibrator, pillow vibrator, or light flasher would be better than an audible alarm. Shop around, and discuss your concerns and options with a company representative before buying a system.

Do you already have a burglar alarm system in your home? Contact the company to see if you can set up a separate zone within your home to sound only if certain doors or areas are violated. You may have the motion detectors or door contacts already—all you may need is a little extra programming or electrical work.

You might also want to replace the loud interior alarm on your burglar system with one that is a little easier on the ears. Discuss this with your alarm company representative. To disarm the alarm after movement has been detected, or to activate the system when you go to bed, you may want to have a keypad and disarming button installed in your bedroom.

If you're planning to install a new burglar alarm system, be sure to discuss with a company representative how to create a separate zone that will notify you of wandering activity. (Refer to the types of perimeters discussed earlier in this chapter.) Some home alarm companies have programs and systems specifically intended to help those with concerns about wandering.

"Last night Mom took a bath and couldn't get out of the tub. We discovered the problem after she had been stuck there for an hour."

How about something simple to allow your loved one to page you when needed? Pagers intentionally activated by your loved one may include a jingle bell or wireless, battery-operated doorbell. A simple button placed next to the bed, night stand, toilet, or bathtub may be very helpful if your loved one is unable to lift herself from the toilet or needs help getting out of bed, etc. Remote doorbells are sufficiently loud yet pleasant-sounding, and will usually pick up their signal anywhere in an average-sized home.

Monitoring Equipment

Monitoring equipment is intended to enable the caregiver to see or hear your family member from a remote location. It is valuable when you need to hear a call for help or see what's going on when you hear a noise (without having to get out of bed).

Wireless baby monitor:

Kids Club, The Right Start, Safety 1st, The Safety Zone, and most stores that sell products for babies.

Some caregivers recommend monitoring devices normally used to listen in on babies from other rooms. These monitors can also be used to let you hear calls for help and alert you to nocturnal activity in your loved one's room, depending on how soundly you sleep. Some receivers can even be worn on your wrist, allowing you to monitor sounds from your family member's room or bathroom wherever you may be in the house.

"Mom, are you all right? I'm talking to you through the intercom."

Intercom systems can also be used to monitor nocturnal activity and to check on your loved one when you hear unusual noises at night. In addition, installing one station in the bathroom and another outside the front door will allow you to find out who is at the front door, even if you are in the middle of helping your family member in the bathroom, without having to leave her alone or risk missing your visitor. Intercom systems also have the added benefit of two-way conversation.

Wireless intercom:

Radio Shack, The Safety Zone, Solutions. Also check home improvement centers and the phone book, under "Intercom Systems."

Locate intercom stations at the front door, in the bathroom, kitchen, your bedroom, your family member's bedroom, and potential future bedrooms (in case you decide to convert a downstairs room to a bedroom for your family member).

Inexpensive wireless intercom systems are available for installation in any home, requiring no costly wiring. They send their messages by radio signals.

Consider installing a surveillance camera in your family member's room, so you can see what your loved one is doing without disturbing her. There are several types on the market. Some are wireless. Several models can be connected to your television set, allowing you to turn to the right channel to check on your family member and what she might be doing. Many of today's surveillance cameras are cleverly camouflaged, intended to monitor babysitters for child abuse. They may serve your needs equally well.

Surveillance cameras:

Alsto's Handy Helpers, Canwood Products, Crest, J. C. Penney Special Needs Catalogue, Radio Shack, The Right Start, The Safety Zone, Vivitar, or home improvement centers.

Distance-Monitoring Equipment

Distance-monitoring equipment alerts the caregiver when your loved one (who wears a special bracelet or anklet) wanders beyond a pre-programmed distance from the system's base unit (usually placed next to the bed). It's useful in all three perimeters. For a stage one perimeter, set the distance at a maximum setting, alerting the caregiver to violations of the greatest allowable distances, perhaps triggered by leaving the home. Stage two may require a distance of only 15 or 20 feet, allowing free movement to and from the bathroom and including certain areas of the home. Finally, stage three will need to alert the caregiver as soon as a short distance is exceeded, so immediate attention can be provided.

Distance-sensitive wander–alerting/prevention systems:

Care Electronics (perimeter system), Guardian Electronics, Wander Watch (Alert 24).

Each company's product is different. Some are adjustable from only a few feet to as much as 300 feet. With others, you actually walk the permitted area. (As you follow the perimeter of the area you wish protected, the unit stores that information.)

The BedNet alarm has some particularly good features, including remote alarms that can be located anywhere in the house, such as the kitchen or caregiver's bedroom. The alarms can be either audible or visual, turning on lights in your father's room or in your bedroom so you can quickly find out what is going on. This system is also modular, meaning that you can buy the basic unit and add features as you need them.

BedNet System:

Guardian Electronics.

Some distance-monitoring systems have tracking features,

Alerting systems that include tracking equipment:

Care Electronics.

so that if your loved one does wander away from home, a hand-held tracker will guide you to him.

Important questions to ask when talking to the manufacturer or company representative about distance-monitoring equipment are:

- Does the bracelet alert the caregiver if your loved one removes it? (It should.)
- Will cellular telephones or garage door openers interfere with the system? (They should not.)
- Is there a battery backup in case of a power failure? (Preferable.)
- For remote alarms, what is the range of the transmitter and receiver? (Minimum 100 feet.)
- Is the bracelet waterproof or water-resistant? Will it still operate if it gets wet or goes under water (for example, when taking a bath or shower)? (Water-resistant is acceptable, waterproof is preferred.)

Child Alert:

LS & S.

Some inexpensive systems are designed to alert mothers when a child wanders too far away. Although these products are designed for children, not adults, they may prove helpful to you.

"Dad is unstable on his feet. We can't turn our backs on him for a minute or he'll try to get up from his chair and fall."

Fall-Prevention Devices

Fall prevention devices immediately notify the caregiver when your loved one tries to get up from her chair, bed, or wheelchair. They work on one of four principles:

String/tab fall-prevention monitors:

Alert Care, Ali-Med, American Health Care Supply, Care Electronics, DAC Technologies, Posey Healthcare, WanderGuard.

The first type is composed of a small box with a string and clip on the end (much like the inexpensive personal security devices discussed earlier). One end of the string is clipped to your family member's clothing and the other has a tab that fits into a hole in the box. The box is attached to the chair, bed, or wheelchair. When your loved one tries to get up, he pulls the tab out of the device, which sets off the alarm.

(Recorded message) "Mother, do not try to get up. I will be right there to help you."

Instead of an alarm, some fall prevention devices offer a recorded message.

One drawback to all of these pull-tab alarms is that they can be set off by tossing and turning in bed or other actions that cause the tab to be pulled from its hole rather than only by attempts to get out of bed.

The second type of fall-prevention device is a pressure-release sensing pad. The sensor strip or pad fits under your loved one's bed sheet or mattress or on the seat of her chair. When your loved one gets up, the pad senses the release of pressure and sounds an alarm.

Here are a few questions (and answers to look for) that you might want to discuss with a sales representative when shopping for pressure-release systems:

- Are the pads protected from damage caused by incontinence? (They should be.)
- How often do the pads or pressure sensors need to be replaced?
    disposable pads that go beneath the sheet (no less than every 30 days)
    re-usable pads that go beneath the mattress (every six months or more)
- How expensive are replacement pads? (Shop and compare prices.)
- Are the chair pads and bed strips interchangeable? Can you just unplug the strip or pad at the bed, take it over to the chair, and plug it into the chair unit? (Preferable)
- Can the system sound a remote alarm in another room, by either a long cord or a signaling device? (A desirable feature, but most do not.)
- What is the range for remote alarms? (100 feet minimum.)
- Is there a time delay to prevent the alarm from going off each time your family member just moves around a little? (Adjustable from 0 to 8 seconds is preferred.)

One company manufactures the Sofa Saver, a pressure-sensitive pad that sounds an alarm when someone steps on it. Many caregivers have told us that it is useful in alerting them of their loved ones' attempts to get out of bed, sounding

String/tab fall-prevention monitors with a speaker and recorded message:

Senior Technologies, Universal Medical Products.

Pressure-release fall-prevention monitors:

Aremco, Bed-Check, Care Electronics, Curbell, Micro-Tech Medical, Secure Care Products, Senior Technologies, Skil-Care, Universal Medical Products.

Cushioned floor mats for next to the bed:

Care Electronics, Distinct Medical Services, Skil-Care.

Sofa Saver:

Abbey Enterprises, R. C. Steele.

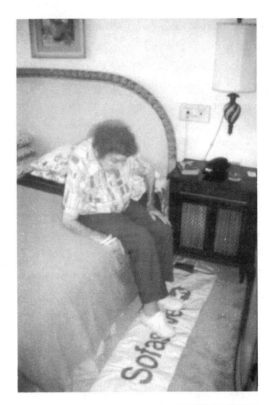

The Sofa Saver can be used to warn you when your family member attempts to get out of bed. Product courtesy Abbey Enterprises. Photo courtesy Juliet Mason.

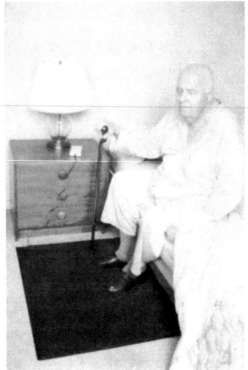

A pressure-sensitive floor mat with a remote chime notifies you when your loved one tries to get out of bed, giving you the opportunity to prevent a fall. Photo courtesy Snyder Electronics.

as soon as their feet touch it. (It is designed to warn pet owners when a pet gets up on the sofa.) (Warning: the Sofa Saver's alarm is attached to the pad, making it easy to step on and possibly break. This can be easily addressed by locating the pad so that the alarm is positioned under the night table. Also to prevent sliding, we recommend securing it to the floor with double-faced tape. Finally, this product can also be slippery to walk on.)

There are also pressure-sensitive floor mats that sound a remote alarm when stepped on.

The third type is a simple device that straps onto your loved one's leg above the knee. As long as your loved one remains seated or lying down and his upper leg remains horizontal, everything is fine, but as soon as he gets up and the leg becomes vertical (or the strap is removed), an alarm will sound.

Finally, distance-monitoring devices can also be used for fall prevention. (See the section earlier in this chapter on distance-monitoring equipment.)

Pressure-sensitive device that slips under one leg of a chair or bed:
Aremco.

Pressure-sensitive floor pads:
Aremco, Secure Care Products, Snyder Electronics.

Leg band wander-alerting device ("Ambularm"):
Alert Care.

Distance-monitoring devices useful for fall prevention:
Care Electronics, Guardian Electronics, Wander Watch (Alert 24).

Be Prepared, Just in Case

Despite your best efforts, your loved one might manage to wander away from home. Do prepare for such an emergency ahead of time. Take advantage of the following suggestions that other caregivers, police officials, rescue personnel, and people dedicated to the field of health care have offered.

Even before someone begins to wander, it's a good idea to register your loved one with both the Alzheimer's Association's Safe Return Program and the Medic Alert Program.

The Safe Return Program helps find and return its members home. Members receive a bracelet or necklace with their name, personal ID number, and telephone number, as well as clothing labels and wallet cards. The program provides accessibility to law enforcement agencies and 24-hour expert guidance to help you and your family through such an ordeal. It is well worth the one-time registration fee for the bracelet or necklace.

These bracelets and necklaces are not just for the patient.

One woman I recently saw with a necklace was a caregiver. Her charm read:

> I am a caregiver for # —— [her husband's ID number]. In case of an emergency, please help by calling —— [the Safe Return emergency number].

This type of tag also provides the caregiver with her loved one's ID number in case he is missing. She can call the emergency number and tell them that "John Smith, # —— [her family member's ID number]" is missing. Also, if something were to happen to the caregiver, *her* bracelet would alert rescue or medical personnel to the needs of the person with AD.

For more information on the Safe Return Program, call or write to:

> The Alzheimer's Association (National Office)
> 919 North Michigan Avenue, Suite 1000
> Chicago, IL 60611-1676
> (800) 272-3900

"Every time we put the ID bracelet on Cousin Marvin he takes it off and loses it. Then we have to buy another one."

One caregiver solved this problem by having a party for his cousin and presenting him with a "wonderful and expensive" bracelet. Everyone raved about it—and now he won't take the bracelet off even when he bathes and displays it with pride at every opportunity!

"Every time we turn our backs, Uncle Allen disappears. He's diabetic and needs his medication."

The Medic Alert program focuses on providing medical information in case of an emergency. A bracelet or necklace includes important medical information, an identification number, and the telephone number of a 24-hour emergency response center. If your family member becomes ill or injured, medical personnel will see the bracelet and call Medic Alert to find out his medical information immediately. You can write or call the Medic Alert Foundation at:

Medical identification bracelets:

Health Enterprises, Medic Alert Foundation, Monroe Specialties.

> Medic Alert Foundation
> 2323 Colorado Avenue
> Turlock, CA 95382-1009
> (800) 432-5378 or (800) 344-3226 or (209) 668-3333

Some caregivers also suggest filling out a police missing person's report form *before* your family member leaves home, just in case. In this way the form is completed ahead of time when your head is clear and you are less apt to forget an important detail. Visit your local police station to pick up a copy. Fill it out and place it somewhere that you are sure not to forget.

If something were to happen to your loved one, you would be able to handle the situation and give the paramedics all the valuable information. But what if something were to happen to you? Who would provide the information to save your life, or whom to contact? What would happen to your confused loved one after the paramedics left? Would he be left alone to care for himself?

Place a non-removable note on your refrigerator door stating:

> In case of an emergency involving —— *[your name]*, EMERGENCY PERSONNEL please notify —— *[friend or relative's name]* at —— *[telephone number]*.
> DO NOT LEAVE —— *[your family member's name]* ALONE.

This note should be placed on the refrigerator door, because that is where emergency personnel are trained to look for medications in an emergency.

If it will not upset your loved one, you might also indicate in the note that he suffers from Alzheimer's disease.

Notify your local 911 emergency system that a person living at your address and telephone number is an Alzheimer's patient. (Call them on a non-emergency number.) Ask them to enter this data in their computer files, so that if your phone number ever comes up on their screen, so will this information.

If your home is connected to a monitored alarm company, you will also want to notify them that your loved one has Alzheimer's. These companies are often the first to be notified of an alarm, and they call the emergency response personnel. If the company is aware of your family member's condition, it can notify the emergency personnel accordingly. (See also the discussion of the RISES PHONE in chapter 4.)

Sew or iron labels to the inside of your loved one's clothing

"Our neighbor had a heart attack last week and had to be taken to the hospital. Her husband, who has Alzheimer's, was left alone and later that evening wandered out of the house looking for her."

Iron-on or sew-on clothes labels:

Identi-Find, Name Makers. Labels are also offered by the Safe Return program.

Self-inking stamp for clothing:

Kids Club, Perfectly Safe.

with her name and an emergency telephone number. If she ever gets lost, this could be helpful.

Take a photograph of your loved one and make copies. Have them available in case you need to show police, neighbors, or others what he or she looks like. Photograph and make a special note of any identifying characteristics, such as a tattoo, birthmark, or scar for easy and unmistakable identification. Make sure that you send a photograph along with your application to the Safe Return Program. You might also make a home video of your loved one, and update it regularly. Each has advantages: Videos are better for television newscasts, and photos can be duplicated, printed, and passed around.

Begin a neighborhood watch program now. Notify neighbors that your loved one is confused. Ask them to notify you if they ever see him or her wandering around the neighborhood alone.

If you live in a development or condominium complex, notify the guard or doorman that your loved one has AD and may wander. If you live in a gated community, provide a labeled picture to be posted in the gatehouse:

IF YOU SEE THIS MAN WALKING BY HIMSELF,
CALL ——— *[your phone number]* IMMEDIATELY.

Take your family member on walks through the neighborhood and introduce him to the neighborhood children. Later you can talk to them, explaining that sometimes your loved one gets a little confused and asking that if they see him wandering alone to either walk him home or come and get you. Purchase some toys or treats to use as rewards—the kids will be sure to talk about them, and the message will be that much more likely to spread.

Finally, if your loved one does wander away from home, consider recent conversations that you have had with her. What delusions does she have? What concerns has she indicated that might give you clues to where she might be headed? Where has she tried to go before? What areas in your community represent immediate dangers? Safe havens?

Proceed in the directions that appear to offer the paths of

least resistance, since people with Alzheimer's disease often seek them. Get out the missing person's report form that you filled out ahead of time, and the photos and videos that you made. Good thing you prepared ahead of time!

Last, but not least, keep a full tank of gas in the car and fresh clothes conveniently laid out, just in case you have to go on a quick tour of the neighborhood.

Wandering is both a complicated and delicate issue. There are good and bad factors to consider. Hopefully, this chapter has given you new insight into the benefits, preparations, and dangers of wandering, as well as the types and possible causes. Arm yourself with this new knowledge and put it to its best use. The benefits will be immense, both in preserving your loved one's freedom and quality of life.

6
Access Denial

Access denial is a controversial subject. The recommendations and suggestions we make must be considered carefully, recognizing they can be upsetting, cause agitation, frustration, or combativeness. Your goal is to provide as much independence and freedom as can be safely and comfortably granted. For example, you wouldn't deprive your loved one of access to a drink of water for fear that she might break a glass or leave the faucet running when you could instead provide a paper cup or a simple, inexpensive device to turn off the water automatically.

This chapter points out different ways to gently, sensitively, and safely deny access where necessary and appropriate—and offers realistic and successful alternatives.

The importance of one's freedom is nothing to take lightly. Wars have been fought to protect it. Your loved one judges her value to her family by how she takes care of her family and home. Denying her access to the kitchen, for example, to protect her from danger, may also be seen as denying her the freedom to take care of her family.

When taking steps to limit your family member's freedom, timing is all-important. Too many locks too soon, and you will cause unnecessary upset. Too little too late could result in an accident. Furthermore, with Alzheimer's disease change is constant. You have to continually observe and react. When certain doors become objects of interest (where dangerous products are stored) or if Mom tries to walk out of the house in search of "home," you must act accordingly. "Acting accordingly" may mean installing locks and alarms on the proper doors and incorporating safe, helpful limitations.

Every idea and suggestion in this book is time-sensitive. There will be a stage in your loved one's life when it is appropriate to incorporate them and a time when it is not.

First of all, control access by recognizing the three kinds of areas in your home: the Respite Zone, Danger Zones, and Safe Zones. (See chapter 1 for more discussion of these zones and chapter 5 for discussion on creating perimeters. Perimeters are helpful in recognizing and establishing a time frame when certain limitations need to be put in place.)

You may feel guilty about denying your family member free access to the entire home. After all, he may have lived in this home for 20 or 30 years, and all of a sudden you are telling him that he cannot go into *his* kitchen, garage, or workshop. It's no wonder if he gets upset.

It is important therefore that among the changes you make in your home there are "creations" as well as limitations. Provide new opportunities for activities that will be interesting for your loved one, and that can substitute for those taken away: special areas for crafts and people watching, garden projects, etc. (See chapter 4.)

"Dad used to be a cabinet maker. Now all he wants to do is go into the garage and work with his power tools. We are terrified that he will hurt himself."

Dementia happens gradually, with periods of clear thought sometimes intertwined in the confusion. Eventually the periods of lucidity become rare, and then nonexistent. In times of clarity, your loved one may feel he is fully capable of performing a certain task, whether it be driving to the drugstore or using the lawnmower. Denying him the dignity and independence of performing what seems perfectly safe to him may be met with anger. Try to balance independence with protection and constantly adjust from day to day.

Substitute related tasks that are more likely to be accepted and completed successfully. For a mechanic, a box of a few large nuts and bolts that can be taken apart and put back together might suffice. Simple productive projects, like picking up leaves in the yard, watering the plants, or pulling weeds in the garden, may fully satisfy the needs of the gardener. Easy-to-assemble puzzles on themes that relate to your loved one's interests may help alleviate the desire to perform more dangerous tasks.

We do not encourage, suggest, or promote any form of physical restraint. If there is any way at all to avoid such brutal and inhumane measures, then by all means take it. Physically restraining your loved one is not only cruel, but dangerous. In the event of an emergency, such as a fire, he might recognize the urgent need to escape and be unable to. Your family member may also resort to extraordinary means to overcome such restraints, resulting in injury to himself or damage to your home. We strongly support a restraint-free environment. For more information contact:

"We don't want to tie Dad up, but sometimes it seems like it would be best for him. He's always wandering away or getting into something. We just can't take our eyes off of him for a minute."

"Untie the Elderly"
P.O. Box 100
Kennett Square, PA 19348
(610) 388-5580

If your family member becomes a threat to the safety of you or your family, professional supervision in an Alzheimer's care facility may be in everyone's best interest. If that is not an alternative, then protecting and alerting yourself to possible danger may be the best course of action. This may include alarms and motion detectors in strategic locations and secure locks on your bedroom and your children's bedroom doors. (See chapter 5 for suggestions on alarms and notification devices of all types to alert you to nocturnal activity and create a safer environment for everyone.)

Locks

Locks are essential tools for restricting access. There is a lock for every kind of door, cabinet, and drawer, including bi-fold doors, medicine cabinets, toilets, refrigerators, and ovens. There are even child-proof locks that can be located inside your cabinets, invisible on the outside, avoiding the cues that might upset your loved one. When looking for locks for unusual situations, consult a locksmith, a local lock or security store, local baby supply stores (for child-proof locks and devices), or your local home improvement center.

Strategies to consider when using locks include:

- Using more than one lock.
- Using different types of locks, requiring different skills to open each.
- Locating the locks in obscure locations, high and low, outside the normal range of your loved one's view.
- Whenever possible, hiding or camouflaging the locks.

Locks not only prevent access, they are also deterrents to loud alarms going off. Place a lock on doors and cabinets that require alarms, and the lock will be the first defense to not only opening that door or cabinet, but setting off the alarm, as well.

Your selection of a lock will also depend on the degree of security you need. Simple inexpensive locks provide basic protection that can often be overcome. Doors and cabinets protecting dangerous supplies or exits from the house will need more secure locks.

One of the simplest and least expensive locks is a hook-and-eye latch. They come in many sizes and are available at any hardware store or home improvement center. Since they are inexpensive and easy to install, you can put more than one on a door, making the unlocking process a little more complicated and less likely to be accomplished by someone with cognitive impairment. Hook-and-eye latches, however, are not very dependable or strong. Someone with strength and determination may be able to force them open or unhook them.

Another inexpensive locking device is a surface bolt, which has a rod that slides into a plate or hole in the door frame, preventing the door from opening. Like hook-and-eye latches, surface bolts can be installed two to a door.

Make sure that you have extra keys for all locks that need them. (You never know when one might disappear!) Label all your keys and store a complete set of spares in a secure, remote location.

A common suggestion to prevent wandering from the home is to place locks on exterior doors. Many of these locks (such as dead bolts) require keys to unlock from the inside. This may not be such a good idea. Keys can "disappear," or you might store them in a remote location. In an emergency you might forget where they are, not be able to get to them in time, or discover that your loved one has hidden the key. At the very least, locate a spare emergency key nearby—maybe on an elastic string that will stretch to the lock, yet be far enough away to make the association difficult for your family member. It would be better if you replaced the lock with one that would be more user-friendly in a crisis, perhaps one that uses a knob on the inside rather than a key (located unusually high or low). For added security, alarm the door.

Don't let yourself be locked out! Many a caregiver has been locked out while going for the newspaper or mail, leaving his loved one in the home, unsupervised and alone. You can carefully hide a key somewhere in the yard in case of such an emergency, or you can give a spare key to a trusted neighbor (and hope he'll be home when you need it). Be very careful when choosing your hiding place:

- Don't put the key where strangers might look for it. Do not hide it under the doormat or a flower pot on the front porch, or over the door. Burglars commonly look for hidden keys in these locations.
- The key that you hide doesn't have to open the door that got locked, or the closest door—any door into your home will do.
- Tell a trusted friend where you have hidden the key, in case you forget.

Also check your home improvement center to see if it sells secure key boxes (with push-button key pads) for storing keys outside.

Cabinets and Drawers

The more safe, remote storage space you have in your secured Danger Zone, the fewer cabinets you'll need to lock in the Safe Zone, where they might agitate and upset your family member. Look for unused space over the washing machine or wall space in the garage for new cabinets. Purchase free-standing lockable cabinets for rooms that are off-limits. Consider getting rid of things you've kept for years to make room for other items that are now more important.

On most cabinets (including kitchen cabinets) you can install locks that require keys. The key can be located near the door, maybe on an elastic string attached nearby that will reach the lock only when stretched.

You can also install child-proof locks on cabinets and drawers. Be aware, however, that your loved one may be far smarter, stronger, and more clever than the child for whom a child-proof lock was designed. Some of the newer and more clever child-proof cabinet locks require a magnetic key. From the outside there is no lock visible. The cabinet door stays locked until the magnet is passed over the lock in just the right spot. (See the discussion later in this chapter on hiding the locks.)

Be sure to install locks on medicine cabinets or remove all dangerous items. Medications can be abused, taken in excessive dosages, improperly mixed with other medications, taken by mistake, or hidden for consumption later. And finally, don't forget the liquor cabinet!

Doors

Restrictions to previously accessible areas may cause frustration, stress, and anxiety. Your loved one may not understand why she is not permitted to go into these areas, even if you have explained it to her a hundred times. The result may be more determination and more persistence to get the door open. Some people will rattle and work on a locked door endlessly, until eventually something gives. It may become the focus of rage or obsession, resulting in shaking so heavy and hard that the door is broken or the handle is pulled off.

Lockable cabinets:

American Health Care Supply.

Child-proof door and drawer locks:

Gerber Products, Perfectly Safe, Rev-A-Shelf, Safety 1st, The Safety Zone, The Woodworker's Store, and baby supply stores.

Medicine cabinet locks:

Brainerd, Safety 1st, home improvement centers, or baby supply stores.

Any lock needs to be installed properly and securely. Some interior wood doors are hollow core rather than solid, making it difficult to properly attach locks. In order to be dependable, locks must be attached to a strong internal framing member of the door, not just the surface finish. A good handyman or locksmith is your best assurance of a secure, reliable installation.

There are also child-proof doorknob covers that fit over knobs and are difficult for children to operate. They may be equally difficult for someone who is confused. Another company offers hidden child-proof door locks that attach at the top of the door.

Child-proof doorknob covers:
Safety 1st, baby supply stores.

Overhead child-proof door locks:
Perfectly Safe.

For rooms that need to be locked while you are inside (perhaps your bedroom, bathroom, Respite Zone, or office), one easy way to restrict access is to replace the passage lock with a privacy lock. A passage lock is a doorknob with no locking mechanism on either side. It allows free access with a simple turn of the knob, coming and going. Privacy locks can be locked from one side only, by pushing and turning the handle, turning a knob, or pushing a button. In case of an emergency, privacy locks are designed to be unlocked by inserting any small, pointed tool (such as a screwdriver or a straightened wire hanger) through the hole in the exterior knob. Wherever you have a privacy lock, you'll need to keep an emergency key nearby, whether it's a screwdriver or modified hanger. (For better advice on locks or what will work as an emergency key, contact a locksmith.)

Another idea might be to install a "secret" hook-and-eye latch on your bedroom or bathroom door. Locate it high up, out of one's normal range of vision, where it won't be noticed.

For doors that need more secure locks, contact a locksmith or handyman. There are numerous types of locks, from inexpensive sliding bolts to more expensive dead bolts. There is a lock for every need and every type of door.

"Stop" and "Do Not Enter" signs:
AliMed, American Health Care Supply, Briggs, Clock's Medical Supply, Posey Healthcare.

In addition to locks, consider labeling doors with signs that read "DO NOT ENTER" or "STOP," reminding your family member not to open those doors or go into those rooms. If you make your own "STOP" sign, be sure it is strong enough to remain in place, and large and colorful enough to be easily read.

"Stop" sign with an alarm and door-mounting kit:
Crest.

The Stopper Kit is an easy-to-attach cloth band that can be used to limit access where a lock is not warranted.

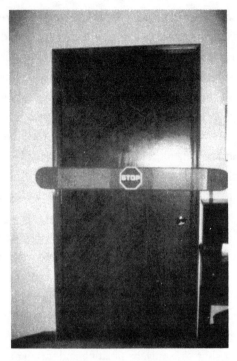

The Stopper Kit:

Clock's Medical Supply.

The Door Stop:

Posey Healthcare.

The Stopper Kit and Door Stop are cloth bands approximately 8 inches wide that go across door openings and attach on both sides with Velcro strips. The band, with a "STOP" sign in the middle, blocks the doorway.

Keep in mind that a "STOP" sign is no substitute for a lock. We have heard stories of family members doing exactly what the sign suggests: They stopped, looked in both directions, and then proceeded through the door. (You might be better off with a sign reading "DO NOT ENTER.")

Dutch doors can also be effective barriers. (Your local contractor can provide and install a Dutch door for you.) It provides confinement and helps define a safe and secure personal space for your family member.

Some caregivers have had success with saloon doors. They are attractive, non-institutional in appearance, and provide a partial barrier that may work in your situation. A simple hook and eye latch will secure the two doors to one another, locking both. Keep in mind that even locked saloon doors can be crawled under. You can discourage this by installing the doors lower.

Another alternative to a conventional door lock is an electric lock operated by a remote button. These can be rather expensive, however. Locate the button away from the door yet within arm's reach, so the door can be opened when the button is pushed. Your loved one will probably not make the connection between the button and the lock. On some models, an alarm sounds when the door is opened. When buying any electric lock, make sure it will allow you to unlock the door manually during a power failure.

Don't forget the garage door. If you have a motorized door, it usually opens by pushing a remote-control button or a button mounted on the wall. Your loved one may suddenly and inexplicably remember it one day. Don't take anything for granted.

There are some doors in your home that you don't want to be lockable. In other words, your family member may be the one denying *you* access!

The most obvious solution is to have an emergency key nearby. Or you can replace the bathroom privacy doorknob and your family member's lockable bedroom doorknob with passage locks. Locks can be used to keep you out, or someone can accidentally lock himself in the bathroom and not realize how to unlock the door. For all doors that can be locked in your home, know how and be prepared to unlock them.

Outdoor Gates

For outdoor gates, go to your local home improvement center for two weather-proof gate latches that lock automatically, using gravity. Two latches will require your loved one to operate both of them simultaneously. Place one at the top and one at the bottom of the gate, spaced so you can just reach both at the same time. Unlocking two latches at once takes skills and coordination that your family member may no longer have. The greater the distance between the latches, the more difficult their simultaneous operation will be.

For additional, more permanent security, gate latches also allow you to install a lock in them, ensuring that the gate cannot be opened.

Electric locks:

Locknetics, Weiser Lock Co., or contact your local locksmith or electrician.

"Arthur watches movies on TV, then thinks the police are coming after him. He goes into the bathroom to hide, locks the door and then forgets how to unlock it."

Childproof key-lockable gate latch and self-closing hinge:
D&D Technologies.

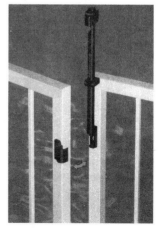

A childproof outdoor gate latch. Photo courtesy D&D Technologies.

A sheet draped over the gate may be an additional ploy to make the gate more difficult to discover—and therefore use.

Finally, don't forget to alarm the gate also. (See chapter 5.)

Sliding Glass Doors and Windows

Don't lock the doors and overlook the windows, especially if you live on an upper floor. Install locks on sliding glass doors and windows that allow them to be opened enough to let in fresh air, but not to allow a person to crawl or walk through. Your family member might try to get out of a window or over a balcony wall, not realizing that he lives on the fifteenth floor. A balcony railing, to him, may seem like a low fence, with freedom on the other side. Install locks on your windows and on doors leading to the balcony.

There are numerous locks and strategies for sliding glass doors and windows. How about inexpensive plastic flip-down locks (available at your local home improvement center)? These hinge-like devices adhere to the glass of the sliding part of the door or window. When the lock is flipped up, the window or door operates normally, sliding right past the lock. When flipped down, the lock's arm blocks the slider from opening.

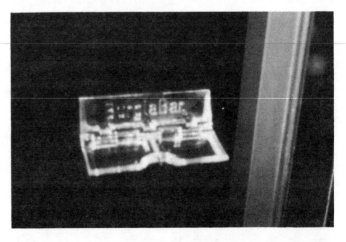

The flip-down sliding door lock prevents the door or window from sliding past it when it is flipped down.

Sliding windows and doors can also be locked by drilling a single hole in the frame and inserting a pin, available at home improvement stores. The hole must be drilled where the two frames overlap. Be careful you don't drill the hole into the glass (inside the frame) and break it. Be sure to drill the hole at a slightly downward angle so that vibrations or shaking won't rattle the pin out of the hole and onto the floor.

Simple clamps that may cost as little as 50 cents at your local hardware store can be easily installed on a window or sliding door track to limit how far the glass can open. Make sure the clamp is installed tightly enough so that it won't be budged by attempts to force open the door. A good set of pliers will help you gain the grip and leverage to ensure a tight and secure installation

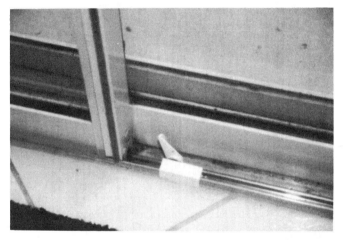

An inexpensive clamp on the track limits how far the door or window can be opened.

Another simple idea for sliding glass doors is to place a wooden dowel in the track. This will prevent the slider from moving, and in most cases will be sufficient to deny access to a confused person. You can either buy a dowel, a Charley Bar, or cut an old broomstick to a length that fits in the track. Painting the dowel silver or black to blend with the track of your sliding glass door will make it harder to see and less likely to be discovered.

Keep in mind that these inexpensive, simple deterrents can be overcome by force or persistence or weaken over time. Periodic testing of these devices ensures that they're still in place, strong enough, and dependable. Better yet, use more than one device so that you have a backup in case the primary fails. Adding an alarm for backup will also let you know if and when the lock is outsmarted. (See chapter 5 for information on different types of alarms.)

The Charley Bar:

Charles-Bar Lok Corp; also check with your local locksmith or home improvement centers.

Sliding window and door alarms:

Alsto's Handy Helpers, DAC Technologies, J. C. Penney Special Needs Catalogue, Perfectly Safe, or home improvement centers.

There are many ways to limit or lock sliding glass doors. Use more than one for backups. Many of these strategies can also be used on sliding windows.

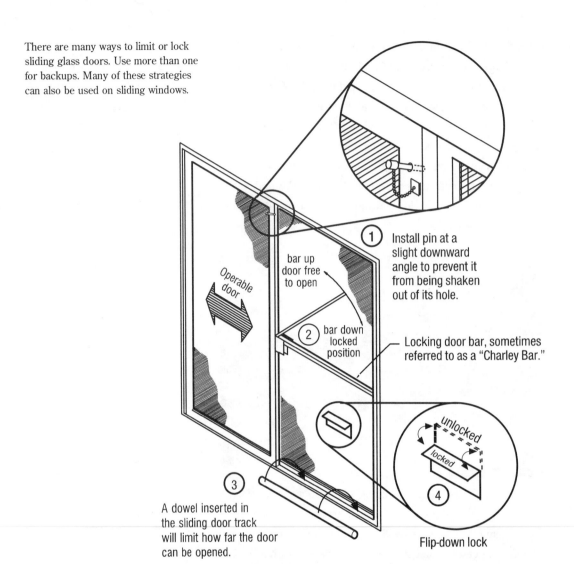

Operable door

bar up door free to open

① Install pin at a slight downward angle to prevent it from being shaken out of its hole.

② bar down locked position

— Locking door bar, sometimes referred to as a "Charley Bar."

③ A dowel inserted in the sliding door track will limit how far the door can be opened.

④ unlocked / locked

Flip-down lock

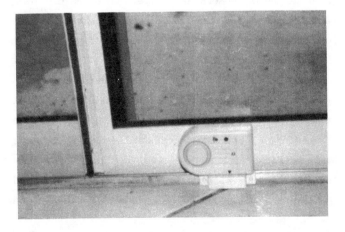

It's wise to add a door or window alarm in case your family member outsmarts the lock.

Special Areas of Your Home

Certain areas in your home may pose more danger than others. There are many ways to create barriers, even for unusual or difficult situations.

Ordinary doors, Dutch doors, folding fabric doors, or gates can be installed in any hallway or opening to create a barrier to the portion of the home beyond. Child-proof gates come up to lengths as wide as 13 feet. Parents use them to keep toddlers out of certain rooms, and they may be just as useful to you.

Install lockable gates or doors in openings leading to areas that may only need to be restricted at night, such as the kitchen. Doors don't have to be expensive. A simple, easy-to-install, cloth bi-fold door, available at most home improvement centers, may suffice. Some people like the idea of installing saloon-type doors locked with a hook-and-eye latch.

Another option may be a curtain to hide the room or door, yet allow access to others in the household.

Adding an alarm to any door will make it safer, alerting you of any unauthorized attempts to open it. It is always wise to install multiple barriers rather than rely on a single strategy, especially when the door leads to a particularly dangerous area.

Finally, you can install a motion detector with a remote alarm (in the caregiver's room) to notify you of activity that gets past your barriers or within specific rooms.

Gates that expand up to 13 feet with walk-through doors:
The Safety Zone.

Retractable horizontal gate (like a pull-down shade, only sideways):
Perfectly Safe.

Stairs

Stairs pose serious dangers for those having difficulty with vision, balance, or remembering how to use the stairs. Your loved one may forget how to negotiate steps or the proper sequence of stepping, transferring his weight, and maintaining balance to ensure a safe transition.

Install a safety gate at the top *and* bottom of your staircases. Gates are sometimes installed only at the top or bottom, allowing a confused person to climb up the stairs, only to find himself confronted at the top by a closed, probably locked gate. He now has nowhere to go but back down the stairs, a task that might be difficult. Also, gates installed at the top of stairs should never swing out over the stairs.

"Daddy goes up the stairs the right way, but comes down the stairs backwards!"

"Mom still thinks her room is upstairs, so she is constantly trying to go up the stairs. We put a gate at the bottom for her safety."

Safety gates:

Kids Club, Perfectly Safe, The Safety Zone, home improvement centers, or baby supply stores.

"We put a shower curtain in front of the stairs to hide them so Grandmother wouldn't go downstairs at night. We never thought that she would lean on the curtain or try to walk through it, but she did."

GFI outlets:

hardware stores or home improvement centers.

Note that gates intended to protect children can be climbed over or forced open by persistent, stronger, and taller adults. Keep this in mind when selecting and installing your gate.

You can always add a lock to your child-proof gate. One that is easy to install and effective is a simple door chain. Attach the chain much the same way you would if it were on a door. When it's time to lock the gate, just insert the end of the chain into the slot attached to the gate post or wall.

Consider installing a sturdy wrought-iron gate. These can be attractive, strong, and if properly installed, unlikely to be overcome by even the strongest adult.

Installing a door in front of the stairs will hide them. If the stairs are "no longer there," your loved one won't be able to go downstairs at night. Make sure that whatever you use to hide the stairs is sturdy, strong, and reliable. Consider locking and alarming the door. You wouldn't want your family member to get through it, only to find a treacherous staircase beyond.

Finally, keep in mind that stairs that are "missing" might also add to your family member's confusion. Searching for the staircase may be a new reason to wander.

Appliances

Access to electrical appliances that may be used inappropriately by those whose judgment and coordination is no longer what it used to be is cause for concern. Two strategies worth mentioning are ground fault interrupted (GFI) electrical outlets and timers to turn off your appliances.

GFI wall outlets have a test and a reset button. By pushing the test button, you'll hear a click, automatically disabling the outlet. Now nothing plugged into the outlet will work. To turn the outlet back on all you have to do is push the reset button.

Before you rely too heavily on this plan, realize that sometimes electrical devices fail. In other words, make sure that once you disable the outlet, it is non-functioning before you rely on it as a "secret" switch. If you have any questions or doubts, ask your local electrician or handyman to check it for you (or to install a new GFI outlet).

Timers that turn lamps on and off at certain times can also

limit when other devices plugged into them can be used. If your coffee maker is plugged into a timer and set to turn off at 8:00 P.M., that coffee maker won't make coffee after 8:00, no matter how much your mother plays with the knobs at night while you are asleep. Tomorrow morning at 9:00 A.M., when the timer comes back on, the coffee maker will again be operable. Visit your local home improvement center for light and appliance timers. (See the photo on page 42.)

The Stove

Quite often nighttime wanderers end up in the kitchen. Your loved one may decide to cook herself a little snack and forget to turn off the stove, or she may hide something under the burners.

Gas Stoves

Gas stoves are inherently more dangerous than electric. They have a live flame that makes it easier to set fire to food and clothing (particularly a bathrobe and pajama sleeves), and they use gas, which comes with its own set of dangers.

The simplest fix is to remove the knobs on the stove. Most can be pulled off with little effort. Keep one knob in a locked drawer to be used as a "key" when you need it or when safe, supervised use is possible.

You can also install child-proof stove knobs. These "bubbles" fit over your stove's knobs, preventing access to the real knobs.

Child-proof stove knobs: Perfectly Safe, Safety 1st, or baby supply stores.

Finally, consider replacing your gas stove and oven with a safer electric model.

Electric Stoves

Again, the simplest way to prevent use is to remove the knobs on the stove.

In addition, you can turn off the stove's circuit breaker at night or after each use. Go to your circuit box or electrical panel, identify which circuit controls the stove, label it properly and clearly, then turn it off each night for a safer night's sleep.

SwitchGuards: Improvements.

Better yet, have an electrician install a hidden, remote switch that must be turned on to operate the stove. You might

Stove timer that shuts stove off after a certain length of time:

Logan Powell Company. This company also offers a device that turns off your stove if it senses extreme heat on or over the stove, such as a fire.

Stove timers set for certain hours:

Grainger Electrical Supply.

Solid burner replacement coils:

Improvements, appliance dealers, the manufacturer's representative for your stove, and home improvement centers.

"Aunt Bessie loves hard-boiled eggs. Last night she tried to make some in the microwave oven. It sounded like the Fourth of July and looked like the parade had been in the oven."

"Last night Mom went into the refrigerator and ate part of a raw chicken!"

locate the switch under a counter or inside one of the cabinet doors. To discourage meddling with a more exposed switch, consider installing a switchguard or cover that hides it. These small plastic boxes have small doors that must be opened before the switch can be seen or turned on or off.

Install a timer that will turn your stove off after a preset length of time. Set it for 60 minutes, and the stove will automatically shut off when the time is up, a task that may be too foreign and complicated for your family member to accomplish. Or you can have an electrician install a timer that will allow the stove to operate only during certain hours. Setting the timer so that the stove is inoperable after, say, 7:00 P.M. would help guarantee a safer night's sleep. Another possibility might be installing a pool pump or water heater timer at your electrical breaker box for your stove. Discuss this with an electrician.

Even if she can't turn on the stove, your loved one might hide something under the burner coils. Whatever she hides there could be ruined, and it might get hot enough to start a fire.

Replace coiled stove burners with solid burners. Solid burners are less likely to be removed, since the cavity below is not visible and probably not a temptation. Out of sight, out of mind!

Microwave Ovens

Microwave ovens can be dangerous also, as discussed in chapter 1.

Microwave ovens are often plugged into a wall outlet. If the outlet is accessible, you can simply unplug it. If not, go to your electrical circuit box and identify and turn off the oven's breaker every night. Label it to make sure that it is not reset by mistake.

At some point making the kitchen off-limits entirely may be safer and in everybody's best interest.

The Refrigerator

The refrigerator is often overlooked as a potential danger until it is too late. Sometimes foods spoil and are not promptly thrown out. Other edible items stored there are intended to be eaten only in moderation, when cooked, or when ripe. Many caregivers have shared stories of a family member going into the refrigerator and eating a jar of mayonnaise or drinking a bottle of pickle juice! An inability to smell or interpret odors may contribute to your loved one's eating inappropriate items.

Install a lock on the refrigerator, especially if it is used to store and keep medications cool. Better yet, eliminate the danger by investing in a small refrigerator for medications. Keep it in the garage, a locked closet, or anywhere in the house that is safely inaccessible. Or keep dangerous medications only in a locked box, stored inside your refrigerator.

Child-proof locks are also available for refrigerators.

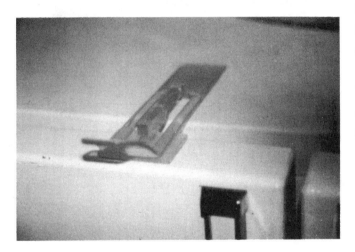

You could also camouflage the refrigerator by changing its appearance. Install wood-grain panels on the front to make it look like a cabinet. These panels are common options available for some refrigerators and are easily installed. If panels aren't available for your model, consider contact paper that looks like wood paneling or decorative wallpaper on rigid cardboard or foam board panels. Look for wallpaper that resembles something that it isn't, such as rows of books on shelves. Attach the panels with double-faced tape.

Most refrigerators have a thermostat located where it can be easily adjusted. Place a small spot of red nail polish on the dial and one on the case so that when they line up the refrigerator is at the correct setting. If one day you notice the dots do not line up, someone has been playing with the dial.

To solve the problem first try removing the knob. If you

Small, compact refrigerators:

American Health Care Supply, Koolatron,* Igloo Products,* Intirion, Marvel, U-Line, or appliance dealers. (*Make sure you ask for the converter that allows you to plug the unit into a wall outlet.)

Lockable cabinet for inside the refrigerator:

Basco or Perfectly Safe. A small, lockable file box, available at office supply stores, is also effective.

Child-proof refrigerator locks:

Gerber Products, Perfectly Safe, Safety 1st.

This child-proof refrigerator lock is located out of sight at the top of the refrigerator door.

Foam board is a composite panel made up of paper and styrofoam. It is available at art supply stores or sign printing companies.

"This morning we opened the refrigerator and for some reason all of the food had spoiled."

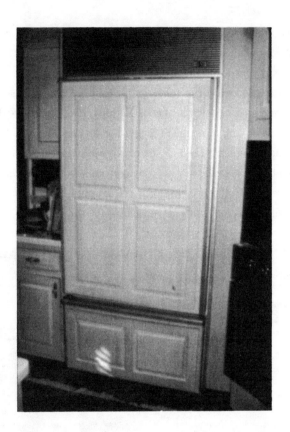

Panels attached to the doors make this refrigerator look more like a cabinet.

have a problem, call the manufacturer, your local dealer, or appliance repair company and ask how to do this for your particular model. As with the stove, removing the knob may be a simple solution. If that doesn't work, try hiding the thermostat. Maybe you could cover it with a cigar box painted white. If the control is in the back of your refrigerator, place a large unmarked box in front of it to make it disappear.

Freezer alarm:

Improvements, Independent Living Aids.

Another way to protect your freezer is a freezer alarm. Though it won't deny access to your freezer, it will alert you when the temperature rises above 15 degrees.

Alternative Methods

Besides locks, there are other ways to deny access. We include a few ideas in this section. Discuss the following thoughts in your support groups. Maybe you'll discover even better solutions that are more applicable to your situation.

Remove the Danger

If a particular closet or cabinet door triggers incessant persistence to overcome a lock, you might solve your problem by storing dangerous items someplace else, so the door wouldn't have to be locked. Over time the desire and urge to open that door may recede, and you may be able to replace the items and lock the door again.

To discover hidden food in your loved one's bedroom, take advantage of the family dog! When your loved one is at day care or on a field trip with another caregiver, allow the dog to check the room. Most likely his nose will alert you to hidden "treasures." He may be her best friend, but when it comes to food, he will likely betray your loved one for a possible treat.

Make Concessions

When you deny access, remember to offer some concessions. It may be best for your loved one to remain in his room at night, for example, but if you can at least give him a view of the outside world, you are not denying him everything. Some special Alzheimer's care facilities do this by replacing bedroom doors with Dutch doors. Opening only the top half (and locking the bottom) allows your family member to see what is going on outside, yet remain safe and secure in his room. His activities can be easily supervised, and he can feel comfortable behind a line of demarcation that excludes others from violating his space. Gates and Dutch doors can be climbed. If this is a possibility for your family member, another alternative may be a screen door. An added benefit will be good ventilation, compared to a closed door.

Use Diversions

Access denial works hand-in-hand with diversion—distracting your family member to cabinets, drawers, and doors that are safe. Take advantage of anything that attracts your loved one's attention: color, light, signage, or attractive drawer handles. Diverting your loved one's attention from a locked cabinet or door minimizes the likelihood that her inability to open it will

"Aunt Martha has an imaginary 'friend' that she visits in her bathroom. It's really only her reflection in the mirror, but last week she started stealing food from the kitchen to feed her 'friend'! Her room smells from rotting food."

result in upset or agitation. (See also the discussion on diversions in chapter 5.)

In addition, never lock all the drawers and cabinets. Always leave a few that are accessible, full of items that are safe for your family member to find and do whatever he feels he must—items that, if removed, won't be missed.

Place something of greater interest near locked doors or cabinets to divert your loved one's attention. One family kept their cat's bed next to the locked door to the garage. Whenever their loved one approached the door, the sleeping cat distracted him long enough for him to forget his desire to go into the garage. Another family created a similar ploy with a bird cage. The cute singing bird was always far more interesting than the locked cabinet next to it.

"Aunt Karen is always playing with the room thermostat. Last week she turned it up all the way and the room got up to almost 90 degrees."

Install a protective, lockable thermostat cover and divert your family member with a false thermostat. Purchase any thermostat from your local air conditioning dealer, your local home improvement center, or even at a garage sale. Attach it to the wall in a prominent location, and cover the other, working thermostat. The new, non-working thermostat can be adjusted to your family member's heart's content, without actually changing the temperature of the room. (False thermostats can be installed in the refrigerator, too.)

Lockable thermostat covers:
Chatham Brass, Honeywell.

Be careful when denying access to the thermostat, however. Your loved one may have a real need to adjust the temperature. (See the discussion of unusual, inexplicable behavior in chapter 3.) Denying access to the thermostat is recommended only for family members living with a caregiver who can monitor the home's temperature properly and make the appropriate corrections when needed. (If the windows and doors are also locked, there is no way to allow cool air in if it gets too hot, or warm air if it gets too cold.)

Freeze alarm voice dialer (a thermostat connected to the telephone that will alert a distant caregiver to high or low indoor temperatures):
Control Products.

Camouflage

The effectiveness of camouflage greatly depends on the stage of Alzheimer's.

Try using paint or wallpaper to hide the thermostat. Find a box that will fit over the controls and either paint it to blend

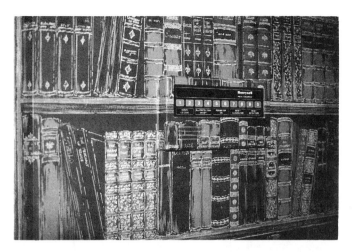

If you look very closely, you will see a thermostat camouflaged to match the wallpaper.

with the adjacent wall or cover it with matching wallpaper. Hinge it on the top with tape, so when you need access all you'll have to do is lift it up.

Camouflage the sliding glass door so it looks like a window. You can easily do this by installing fake mullions (vertical and horizontal strips) over the glass. (See the photo in the section on doors in chapter 1.)

Fake mullions for sliding glass doors or windows:
New Pane Creations.

There are all kinds of creative ways to "hide" a door. One story I heard involved a canvas on which a relative painted a beautiful landscape. It was hung over a door, with a flap for the doorknob. It became a favorite piece of artwork for the person with AD and an effective camouflage of the door behind it. This can also be done with mural wallpaper applied to the door, painting the door the same color as the adjacent wall, or just applying a decorative piece of fabric. Other caregivers have simply placed a curtain (or sheet) in front of the door, or installed a pull-down shade.

Door murals:
Tamarac Development Group, local wallpaper and paint stores, home improvement centers.

Camouflage cabinets by removing the clues that identify them. Among those clues are their handles or knobs. Without them, your family member may not realize that she is looking at an operable door. Try making the cabinet handles harder to see, or remove them altogether. You could paint the handles to match the face of the cabinet. On the other hand, make sure that handles or knobs on safe cabinets are large, easier to use and see, bright, and more likely to attract attention.

Don't depend too heavily on deception as a means of access

denial. It is not unusual to hear stories of sudden periods of lucidity or when someone mysteriously figures out a clever caregiver ploy.

Hide the Locks

Locks are harder to defeat when they can't be seen. Many people with Alzheimer's disease tend to see through a narrow window, a form of tunnel vision that does not include high or low areas. Since locks or bolts are not usually located at the top

Tunnel vision may or may not be a visual impairment. The result, however, is a visual field limited to that which is directly in front of a person.

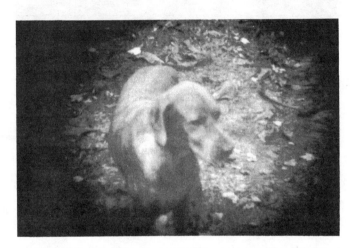

"There's a cabinet in the kitchen where we keep knives. Dad got so angry when he couldn't open it last night that he ripped the handle right off the door."

or bottom of doors, your loved one is less likely to look for them there. Some caregivers have taken advantage of this by placing locks or child-proof devices on doors closer to the top and bottom rather than in more typical locations. Make sure, however, that you can comfortably reach and operate these locks yourself.

Combine a magnetic lock with a spring-loaded latch and remove the cabinet's doorknob altogether. This does several things for you, inexpensively. It hides the lock (now only visible from the inside), removes any knob to grasp and pull, and it hides the cabinet by eliminating the doorknob as a cue. All that remains is a blank panel with nothing to grasp. When you want to open the cabinet, simply attach the magnetic key, gently push the face of the cabinet door, and it will pop open. Remove the magnetic key and the cabinet will remain locked, no matter how much you push or pull.

Invisible magnetic locks:

Perfectly Safe, Rev-A-Shelf, the Woodworker's Store.

Spring-loaded latches are available at home improvement centers and can be installed on the inside of just about any cabinet door.

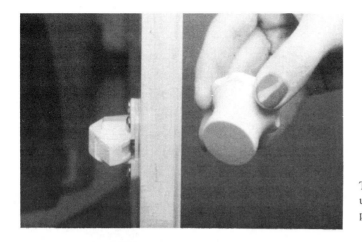

The Tot-Lok is a childproof lock that uses a magnet for a key. Photo and product courtesy Rev-A-Shelf.

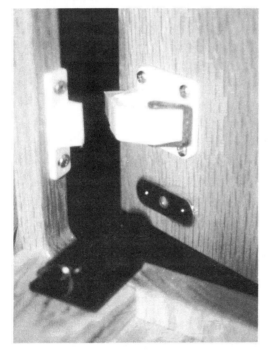

Add a spring-loaded latch to the Tot-Lok and remove the doorknob. Without the knob as a cue, your loved one is less likely to realize that it's a locked cabinet, but you can easily open it with the magnetic key.

You can also install a drawer lock that can only be accessed by opening the cabinet door next to it. This can be something as simple as a bolt mounted horizontally on the inside of the vertical stile next to the drawer. To lock the drawer, slide the bolt into a hole drilled in the side of the drawer. The only way to unlock it is to open the adjacent cabinet door, and unslide the bolt. This may sound complicated, but any good handyman with a drill and a screwdriver should have no problem.

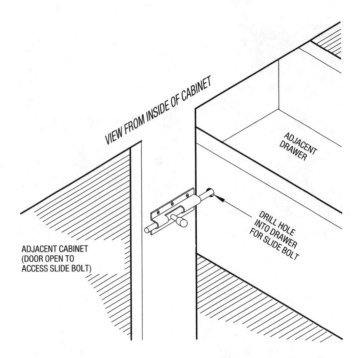

A slide bolt is mounted on the inside face of an adjacent cabinet to lock a drawer.

Child-Proofing Devices

The analogy is often made to safety-proof the home for a person with Alzheimer's in much the same way as you would for a two-year-old child. Although the dangers are much the same, the resources an older person has may be much greater than those of a two-year-old. Your family member, though confused, may still recall what it takes to unlock a door. He also is probably much stronger than a small child—and willing to use this strength to get what he wants.

For these reasons, use child-proofing devices with caution. Don't rely on them too heavily. They were designed for children, not adults.

Nonetheless, some child-proofing devices may be useful in your situation. They may succeed in denying access entirely, delaying entry long enough for the caregiver to arrive on scene, or by alerting the caregiver of new areas of interest.

Child-proof locks and devices are available for:

medicine cabinets	drawers
toilet seat covers	electrical outlets
doorknobs	refrigerator doors

Simple child-proof locks:

Alsto's Handy Helpers, Brainerd, Fisher-Price, Gerber Products, OFNA Baby Products, Perfectly Safe, Rev-A-Shelf, Safety 1st, The Right Start, The Safety Zone, and baby supply stores. For more secure locks, contact a locksmith.

windows	stove knobs
sliding glass doors	gas fireplace valves
pool gates	fireplaces
ovens	cabinets
bi-fold doors	

Multiple Barriers and Locks

Areas that are particularly dangerous for your loved one may warrant multiple barriers, so that if she manages to get by one, there will be backups. Examples of multiple barriers are:

- a drawer, cabinet, door or gate with a sign, an alarm, *and* a lock;
- requiring a person to get past more than one locked door or gate en route to an area of danger or outside;
- multiple locks on a door, cabinet, or gate, requiring one to achieve the proper combination of locked and unlocked devices (even as few as two locks have four possible combinations—open/open, open/locked, locked/open, and locked/locked— with only one allowing entry);
- sliding windows or sliding glass doors with a dowel, pin *and* a flip-down lock.

When using multiple locks, installing different kinds is better than using the same type. Different locks require different skills and cognitive abilities, minimizing the possibility that your loved one, now having figured out how to defeat one lock, will be able to use the same skills to defeat the other.

Passive Barriers

Passive barriers restrict or detour access by using an inoperable, non-mechanical factor or feature of the environment rather than locks or alarms. Diversions, like the cat's bed next to the garage door, can be a passive barrier. A soft, comfortable easy chair that is difficult to get out of is a means of access denial (passive restraint), as can be "visual cliffing."

Some people with AD experience visual cliffing, the misin-

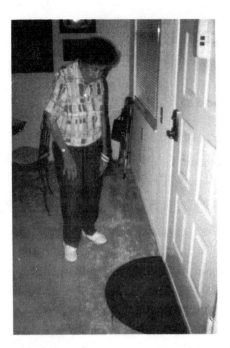

The caregiver has taken advantage of visual cliffing to create a passive barrier. Photo courtesy Juliet Mason.

terpretation of a difference in color or brightness as a difference in depth. You may be able to take advantage of this condition. Try adding a dark strip or a non-slip floor mat in front of a door that you don't want your loved one to use. Your family member may avoid the door, preferring not to attempt to cross the dark "trench." (Observe your loved one carefully. If she tries jumping over the mat or taking long, unsafe strides to cross it, it may be more of a danger than a barrier.) (See also the discussion of visual cliffing in chapter 2.)

You can easily create a visual cliffing barrier on a smooth or carpeted floor with a dark mat. Some caregivers have had success with using colored electrical tape to create a series of "confusing bars" on the floor—a deterrent that their loved ones did not want to cross.

Have a Backup Plan

Be careful how you employ passive barriers. They are inexpensive and often effective. But everybody is different, not only from other individuals but also from one moment to the next and one day to another. What worked for others may or may not work for you. What works today may not work tomorrow. Always take into account that your loved one may figure out your best ploys and strategies. If you use passive barriers, have a backup plan.

Dementia-related disorders, and those who suffer from them, are unpredictable. Some people at times are completely incoherent, without any evidence of rational thought whatsoever—and at other times are remarkably clever and coherent. A person can walk slowly, dragging his feet and taking every step carefully—then the minute you turn your back he's out the door and down the block!

There is no substitute for loving, devoted, caring supervision.

Don't take anything for granted, too much is at stake. Backup plans with multiple methods of access denial are essential. Use your best judgment and keep adapting your plans to match your family member's unique and ever-changing capabilities.

7

Incontinence

While often viewed as a distasteful task, most caregivers deal with incontinence with love and devotion. They overcome the difficulties and rise above the unpleasantness, taking great pride in a job well done and the comfort and dignity they can provide for their loved one.

Hopefully, this chapter will give you insight into some of the strategies and products that are available to help you deal with these difficulties. Perhaps you may even emerge with the hope and realization that the challenges of incontinence can be overcome and are possibly even minor, compared to the blessings of caring for someone whom you love so much.

Realize also that incontinence is often a medical problem. The suggestions in this chapter are not intended to take the place of medical advice. Seek the wisdom of your doctor.

The problems that Betsy and Uncle Ken are experiencing have more to do with the confusion that Alzheimer's creates in its victims than with a medical condition. It would be irresponsible for us not to recognize that confusion alone may be the cause. There may be times when your loved one has an accident that almost appears intentional. When this happens, the best you can do is deal with the consequences. Clean up as best you can. No modification to your home can solve this type of problem. For this reason, caregivers dealing with incontinence often suggest

"Betsy knows when she has to go to the bathroom, but won't tell anybody, she just goes—right where she's sitting."

"Uncle Ken can't find the bathroom. He's lived in this house for more then 25 years, but suddenly he can't find his own bathroom."

that you remove carpeting or invest in a vacuum cleaner that handles both wet and dry problems.

We do feel, however, that there may be other reasons for incontinence that have little to do with medical conditions. You can prepare your home to help deal with them. We identify three types of non-medical incontinence:

- environmental incontinence,
- incontinence due to poor judgment or balance, and
- cognitive incontinence.

Environmental Incontinence

Environmental incontinence is caused or affected by a factor of the environment. Perhaps your loved one's easy chair makes it too difficult to stand up or the white toilet in the white bathroom is hard to see. Maybe the bathroom is just too far away, or perhaps there are physical barriers that make it impossible to get to the bathroom in time.

"Mary just sits in the den most of the day in her favorite chair. She seems to know when she has to go the bathroom, but doesn't."

The "Easy" Chair

Maybe Mary can't get up from that chair. Chairs that are too low or have sunken, worn seats are difficult for older people. Check the angle of your loved one's upper legs. If the angle is sloping down toward her hips, she may be sitting too low. Her upper legs should be parallel to the floor, not sloping, and her feet should reach the ground.

Examine the chair seat for signs of sagging or pockets. Much like an old baseball glove, seats can get softer and deeper over time as their stuffing compacts, flattens, or migrates to the sides. If the cushion has shrunk, replace it.

Maybe the seat supports have worn over time and are now broken or sagging. Remove the chair's cushion and take a look. If so, add a piece of 1-inch thick plywood beneath the cushion. Have your handyman cut it to fit the entire seat so that it will span the depression and offer full support. Or you can order the Sav-A-Sofa, which fits under your sofa or chair cushion to reinforce it.

The Sav-A-Sofa seat reinforcer:

Santa Barbara Promotions.

For a chair that is just too low, build a platform under it to elevate it and reduce the travel distance when sitting down and standing up.

- Make sure the chair cannot slip or slide off of the platform. Attach the legs of the chair to the platform.
- Don't make the platform too high. Two or three inches is probably all that you need. Any more, and your loved one might be afraid to sit in the chair because of its height.
- Make sure that your family member's feet reach and sit comfortably on the ground. A portable foot rest or ottoman may be just what the doctor ordered for complete comfort.

Chair and bench anchors:

(brass anchors) Smith & Hawken; or check your local hardware store for plain metal angles that will serve the same purpose.

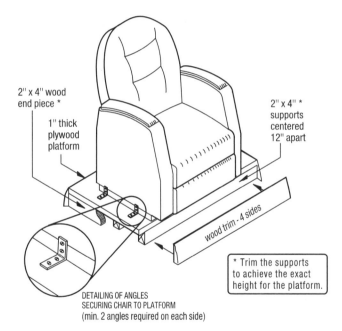

2" x 4" wood end piece *

1" thick plywood platform

2" x 4" * supports centered 12" apart

wood trim - 4 sides

* Trim the supports to achieve the exact height for the platform.

DETAILING OF ANGLES SECURING CHAIR TO PLATFORM
(min. 2 angles required on each side)

Many chairs are comfortable to sit in, but too low to stand up from easily. Building a platform to elevate a chair makes it much easier to sit down and stand up. The width of the platform should be wide enough to fit the chair base, plus the angles attaching it to the platform. The depth of the platform should be no deeper than the depth of the chair base, allowing your loved one's feet to reach and rest comfortably on the floor.

Consider an automatic lifting chair equipped with a motor to raise and lower your family member slowly and gently. (See chapter 8.) Pay close attention to the color of the chair and consider how well it will hide stains.

Finally, chairs that do not have arms extending far enough forward or space below and in the front, allowing feet to get underneath the body, may not offer your loved one the leverage she needs to raise herself.

Install poles with grab handles next to the chair to give your loved one something to hold when pulling himself up. (Have a physical or occupational therapist show you exactly where to locate these poles and their handles for maximum leverage.)

Or perhaps it would be best to replace a problem chair with one that is easier to use. Refer to the drawing below for suggestions on what to look for.

These are some features to look for in a chair. This drawing illustrates the Laurel armchair by Senior Style.

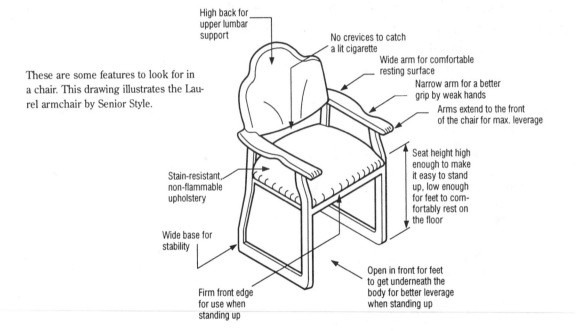

High back for upper lumbar support

No crevices to catch a lit cigarette

Wide arm for comfortable resting surface

Narrow arm for a better grip by weak hands

Arms extend to the front of the chair for max. leverage

Seat height high enough to make it easy to stand up, low enough for feet to comfortably rest on the floor

Stain-resistant, non-flammable upholstery

Wide base for stability

Firm front edge for use when standing up

Open in front for feet to get underneath the body for better leverage when standing up

The Bathroom

If you can't FIND the toilet, GET to the toilet, or SEE the toilet . . . You can't USE the toilet!

Since the culprit in many cases is the bathroom, start by making sure the bathroom:

- is accessible (whether using a wheelchair, cane, or walker or just walking slowly),
- is easy to use,
- is safe,
- is comfortable, and
- protects your loved one's privacy and dignity.

In addition, when dealing with incontinence there are four more factors that will make the caregiver's job easier:

- creating a bathroom and home that are easy to clean and maintain,
- making it as easy as possible to do laundry (as most caregivers know, along with incontinence comes a lot of laundry: heavy, wet sheets and towels that somehow have to be carried to the laundry room),
- controlling odors, and
- ease of cleaning your loved one and keeping her comfortable. (See chapter 4.)

Accessibility

The route to the bathroom needs to be unobstructed, direct, short, and clear.

- Remove obstacles and modify furniture arrangements to simplify the trip to the bathroom.
- Check to see that his comfortable chair is easy to get up from and located as close to the bathroom as possible.
- Make sure the bathroom is easy to find and identify. (Refer to the section on cognitive incontinence later in this chapter.)
- Remove distractions along the way that could stall your family member, giving him time to forget where he was going, while the urge and need persist.
- Provide a place for his cane or space for a walker close to his favorite places, so a separate trip to get it isn't necessary.

Sometimes the trip to the bathroom is just too difficult to make the effort. Make the journey to the bathroom as easy and comfortable as possible, and most likely to result in success. If it is too difficult or likely to result in failure, it will be avoided. Remember those with Alzheimer's often seek the path of least resistance. Sometimes that path may be just remaining in place and not doing anything.

"Uncle Earl wets the bed almost every night. I know he wakes up, but he just doesn't get up to go to the bathroom."

Photocell night lights:

Aids for Arthritis, Home Trends, Westek, home improvement centers, hardware stores.

Motion detector night lights:

BRK Brands, HITEC, Improvements, The Safety Zone.

Motion-detecting wall switch:

BRK Brands, Improvements, home improvement centers, hardware stores.

Motion detector light adapter:

Alsto's Handy Helpers, The Safety Zone, BRK Brands, home improvement centers, hardware stores.

Motion detector with lamp adapter:

Improvements.

Motion detector & electrical plug interface:

Steinel America (will turn on a remote lamp).

Remove obstacles that might get in the way of someone urgently trying to get to the bathroom—perhaps for someone who has difficulty walking, even without an impending emergency. Throw rugs or low tables may make your family member anxious about falling or tripping and inhibit him from attempting the journey.

Verify that routes are short and direct. Your loved one should never have to walk around a piece of furniture if it is not necessary.

Check the lighting en route to make sure it is sufficient to illuminate objects that may be difficult to see. Consider the typical paths of travel: from the bed to the bathroom, from the easy chair to the bathroom, etc. These paths might be taken at times when speed is more important than safety.

Install night lights with photocells or motion detectors in the bedroom, the bathroom, and in the hallway to the bathroom that turn on automatically at night.

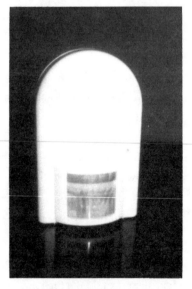

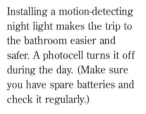
Installing a motion-detecting night light makes the trip to the bathroom easier and safer. A photocell turns it off during the day. (Make sure you have spare batteries and check it regularly.)

Provide a continuous railing to assist and lead your family member to the bathroom (and back to her room or bed).

If fear of falling is an issue, consider installing a fall prevention device to notify you of attempts to get out of bed so that you can help. (See chapter 5.)

Make the bathroom accessible, not only for your family member, but also for the caregiver, just in case there is an emergency and help is needed. Replace the bathroom door lock with a passage lock, rather than a privacy lock. A passage lock cannot be locked from either side and allows free entry at any time. You can also remove the door and replace it with a heavy shower curtain, both to preserve privacy and allow free and immediate access.

If there isn't a bathroom nearby, you might be able to convert a nearby closet into a small bathroom that is closer to your dad's favorite chair. You can either call a plumber and discuss the possibilities with him for a conversion or remove the hanging coats, add a good light, and a portable "john." This room will probably require some assistance, as it is new and may not be remembered. A sign on the door that reads "Bathroom" will certainly be helpful and a nice curtain to replace the door may make the room less confining, as well as accessible.

Ease of Use

Install a bell, call button, baby monitor or intercom next to the toilet, in case you're needed in the bathroom. Any of these can be used to call you when your family member is finished, if there is no toilet paper, or in an emergency. For those who may have difficulty using a pager or bell, try placing a sign next to it—"Dad, if you need help, press this button and call for Joan."

An added benefit of some intercoms is that they have a "listening" feature allowing you to monitor your loved one in the bathroom or have a two-way conversation, while maintaining privacy. Wireless intercoms do not require any expensive electrical wiring and are easy to install.

Or you could install a remote doorbell button next to the toilet. Remote doorbells send a signal to a plug-in or battery-operated chime that can be located or carried anywhere in the home.

Is the toilet seat too low, making it difficult for your family member to sit down and stand up? Raise it. Install a toilet seat extension, replace your toilet with a higher, handicapped-accessible toilet, or elevate your toilet on a pedestal. For weaker mus-

Wireless intercom:

Radio Shack, The Safety Zone, Solutions, or home improvement centers.

Remote doorbells:

Home Trends, Joan Cook, Radio Shack, hardware stores, home improvement centers.

Elevated toilets are available through your plumber or at home improvement centers.

cles or painful arthritic joints, a higher, elevated toilet makes the trip up and down shorter, easier, and more comfortable. Make sure the toilet is at an appropriate height. Your family member's feet should comfortably reach the floor, otherwise the circulation in her legs might be cut off, or she might just feel uncomfortable and insecure sitting so high up. Make sure the toilet is at a height appropriate for others who will also be using it. You may need to add a portable foot rest for certain family members. (See chapter 8 for more ideas on elevating the toilet.)

A toilet platform is a pedestal that goes underneath and raises your existing toilet. Installing one is not a simple project to undertake by yourself; you will need a plumber. The result will be a toilet that is higher and easier to use. It will be more stable than a toilet with an inserted seat extension, and you can keep your old toilet.

Toilet platforms:

AliMed, Medway Corp., North Coast Medical.

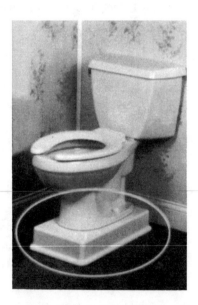

A toilet platform raises the entire toilet. It should be installed by a plumber. Photo courtesy Medway Corporation.

Mechanical toilet seat lifts:

Home Care Products LLC, Stand-Aid of Iowa, Transfer Master Products, Ultimate Home Care.

Another option is a mechanical toilet seat lift. In its ready position, the seat is elevated and tilted forward. Your family member sits on it, holding the arms or grab bars. At the push of a button, the seat slowly lowers him to a sitting position. Pushing another button slowly raises the seat and tilts it slightly forward, so that it is easier to stand up and walk away. When not in use, the seat can be folded up, so that others can use the toilet normally.

A higher toilet also needs arms or sturdy grab bars on both sides. This will help your loved one considerably, whether sitting on the toilet, standing, or just relying on the bars for a little extra security. (See also chapter 8.)

As mentioned earlier, some bathrooms look like a polar bear in a snowstorm. When the color of the toilet matches the color of the floor, Benny may not be able to see the toilet when standing over it. This is especially true if the situation is complicated by a visual impairment.

"Benny makes it to the bathroom just fine, then he urinates all over the floor."

A possible solution to this problem might be to:

- Raise the toilet. A higher and therefore closer "target" will may make it easier to see and hit.
- Next modify the colors of the floor, toilet, or wall to make the "target" easier to see.

Try placing a contrasting-colored floor mat around the base of the toilet. This will make the toilet easier to see and, after those near misses, the mat can be easily cleaned.

Floor mats for in front of toilet:

Kids Club or bath supply stores.

You can easily make such a mat yourself. To make your own, start with a rubber floor mat. First create a template as illustrated below.

Floor mats:

Consolidated Plastics, Rubbermaid, or home improvement centers.

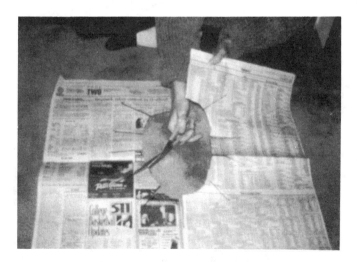

In a piece of newspaper cut a hole a little smaller than the base of the toilet (estimate it). Make 3-inch cuts radiating out from the center of the hole about 4 inches apart. A cut from the top of the hole to the edge of the newspaper will allow you to place the paper on the floor around the toilet.

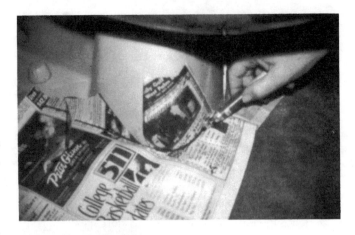

Place the template on the floor around the base of the toilet and press it snugly to where the base meets the floor. Trace the base closely, section by section, folding the sections to create a tight, snug outline of the toilet base. Cut out the extra pieces, section by section, following your outline on the newspaper.

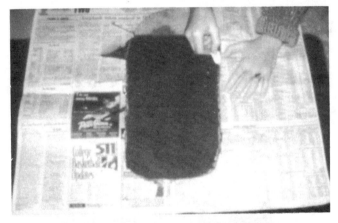

Transfer the outline of the newspaper template to the rubber mat. Adjust the location so that the hole is right where you want it to be. Use a sharp piece of soap as a marker.

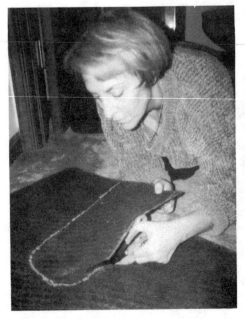

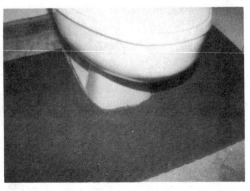

Now you have a floor mat that will fit snugly around the base of your toilet.

Cut out the rubber mat, following your outline.

Here are some other ways of making the toilet stand out and easier to see:

- Use colored electrical tape to outline the rim of the bowl.
- Paint a "target" in the toilet bowl. (One caregiver painted a bull's-eye in the toilet bowl for a man who was having trouble hitting the bowl. It worked! If you like this idea, empty, clean, and dry the toilet before painting it. Use waterproof, enamel paint that will hold up underwater.)
- Buy a new toilet seat that is a different color and contrasts to the floor. Check the selection at your local bathroom supply store or home improvement center.

One caregiver that we know removed the toilet seat, took it outside and spray-painted it blue. It's hard to miss now!

A potential drawback to this approach, for men, is that the toilet seat remains down while in use, creating a smaller hole and target.

- For a light-colored toilet, add colored disinfectant tablets that go into the toilet tank and tint the water blue or green.

Provide plenty of light in the bathroom. I can't overemphasize the need for sufficient lighting, especially in the bathroom, whether it is to find a white pill that has dropped onto a white floor, see a white toilet bowl against a white background, or have enough light in the shower to comfortably bathe. In addition to general lighting, you'll need light to guide your family member to the bathroom on those nights when he is a little drowsy or has forgotten which room is the bathroom.

Finally, the type of clothing worn by your family member (and how easy it is to remove) will also play a role in his ability to use the bathroom. Seek the advice and recommendations of your occupational therapist for sources and the best types of clothing for your family member.

Safety

Without question the bathroom needs to be safe. (See chapter 9 for more ideas on this important subject.)

Make it possible to get to your loved one fast and easily (for example, not hindered by any doors that might have been locked for privacy or out of habit). Replace privacy locks with passage locks, or doors with shower curtains.

Furnish assistive devices, such as grab bars, wherever they might be helpful. Install them on both sides of the toilet to use with both hands while sitting or standing, helping your family member with balance so he doesn't wobble while standing to urinate.

Provide convenient storage for items frequently used or needed in times of crisis, such as:

Toilet games to keep your family member occupied:

Harriet Carter (fishing game and golf game placed on the floor in front of the toilet).

- his walker or wheelchair
- towels
- fresh clothes
- extra toilet paper, soap, etc.
- medical supplies
- lubricants and rubber gloves
- a warm blanket to wrap around your family member sitting on the toilet on cold days or nights.

Making sure these supplies are readily available ensures that your loved one will never have to be left alone—even for just a few seconds—while the caregiver gets them.

Comfort

Interesting wall murals:

Tamarac Development Group and wallpaper stores.

Music from the "good ol' days":

Collectors' Choice, Elder Books, ElderSong Publications, Hammatt Senior Products, HeartWarmers, Nasco, Senior Products, Sound Choice, Wireless.

Incontinence doesn't just mean the inability to control oneself; it also means that more time will be spent in the bathroom. You will want to make this room as pleasant and comfortable as possible, providing things to do and look at while on the toilet. Take advantage of the space on the wall or door across from the john (perhaps for an interesting poster or lithograph, reminding your family member why she is in there).

Make the bathroom homey with pretty colored towels, curtains on the window, and attractive wall finishes. Add music with a battery-operated radio or a cassette tape player for favorite hits or calming music. Make sure that the room temperature is comfortable for your family member. (See also chapter 1 for more ideas on making the bathroom comfortable.)

Your bathroom may be too busy and confusing. Though your father may have used this bathroom for thirty years without a problem, its floral or patterned wallpaper may now be too much for him. Just walking into the bathroom may be overwhelming if there are flowers on the wall, hundreds of objects repeated in the wallpaper, decorative items on shelves, magazines on the floor, along with all the other items normally found in the bathroom.

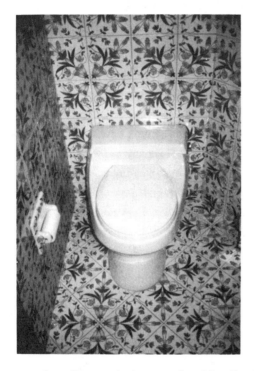

Clutter and busy patterns create confusion. Keep the decor simple.

Make sure the toilet seat isn't uncomfortable. Check your local home improvement center for soft, cushioned toilet seats.

Privacy and Dignity

As the disease progresses your loved one will eventually be unable to take care of himself and even perform simple tasks. Though his abilities may be declining, his sense of pride, dignity, and self-esteem will probably remain well intact.

Privacy and dignity can make the difference between using or not using a bathroom. Some people simply choose to soil themselves rather than use a bathroom in front of someone or be assisted while toileting. Making a bathroom as private and dignified as possible can make it far more inviting and acceptable and reduce the number of "accidents."

Given some of the unique problems accompanying AD, preserving privacy may include removing or covering the bathroom mirror—to eliminate the "stranger" that "keeps following me into the bathroom."

Lack of Balance and Incontinence

"My husband has to put one hand on the wall to balance himself while urinating. Then he still goes all over the floor."

A problem men sometimes have is dripping on the floor while standing over a toilet, sudden rushes of urine, splashing, or just poor aim. The floor in any public men's room offers plenty of evidence to this. Instability when standing over a toilet or difficulty performing several functions at a time (urinating, aiming, standing, and holding onto a grab bar) can also contribute to accidents. These are not symptoms of incontinence at all. Though they may be complicated by conditions associated with AD, they should not be matters of great concern, just reasonable concern for cleanliness.

As discussed earlier in this chapter, you can install a waterproof mat around the base of the toilet. Also consider installing a toilet seat extension, a higher toilet, or elevate the toilet on a pedestal. A closer "target" is easier to hit.

A well-placed grab bar may also offer support in just the right location. Discuss this with your occupational or physical therapist.

Cognitive Incontinence

"Arnie starts to walk into the bathroom, then turns around and walks out. Then he goes over to the corner of the bedroom and urinates."

Cognitive incontinence results from confusion or, as in the case of Alzheimer's disease, failure to process all the information necessary to make appropriate or correct decisions—difficulty finding the bathroom or confusing a wastepaper basket for a toilet, for example. Sometimes simple solutions or additional information can provide good results.

Is there "someone" already in the bathroom? What is the first thing we usually see when we walk into a bathroom? Is it the mirror and our own reflection? For Arnie, perhaps that reflection is another person in the bathroom. If the bathroom is occupied, turning around and leaving may be a logical action to take. To eliminate the "occupied bathroom," cover or remove the mirror. A simple pull-down shade mounted above the mirror will make it accessible for grooming, yet cover it when Arnie needs to use the bathroom.

Making the Bathroom Easy to Find

For the person with Alzheimer's, the memory of her current home and its layout may gradually disappear. Though the bathroom has always been "the first door on the right," now that fact may no longer be recalled, and your loved one may have to look for other clues to help her find the bathroom. Alzheimer's disease erases memories, and one of them may very well be where the bathroom is or how to recognize it.

"Grandma Casey can't find the bathroom at night."

In order to make it easier for your family member to find and identify the bathroom, multiple or redundant cuing is essential. You'll need to provide as many cues and signals as possible to help her find and recognize that room. Make the toilet visible by keeping the door open and a light on at night. Install signs and arrows to point the way to the bathroom. This will help make the journey to the bathroom more successful and eliminate unnecessary delays that come with failures to recognize the bathroom in time. (See chapter 8 for more suggestions and ideas.)

Maybe your family member can't see the toilet, even when the bathroom door is open. That would definitely make the

For those with normal vision, the standard white-on-white bathroom poses no challenges.

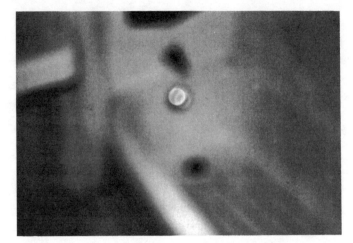

For those with visual impairments, the same white-on-white bathroom may be very hard to see and understand.

bathroom harder to find. So many bathrooms are decorated monochromatically: with a white toilet, white wall behind it, and a white sink, tub, shower curtain, grab bar, and towel bar.

Try painting the wall behind the toilet a contrasting color, or placing a panel behind it to make the toilet more visible. Replace the toilet seat with one of a different color (it will help whether the seat is up or down). Also, make sure your bathroom has sufficient lighting so that your family member can see the toilet when she goes by or is in the bathroom.

"The other night Dad was in the hallway. He just turned, unzipped his fly, and urinated in the flower pot. When he was finished he seemed to realize what he had just done and was so embarrassed."

Not only trash cans but also purses, pillowcases, planters, hampers, and anything that resembles a container have been mistaken for a toilet. A flower pot is as much a receptacle as a urinal. To someone with AD, it may seem perfectly logical to use it as a urinal. Another possibility is that people with Alzheimer's often retreat to their childhood, perhaps when their families might not have had indoor plumbing. In those days they may have used cans, bottles, or maybe an outhouse. They may have kept a can or bottle next to the bed at night. Now, when they're unable to find their "outhouse" or "can" they may resort to something else, such as a flower pot.

"Uncle Earl keeps going to the bathroom in the trash can in the bathroom. It's right next to the toilet, but he won't use it."

Try relocating the wastepaper basket inside a cabinet, making it out of sight and out of mind. Your family member will have to seek other places to urinate or throw the toilet paper, and maybe she will come up with the right solution on her own. There are also hampers with lids and child-proof locks.

Child-proof hampers:

Safety 1st.

Make sure your loved one can see and find the toilet. If your bathroom is one where everything in the room is one color (except the waste basket), maybe that's the problem. The waste basket is the only receptacle that your loved one can find, therefore that's what he uses!

Dealing with the Consequences

Unfortunately, modifying the home may have little to do with the causes of incontinence. But you can prepare your home to help you deal with the consequences. As is true for any difficult situation, foresight and preparation make problems much less stressful and difficult for everyone. After all, your loved one didn't choose to be this much trouble and may be concerned about being a burden. Do what you can to minimize her concerns, not only for your convenience, but for your loved one's peace of mind as well. (Refer also to the section on toileting in chapter 4.)

Bedwetting alarms:

Care Electronics, Health Sense International, Starchild Labs, The Take Care Store.

Creating a Home That Is Easy to Maintain

Make it possible to clean up accidents quickly and easily. The longer the reminder is present, the more time your family member has to grieve over her situation or the difficulty she may be causing.

Invest in a wet/dry vacuum cleaner that will clean up both dry and wet accidents. Among other advantages, you'll be able to use wet household cleaners on carpet and vacuum them up, leaving carpeting cleaner and faster-drying.

Fans and air purifying equipment maximize air flow and help dry damp carpeting, accidents, and wet floors. (Refer to the section on odor control later in this chapter.)

Add an incontinence chair pad to your family member's chair (and bed) that absorbs and retains moisture, preventing it from reaching the cushion (and mattress) underneath.

Place a waterproof mat around the base of the toilet. (Refer to the discussion on making the bathroom easy to use earlier in this chapter.)

Small, portable carpet cleaner:

Alsto's Handy Helpers, American Health Care Supply, Bissell, Eureka, Hoover Company, Improvements.

Incontinence bed and chair pads:

Accent on Living, Enrichments, Mature Mart, M.O.M.S., Sammons Preston, Sears Home HealthCare Catalogue.

If you're adding or renovating a bathroom:

- Use materials that are easy to clean and won't absorb or retain fluids, such as ceramic tile. Make sure also that the tile that you choose is slip-resistant.
- Provide a drain, either in the bathroom floor or in a roll-in shower, to allow water on the floor to drain. (See chapter 8 for more information on roll-in showers.)
- Cleaning your loved one after an accident may be both difficult and unpleasant. This is a good reason to have a roll-in shower rather than a bathtub. (See also chapters 4 and 8.)
- Avoid carpeting in areas where "accidents" are more likely to occur, the bedroom and bathroom. Most caregivers we interviewed recommended not using carpeting at all in homes dealing with incontinence.

SpillBlock:

DuPont.

Nonabsorbent, anti-microbial carpeting:

Collins & Aikman Floorcoverings, Lowe's.

Waterproof seat cushions:

AliMed, Enrichments, HNE Health-care, Jay Medical, Neuropedic.

"Theresa doesn't always tell us when she has to go to the bathroom; she wears the absorbent pants, but they don't always do the trick. Her chair is starting to smell pretty bad."

If you do install carpeting, inquire about SpillBlock backing. This goes on the underside of carpeting and prevents liquids from penetrating and being absorbed by the padding underneath. SpillBlock makes it much easier to clean and vacuum up liquids. Also inquire about carpeting that does not absorb liquids. These preventive measures, combined with a wet/dry vacuum cleaner, can be very effective in cleaning up accidents and preventing odors.

Waterproof your carpet and cushions. Use nonabsorbent materials for the cushions as well as Scotchgard fabric treatments (available at your local hardware store in spray cans). You will have to re-treat the material periodically according to the instructions on the can to maintain its moisture resistance.

Replace the easy chair cushion with a durable, waterproof patio chair cushion. An added advantage will be that patio cushions are usually firmer and will make it easier for her to get up. Home improvement stores carry styles and colors galore.

Making It Easier to Do Laundry

Incontinence creates the need to launder heavy, wet sheets frequently. This would be so much easier if the washing machine were located conveniently (instead of in the basement or on the other side of the house). To avoid carrying laundry to these remote locations and possibly down treacherous steps to the basement, install a compact washer/dryer closer to the source of the laundry—the bedroom and bathroom. Make sure the washer/dryer is heavy duty or of sufficient quality not to get thrown out of balance by heavy, wet towels.

If you must carry laundry to and from the laundry room, make sure the trip is safe.

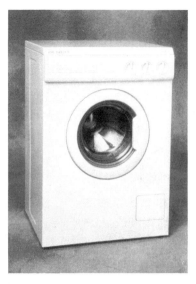

A compact washer/dryer combination installed close to the bedroom saves many steps. Photo courtesy Bendix Corporation.

- Install railings to hold onto in hallways and on both sides of the stairs.
- Repair what needs to be repaired. Over time, steps can wear, and railings can be dangerous if they are not installed properly or have loosened.
- Make sure your steps are slip-resistant and you can easily tell when you reach the last step, on the top and on the bottom. (Refer to chapter 9.)
- Provide plenty of light on the stairs, especially the top and bottom, so you can see where you are going and obstacles in the way.
- Make sure that you have light switches at both the top and bottom of the stairs, so that you will never have to go up or down a dark set of stairs because the switch was at the other end. (See chapter 9.)
- Install a telephone at the bottom of the stairs (near the floor), just in case one day you have an accident and need to call someone. If you already have an electrical outlet there, this may not require expensive wiring or a visit from the telephone company.

Combination washer/dryer that requires no venting:

Bendix, Equator. Also check with appliance dealers. Many carry small, compact units designed for apartments.

Wireless remote telephone jacks that plug into electrical outlets:

Brookstone, Comtrad Industries, Hear More, Phonex, Radio Shack.

Controlling Odors

Odors cause embarrassment and discomfort. They get absorbed into carpeting, clothing, and room materials.

In addition to good cleaning practices, controlling odors in your home requires three additional approaches:

- disposing of soiled incontinence briefs in airtight containers, not allowing them to contact the air;
- providing good ventilation; and
- cleaning the air.

Confidante:

Mondial Industries, Sears Home HealthCare Catalogue.

Many caregivers have taken a lesson from mothers of small children. They suggest a product called the Confidante, which seals soiled adult briefs in a plastic wrapper, thus eliminating their odor and making them easy and convenient to handle.

Air stagnates. Nonmoving air allows airborne particles to settle, concentrate, and accumulate in your carpeting and soft upholstery. You will also want to replace stale air with fresh air whenever possible.

- Add a ceiling or wall exhaust fan in the bathroom to help remove odors to the outside.
- Install ceiling fans, especially in the bedroom, for better air circulation and to facilitate the drying of damp or recently cleaned areas.

Pole-mounted ceiling fans:

The Safety Zone.

Activated carbon air conditioning filters:

Air Sponge Filter Company, Farr Company, Natural Hardware Store.

If the ceiling fan is causing a draft that is bothering your family member, a simple solution is to reverse the direction of the blades. This will cause the fan to suck the air up rather than blow it down. Most fans have a switch that allows you to reverse blade direction.

Air filtering machines w/ HEPA filters:

Absolute Environmentals, American Health Care Supply, Austin Air, Brookstone, Enviracaire, Graham Field, Hammacher Schlemmer, Holmes, J. C. Penney Special Needs Catalogue, McKesson, The Safety Zone, Sears Home HealthCare Catalogue, Vornado Air Circulation Systems.

- To avoid installing permanent fixtures in the ceiling, consider pole-mounted fans for those locations where more air circulation is desired but there is no shelf or wall bracket.
- Open windows to allow fresh air in and force stale air out. See chapter 6 for information on locks that allow windows to be opened safely.

Consider activated carbon filters for your air conditioner. For maximum efficiency, these filters should be changed regularly. You might also want to use an air-filtering machine with an HEPA filter that cleans the air, removing odors. Two suggestions that we make regarding machines using HEPA filters are to make sure they have a minimum capacity of 300 cfm and that their inlet and discharge are on opposite sides of the unit. This way you can be assured that your machine is providing the best air circulation rather than just cleaning the air around the machine.

Finally, you may want to install automatic air freshening machines that disperse a nice-smelling air freshener periodically. Be sure to read the labels and ask questions. Look for air fresheners that neutralize odors, rather than mask them. In addition, add some potpourri to the bedroom and bathroom. Locate the bowl out of reach and out of sight so that the contents are not eaten or mishandled.

Air freshening machines:

Alsto's Handy Helpers, American Health Care Supply.

Incontinence is certainly a difficult problem that no one wants to confront. Hopefully, this chapter has given you some constructive solutions and ideas that hit directly on the difficulties that you are facing.

Alzheimer's disease is truly a mystery in itself, and every case introduces new challenges and unique concerns. Patience and creativity are called for when addressing difficult problems. Don't rely only on your own resources to solve all of your problems. Bring up these issues in your support group. Ask questions and discover what other creative folks have done in similar situations.

8

Mobility

As Alzheimer's disease continues to affect your loved one's abilities and disrupt the signals traveling throughout the brain, mobility will become a problem. At first the obstacles may be cognitive, getting lost or failing to recognize the drug store. As time goes on the problems begin to manifest themselves in more significant and physical ways: walking, using the stairs or a walker, until eventually even getting out of bed becomes too risky.

In this chapter we will examine mobility impairments, difficulties associated with them, and ways in which a caregiver can stay one step ahead. We will begin with independent movement and progress through the full range of declining mobility.

Disorientation and Wayfinding

Episodes of forgetfulness or absentmindedness will be among your family member's earliest mobility problems. At first they may seem insignificant—perhaps momentarily forgetting where one is going, or maybe losing orientation within the home. These episodes, over time, will become more frequent, upsetting, and difficult to resolve. Your loved one may become lost within a single room and unable to find the way out. As time goes on she may not even recognize her own home, from either the inside or the outside. A simple trip to get the newspaper can turn into a terrifying experience when, upon turning around, your family member is unable to retrace her steps back inside.

When well-known cues and landmarks are no longer familiar, you'll need to create new ones. If you add a sign at the door, for example, that reads "The Smith Residence" or "Mabel Jones's House," maybe your loved one will recognize her name. Use a name she will remember. If your mother no longer relates to her married name, use her maiden name. If she is more comfortable with a foreign language, try "Casa de Mabel Jones."

When a choice needs to be made among several doors, make the "right" door unique and call attention to it. At the same time, remove and minimize environmental factors that may distract your loved one or overwhelm him with too many details. For example, in a room where is it important to clearly see and identify pathways, avoid upholstery, carpet, and wallpaper with flowers, plaids, and other repetitive, busy patterns. These only add to the confusion of a room, instead of helping to create one that is easy to understand.

"The other day when I came home from work I passed my mother walking in front of the house. She was alone and crying. When I asked what was wrong she sobbed that she had gone out to get the mail and when she turned around our house was gone."

Cues and Landmarks

Several years ago I attended a conference on aging. I was one of only a few architects there, and the only one participating in this particular exercise. I was given blurry, dark glasses (to simulate visual impairments) and told to walk around the lobby. A whole new world opened up to me. What was so impressive were the different cues and landmarks that suddenly revealed themselves. For example, I no longer could identify the lobby by seeing the reception desk—but I knew I was in the lobby just the same by the conversations that I could hear and the bright light coming in through the large bay windows. The elevators gave themselves away by the bells that sounded when the doors opened, and I could follow music coming from a piano to get to the restaurant.

Your loved one doesn't wear dark, blurry glasses, but her ability to perceive and identify things is nonetheless impaired, by the disease. If she no longer recognizes the bathroom as "the first door on the right," maybe she will recognize it from other environmental cues. Perhaps she will find the room with the toilet, the pink wallpaper, or maybe she will be drawn to it by a nightlight.

A landmark is an obvious and conspicuous environmental feature that helps to locate, guide, or orient a person. We use landmarks, consciously or not, moving from point to point until we finally reach our destination. For example, in order to get from the rear of the backyard to the door we might follow a path that first goes to the garden, then to the bird feeder, and then finally to the door. Landmarks are especially important cues for people with AD seeking to navigate in an increasingly baffling environment.

Cues trigger a behavior, make distinctions, or help your loved one understand something. They provide information, whereas landmarks are features used more for navigation and guidance. Sometimes items can be both landmarks and cues. The dining room table not only helps your family member identify the dining area (cue), but also offers something to walk toward en route to that room.

Examples of environmental landmarks and cues in your home include:

room colors	the dining room chandelier
wallpaper	the dog's bed
cooking odors	the picture on the television
distinctive paintings	music from a radio
light through windows	changes in floor materials
tile in the bathroom	breezes from vents or fans
large potted plants	wind chimes
distinctive door trim	pieces of sculpture
signs	the living room sofa

Use landmarks and environmental cues to attract your loved one in the right directions and to help her make correct decisions. At the same time, to reinforce the cues' usefulness, remove distractions and causes of confusion.

Outside the home, colorful flowers, paint, canopies, and decoration can be used to grab attention—the bolder and

"Mom goes outside to work in her garden and then can't find the door to get back in. So we put a statue of a small dog in front of the door. When she turns around looking for the door she is attracted to the dog and goes over to pet it. When she's done, she finds herself right in front of the door to come inside."

more primary the color, the better. In a plain yard, place a colorful piece of sculpture or a bench to sit on near the door to lure your family member closer. Paint that back door an attractive color and place large pots with red flowers (real or artificial) on both sides. How could you not notice and be drawn to such a door?

Take advantage of this principle inside the home also to help distinguish rooms and sections of the house. Imagine a symmetric home with a door leading to a bedroom on *each* side of the living room. Cues could be used to distinguish the two bedrooms, making each unique and less confusing—maybe by placing a sign or a plant next to the door to one bedroom and a colorful painting next to the other.

Certain rooms have natural cues and landmarks. The living room may have an easy chair, the kitchen has the stove, and the dining room has the dining room table. Recognize and emphasize these distinctive features wherever you can.

Use cues to remind your loved one of what activities go on in each room or area. Display projects in the crafts area, a picture of a child using the toilet in the bathroom, pictures of pies and food in the kitchen, etc. Contact your local art store or picture framing company to see if they have catalogues of pictures to choose from and order.

Locate cues where they are most likely to be seen. Because people with Alzheimer's often see only what's directly in front of them, it is best to place cues right where your family member is likely to see them, not to the right or left, and especially in the places where he would most likely look if he were lost or confused.

Make sure your cues are in plain view. If you have a great painting or lithograph of a bowl of fruit in the kitchen, make sure the silk plant in front of it isn't blocking the view! If you hang a sign to help your loved one identify the bathroom, locate it *next* to the door, not on it, so that the sign will be visible whether the door is open or closed.

Redundant Cuing

If one cue is good, three may be better! For example, smells from dinner cooking, music coming from the radio, *and* signs pointing the way are multiple clues that can help identify or guide your loved one to the kitchen.

This strategy is called "redundant cuing"—the use of multiple cues and multiple senses, rather than relying on just one to get across a single message. Alzheimer's disease hinders the normal transfer of information from one part of the brain to another. Where one informational path doesn't work, redundant cuing offers others that might. For example, the bathroom could be identified by:

- tile on the wall (sense of touch)
- scents (sense of smell)
- sound of running water (hearing)
- a sign on the wall (sight)
- colorful towels on the wall
- a view of the sink, toilet, or tub
- a pretty shower curtain
- light from an open doorway

Keep in mind that Alzheimer's disease may affect some senses more than others, particularly smell and taste. As people get older their sense of smell often decreases, affecting their sense of taste. This may be particularly true for those with Alzheimer's, providing some insight into why one would drink from a bottle of vinegar and think nothing of it.

Too many cues, however, can overwhelm a person with AD, lessening the value of any one. In other words, you don't want to create a panorama of pictures, signs, colors and patterns that will only distract your loved one from the message you had hoped to send.

Don't add to the confusion by introducing conflicting environmental cues either. Imagine how perplexing it might be for a person who is already confused to come across realistic plastic fruit in a bowl, two clocks in the same room showing different times, or a wall mural of a beautiful winter scene in the middle of summer. What would be the right clothes to put on that day?

Minimizing Errors

Remove distractions that might cause your loved one to forget his mission or destination. Anything from mirrors to paintings to wallpaper with curious little figures on it can be distractions. His span of attention may be short, and it may not take much to divert his attention just long enough to forget what he is doing or where he is going. If he's distracted, he might find himself stuck, standing in the middle of a room and not remembering why he's there.

Limit the possibilities for making mistakes. For example, if your mother gets up in the middle of the night to go to the bathroom, she might walk into the hallway only to be dazzled by the number of doors. You might limit her choice (and improve the odds of her choosing correctly) by installing a gate just beyond the bathroom door. Now, instead of lots of doors to choose from, there may be only two.

Pathways

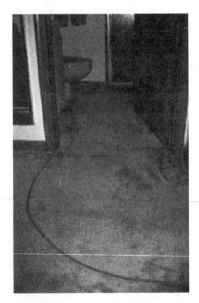

Simple, inexpensive colored electrical tape can create an easy-to-follow path to the bathroom and back to the bedroom.

Colored tape for floors:

Senior Products, home improvement or hardware stores.

Clear pathways are cues in themselves. If you were walking through the woods, wouldn't you prefer to follow a path rather than cut through the briar and the bramble to get where you were going? (See also chapter 5 for more discussion of pathways.)

People with AD are especially attracted to the paths of least resistance—representing safety and the likelihood of success. Incorporate features that reinforce these feelings—good lighting, railings, and furniture arranged to guide your loved one in the right direction.

Make pathways *simple, safe,* and *straight.* Try to maintain momentum wherever you can. Make routes so apparent that success is only a matter of continuous or renewed motion.

Line and define paths with larger, heavier pieces of furniture that can be used as supports along the way, subtly guiding your loved one in the right direction.

Paths can be defined and emphasized on the floor with color. (Many airport terminals use this concept to guide us to the correct concourse.) Colored electrical tape will adhere to any flooring material, including carpeting. Place two strips about two feet apart on the floor marking the route through a room or to an important destination (bedroom to bathroom, for example). Check the tape periodically to make sure it hasn't become detached (a possible tripping hazard).

Walls also define pathways, yet if the color of the wall matches the color of the floor, it can be difficult to tell where one begins and the other ends. It's not unusual to see people who are confused (and perhaps have visual impairments as well) accidentally bump into a wall, not realizing that it was there, or, in the course of a fall, reach for a wall several feet away. The color of your walls should contrast with the color of your floor. If painting the wall is out of the question, try painting only the base molding in important locations—the hallway, for example.

Instability and Falling

At first, your family member may occasionally stumble or trip, then there may be a few falls. Eventually it becomes apparent that she needs assistance walking. Certain home modifications will assist both you and your loved one in dealing with this problem.

Make sure your furniture is reliable and supports your family member's weight without moving, tipping, or sliding. Also

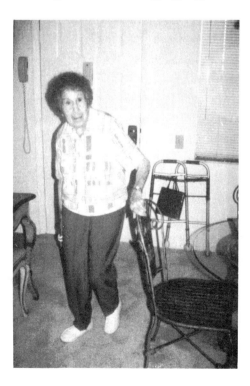

Seniors often abandon walkers and use furniture for support. This is especially true for those with AD. (Note the walker in the background.) Photo courtesy Juliet Mason.

make sure that your family member can easily see each piece of furniture. Color, size, and location make furniture easy to see, reach, and depend on when that little extra support is needed.

Check to see if the gaps between pieces of furniture are small enough to make it easy to get from one to the other without traveling unnecessarily long distances, unassisted and without support.

When your loved one needs help walking, make sure that pathways are wide enough for two people, one assisting the other—at least four feet wide, with no obstacles, is ideal. (Later, when a wheelchair is needed, four feet will be convenient.)

Falls can be caused by features of the home, side effects of medications, dysfunctions related to Alzheimer's disease, and other age-related conditions. AD is associated with some unusual causes for falls, in addition to the more conventional ones.

Some people with AD experience unusual and inexplicable occurrences. Once in a while, they complain that the room or floor suddenly moved, forcing them to lose their balance and grab onto the nearest railing, wall, or piece of furniture. This feels like an earthquake that only the person with dementia experiences. They may be a form of hallucination or a loss of balance that can be communicated in no better way. We call these episodes "quakes."

"Stalling" is another phenomenon that sometimes occurs with dementia-related disorders. Your family member may be happily moving through a room or down the hallway, when she inexplicably and without warning comes to a sudden halt. Her feet stop, but her body and momentum continue. The result is often a fall.

Like most occurrences where most of the information resides solely in one's mind, there is little you can do to anticipate it or stop it. But if your loved one stalls repeatedly in the same spot, there might be something in that location triggering this behavior. Now it is your job to find, camouflage, or remove it. In addition, realizing the likelihood of a fall at this location gives you a good reason to add a railing and other strategies to minimize injury when these falls occur.

Drugs and medications can also cause falls. Common side effects are dizziness, drowsiness, and blurred vision. Your family member may or may not be able to communicate any of these to you, and a fall could occur. Discuss your loved one's medications and possible side effects with the doctor and pharmacist. And make sure your home is as safe as possible, just in case.

Don't overlook other age-related conditions. Problems relating to the inner ear can cause difficulty with equilibrium, and visual impairments can affect the ability to see obstacles or dangers. Diabetes can affect sensation in the feet, making it difficult to feel when the foot touches firm ground. Discuss these and other age-related conditions with your loved one's doctor.

As the disease progresses, your family member's ability to react to falls or losses of balance will also decline. To regain one's balance or protect oneself in a fall requires a complex series of movements. People with AD are often unable to perform a series of actions. Even something as simple as extending her arms in front of her in time to break a fall may be too complicated for your family member.

Grab bars and railings are among the most valuable home additions to prevent such falls. Locate them everywhere and anywhere they might be helpful. (Refer to the section on grab bars in chapter 9.)

Numerous falls occur at night, while wandering, getting in and out of bed, or just going to the bathroom. Is it any wonder? At night your family member may be alone, possibly drowsy and on medications. Turning on the light may temporarily blind him—and who really waits until his eyes fully adjust before beginning the journey to the bathroom? (See chapter 9 for some ideas.)

Single steps and sunken living rooms frequently cause falls. Your family member, no matter how long she has lived there, may no longer anticipate or see single steps. (See chapter 9 for more discussion of steps and stair safety.)

In the later stages of the disease any attempt to walk unassisted may put your loved one at risk of a fall. By this time you will want to make sure your family member cannot get up without you knowing. To alert you of attempts to get up from her chair or bed, add a fall-prevention device. (See chapter 5 for more information on fall-prevention devices.)

You may want to use furniture to subtly and humanely discourage your family member from getting up on his own. A cozy, soft easy chair is not only comfortable, but often difficult for elderly persons to get up from without assistance.

As we have stressed over and over in this book, creating the safest possible home, softening it to minimize injuries when falls do occur, removing potential causes for falls (real and imagined), and making it possible to see hazards that cannot be removed will go a long way toward preventing falls and reducing the injury they might cause. After all, you can't be everywhere and see everything, all of the time.

Bed Railings

Bed railings:

Activeaid, Aids for Arthritis, AliMed, American Health Care Supply, Carex, Graham Field, Larkotex, Lumex, McKesson, Medreco, PCP-Champion, St. Louis Medical Supply.

Mattresses with supportive edges:

American Health Systems, Kelly Medical Group, Sunrise Medical.

Bed railings serve several purposes. Certainly they can be helpful if your loved one is active and has a tendency to fall out of bed. But they can also provide support for either your family member or the caregiver when lifting or helping him sit up.

Bed railings may or may not be necessary. To prevent your loved one from falling out of bed on one side, move the bed against the wall. You might also consider a special mattress with firm elevated edges that will help prevent your loved one from rolling out of bed at night.

Use bed railings with caution. There are partial and full bed rails (spanning one-third, one-half, or the full length of the bed). Obviously the longer the railing, the more the protection. Yet all three leave the foot of the bed open. Your loved one may try to climb over the side railings or over the foot of the bed. This is not uncommon and can lead to serious injury. If any attempt to climb over the railings or foot of the bed is observed, it might be best to remove the railings and look for safer methods to prevent falls from the bed, such as lowering the bed to the floor, thus minimizing the possible injury by reducing the distance your loved one can fall. Note, however, that a lowered bed will be difficult for your loved one to get up from, and weigh the possibility of a fall occurring when getting *into* a bed in this lower, unfamiliar position. (With beds that rise and lower, you can elevate the bed when helping your loved one get in and out of it, and then lower it to the floor to minimize injury.)

Another precaution is to provide a soft pad on the floor next to the bed. Be careful not to create an additional problem by placing something next to the bed that someone might trip over. (See also chapter 5 for more information on fall-prevention devices to warn you of attempts to get out of bed.)

Bed rails can also be dangerous if the mattress does not quite fit the bed, leaving a gap between the mattress and the railing. Some older people have buried their faces in this space while asleep and suffocated. If you use bed railings, make sure your mattress fits the bed properly, especially if the railing did not come with the bed and mattress.

Check to make sure that your loved one cannot get his head caught in the railings' openings and that the railings won't come down if he struggles to get out. You can install protective cushions designed to close the gaps between the railings, making it difficult for arms or legs to go through.

Beds that rise and lower:
Carroll Healthcare, Hertz Supply Co., NOA Medical Industries, Ultimate HomeCare.

Soft, protective fall mat for next to the bed:
Care Electronics, Distinct Medical Supplies, Skil-Care.

Protective bed railing cushions:
AliMed, American Health Care Supply, Briggs, M.O.M.S., Posey Healthcare, Skil-Care.

Canes and Walkers

When your loved one reaches the point when she needs a walker or cane, she may have to learn a whole new set of skills. The use of a walker requires coordination, timing, judgment, and balance. It's almost like learning to ride a bicycle—and at this point learning may be difficult for your loved one. Furthermore, as time goes on your family member may have difficulty using the walker, forget what it's for, or even forget how to use it.

There are a number of steps, however, that you can take to make your home easier to get around in with a walker or cane:

- Widen pathways so that there is plenty of space for your loved one, who may need a little more room, especially while learning to use a new device.
- Make sure pathways are clearly defined and easy to see.
- Remove low, hard-to-see objects that might snag

the cane or walker (planters at the *sides* of hallways, for example).

- Make sure outside pathways are firm and not
  made of gravel, sand, grass, or mulch, which can
  dangerously move under pressure from a cane or
  walker.
- Fix any hazards, such as bumps, and call attention
  to uneven surfaces (steps) along paths.
- Provide ample space to store walkers near the bathroom, the dinner table, your family member's favorite chair, the bed, and at the top and bottom of
  stairs.
- Remove throw rugs that can move unexpectedly.
- Repair carpeting that is worn or has folds that
  might catch the ends of canes or walkers.
- Look out for other "trippers" that might catch the
  tip of a cane or leg of a walker—potholes, cracks in
  your driveway, storm drains in your parking lot.
- Provide sufficient lighting throughout the home.
- Soften the environment in case of a fall.

"Last night we had dinner at one of our favorite restaurants. The weather was nice so we dined outside, facing a ramp. While eating, I watched an older man with his walker use the ramp. The walker had wheels, and the ramp sloped a little more steeply near the end to meet the asphalt below. Suddenly and unexpectedly, the man's walker slid forward and out from under him. Fortunately, his caregivers were alert and caught him in time, before he fell."

Ramps and slopes should be uniform. Any sudden change
in slope can catch your family member off guard, and a walker
(especially if it has wheels) can slip away or tip over. Your
family member may not be able to react quickly enough to
this surprise, and a fall may result. Ramps should also have
railings, just in case.

Changes in sidewalk slopes can be caused by tree roots or ice
formed underneath and lifting the slab (year after year). Maybe
the walkway was just built unevenly years ago and has never
been a problem—until now. Examine your home carefully and
correct any such flaws in your sidewalks or outdoor paths.

"I couldn't help but notice an elderly lady walking into the room when I visited an Alzheimer's care facility not long ago. I watched with fascination as she gave up her walker to use a flimsy table to get to a nearby chair."

Your loved one may abandon or refuse to use a walker or
cane, perhaps due to cognitive impairment, denial, reluctance
to depend on a prosthetic device or be reminded of the disease. With this in mind, recognize the added importance of
providing strong, stable furniture in your home that can be
depended on for support, in lieu of the walker or cane. Orga-

nize and arrange your furniture so that it provides continuous support on the way to important destinations.

Your family member may forget how to use the walker or cane, or forget its purpose. Subtle reminders may help. Try putting up a picture of someone using a cane or walker on a wall where your family member will see it. Look in magazines, or try calling the walker's manufacturer to request one.

Often people resist using any prosthetic device, including grab bars. Whether it's from denial or fear of attempting a task that is too difficult, walkers and canes are often left behind and journeys attempted without the aid and safety of the device.

One ploy I've seen used with some success is getting or creating a walker that looks *really* fancy. Instead of a prosthetic device, turn the walker into an item of pride. Decorate it, paint it, put ribbons on it—whatever it takes to convert that walker into a one-of-a-kind, first-rate item that others might admire or envy, diverting attention from its real purpose.

Transferring, Lifting, and Getting Up

As mobility declines assistance may be needed both when walking and when transferring your loved one from one place to another—standing up from the bed, from a chair, getting into a tub or shower. It can be difficult to lift another person, no matter how strong you may be—especially if you, the caregiver, are smaller or have a bad back or arthritis. And caregiving requires a lot of lifting.

From a Chair

Eventually, two pieces of furniture in your home will become important for you and your family member: his bed and his favorite easy chair. You'll need to make sure that he is able to easily get to, sit down in, and get up from both.

That said, what important features should you look for in a chair? (See also the drawing on page 282.)

- Is the chair soft and forgiving, so it will minimize injury in a fall?

- How high is the seat? Does it assist or hinder the process of sitting down and getting up?
- Is there space underneath the chair with space in front so that feet can be placed under the body for leverage when standing up?
- Are the arms easy to hold, or are they slippery or too big for weak, frail hands to grasp?
- Do the arms of the chair extend to the front of the chair, or do they stop halfway?
- Is the chair stable, or does it move or rock under weight and stress?
- Does the chair have wheels that might let it "slide away"?
- Is the chair in good repair, or are the legs loose or the arms wobbly?
- Is the seat firm and high, or has it developed a pocket over time?
- Is the support under the cushion sagging or broken?
- Is the chair a solid color, or is its upholstery a busy pattern that might confuse and distract your loved one?
- In case of incontinence, will the chair absorb odors? Can it be made water-resistant?
- What color is the chair and how well will it hide stains?

There may be several approaches to making your easy chair easy, some surprisingly simple. Here are just a few.

Examine your easy chair for signs of wear, and consider how difficult it might be to sit down or get up. Over the years, favorite chairs often develop pockets, much like an old baseball glove, resulting in a lower, hard-to-get-out-of seat.

Waterproof seat cushions:

AliMed, Enrichments, HNE Healthcare, Jay Medical, Neuropedic.

Raise the seat by adding another cushion. Some companies offer seat cushions that will not absorb liquids (to help with incontinence). You might also check your local home improvement center for weather-proof cushions intended for outdoor patio furniture. Or you can elevate chairs by building a platform underneath them. (See chapter 7.)

Install poles with handles next to the chair for your family member to grasp and pull herself up, or for the caregiver to hold on to while lifting her.

Replace a worn-out chair with one that is easier to use. Make this an event celebrated by the whole family, rather than a loss of "Ol' Faithful." (Wow! A brand new chair!) Consider a mechanical, motorized lifting chair, which will do all the lifting and lowering for you. Any resistance to a "fancy," motorized chair can be avoided by simply hiding the controls (when not in use) and using the chair like any other easy chair.

Many motorized chairs offer hand-held controls. They may be still wired to the chair and potentially hazardous. To avoid a shock in case of incontinence or a spill, make sure the chair's electric controls are low-voltage and water-resistant. Discuss this and other safety features with the chair manufacturer's representative or sales person.

Before you buy a lifting chair, sit down in it yourself and, if possible, allow your loved one to try it, too. Check out the chair's elevation (how high will it raise you?) and speed of movement up and down (too fast or too slow?) Ask yourself: Will this frighten my family member?

You can also convert your existing easy chair to a motorized lifting chair by installing a motorized lifting platform under it.

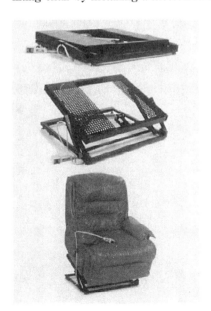

The Enhan-Sit is a motorized lifting platform that attaches to the base of an easy chair to raise and lower the occupant. Photo courtesy ADI.

Poles with handles that attach to the floor and ceiling:

HealthCraft Products, Independent Living Products, M.O.M.S., North Coast Medical, Sears Home HealthCare Catalogue.

Motorized lifting chairs:

Care Catalogue, Enrichments, Golden Technologies, Graham Field, J. C. Penney Special Needs Catalogue, Leisure Lifts, Maxi Aids, McKesson, Med-Lift, Ortho-Kinetics, PCP-Champion, Pride Health Care, Sears Home HealthCare Catalogue, Shamrock Medical Equipment, St. Louis Medical Supply, Wheelchair Warehouse.

Motorized lifting platform for an easy chair:

Access One, ADI ("Enhan-Sit"), Better Living.

Comfortable chairs for seniors:

ADD Interior Systems, Adden, HumanCaré, Sauder, La-Z-Boy Healthcare, Senior Style, Sunrise Medical.

For chairs other than easy chairs, some companies manufacture simple chairs specifically for older adults and others who may need extra support and help getting up. These might be useful in areas where a big, soft easy chair isn't really appropriate, but comfort and ease of getting up is, such as at the dinner table or in the bedroom.

From the Bed

"My husband weighs 180 pounds, and I weigh only 102. I can't lift him out of bed or even up to a sitting position. What can I do?"

Falls from the bed can be caused by your loved one trying to get out of bed by himself, or by a caregiver underestimating the burden of helping to lift him from the bed. Many falls occur at the bed, a place one would think is safe.

You actually have several options or combinations:

- a grab bar for both your family member and the caregiver
- a "bed bar"
- a pull rope
- a "trapeze" bar
- a motorized, mechanical bed

Bed bars and handles:

AdaptAbility, Aids for Arthritis, Ali-Med, American Health Care Supply, Assist Equip., Bed Handles, Brown Engineering, Easy Street, Graham Field, J. C. Penney Special Needs Catalogue, Larkotex, LCM Distributing, Mobility Transfer Systems, North Coast Medical, Sammons Preston.

Grab bars are not just for your loved one. They're for the caregiver too. When lifting a person, you need to be able to rely on something to transfer both your weight and his, and to stabilize yourself. A properly located grab bar (or bed handle) can be helpful.

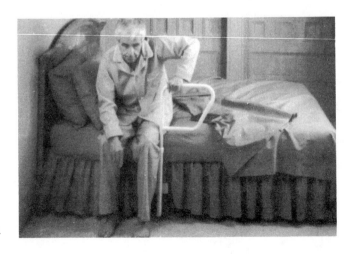

The Bed Bar provides support for both the caregiver and the person with AD. The Bed Bar is available through Sammons Preston, a BISSELL® Healthcare Company. Photo reprinted with permission.

Bed bars or handles attach to the bed, where the caregiver or your family member can rely on them while lifting, transferring, or sitting up. These are very different from bed railings.

If helping your loved one sit up in bed is a problem, you might consider providing a thick rope with a series of knots or handles. Attach it to the foot of the bed for your family member to use to pull himself up to a sitting position. You can easily make one of these yourself, or buy one.

Trapeze bars also enable people to pull themselves up to a sitting position. They go over the head of the bed and are composed of a mounting bracket, a chain, and a handle shaped like a coat hanger. Trapeze bars are mounted to either the bed or the wall.

Mechanical beds assist your family member to a sitting position from which she can more easily turn, hang her legs over the side, and stand up. They can be either motorized or manual (operated by a crank).

Maybe your family member's bed is too low and, though she can sit on the edge, she just can't stand up. Raising the mattress will make it easier for her to stand up—making the caregiver's job more comfortable and less stressful on the back. The following illustrate a few ways to change the height of the bed.

One of the easiest ways is to raise the bed is to add another mattress. Warning: Raising the bed also increases the distance of your family member from the floor. If he falls out of bed, he's more likely to seriously injure himself. (Refer to the discussion on bed rails later in this chapter.)

If the bed is at one height and the wheelchair at another (usually lower), transferring is more difficult. To solve this problem you can lower the bed or build a ramp and platform for the wheelchair next to the bed. This may not be as difficult as it sounds. (Refer to the section later in this chapter on ramps for sources of prefabricated ramps and platforms.)

The NOA Riser Bed might solve all of your bed-too-high or bed-too-low problems. This motorized bed can be raised and lowered from 7 inches to 23 inches above the floor (plus the thickness of the mattress). You can raise the bed to make it easier to get out of or into bed, lower it to line up with the

Bed pull rope with handles:
AliMed, Enrichments, Maddak, North Coast Medical, Sammons Preston.

Trapeze bars:
AliMed, American Health Care Supply, Graham Field, Lumex, McKesson, Sammons Preston.

Manual mechanical beds:
American Health Care Supply, Care Catalogue Svcs., McKesson, Sears Home HealthCare Catalog, Sunrise Medical, health-care supply stores.

Motorized mechanical beds:
American Health Care Supply, Barr Mobility, Electropedic, Golden Technologies, Invacare, J. C. Penney Special Needs Catalogue, McKesson, Medreco, Sears Home HealthCare Catalog, Sunrise Medical, Ultimate Home Care, health-care supply stores.

Truman Bed Buddy—converts a bed to a mechanical lifting bed:
Princeton Products.

Wheelchair seat cushions:
AliMed.

Beds that rise and lower:
Carroll Healthcare, NOA Medical Industries, Ultimate Home Care.

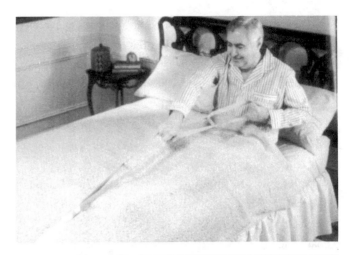

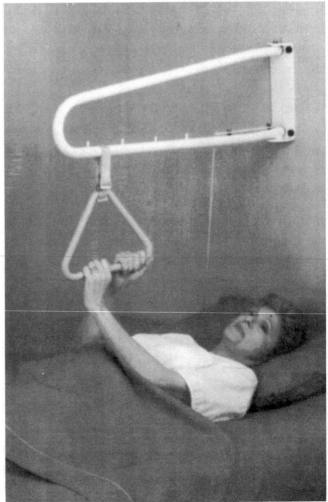

With a bed pull rope (top) or trapeze bar (bottom), your loved one can pull himself up to a sitting position. Photos courtesy Sammons Preston, a BISSELL® Healthcare Company. Reprinted with permission.

wheelchair, or lower it all the way to the floor to minimize injury if your loved one rolls out of bed during the night.

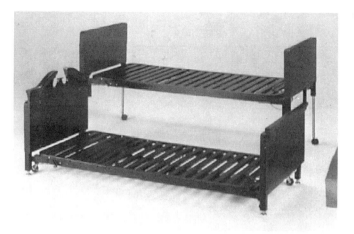

The Riser Bed can be raised or lowered to any height you need. Photo courtesy NOA Medical Industries, Inc.

For transferring from a bed to a wheelchair (or vice versa), the options include: just sitting on the edge of the bed and transferring directly into the wheelchair; a lift (refer to the discussion on lifts later in this chapter); or a transfer board. A transfer board smoothly spans the gap between bed and wheelchair, allowing your loved one to slide from one to the other. They are portable and useful at other locations, as well.

Bed transfer boards:

AliMed, American Health Care Supply, Bailey, Enrichments, Graham Field, Maddak, Sammons Preston, Smith & Nephew, health-care supply stores.

Using the Toilet

To lift someone from a toilet, a caregiver normally stands in front of the person, grasps her (often under the arms), leans back, and lifts (using her own body weight). This requires space in front of the toilet, a good four feet. However, to help someone go from a toilet to a wheelchair, you need space *next* to the toilet. If you're planning a new bathroom, it would be wise to anticipate both situations and provide room for them.

It doesn't take a bathroom the size of the Taj Mahal to accomplish this. Locating the toilet facing the door provides you with more than enough space in front (by opening the door!). Installing a roll-in shower next to the toilet serves two purposes: it provides you with an accessible shower and additional room next to the toilet to transfer from a wheelchair. Existing bathrooms can be converted to a more accessible

Roll-in, wheelchair-accessible shower kits:

Aqua Bath, Clarion, Concept Fibreglass, Fiberglass Systems, Invacare Continuing Care, Kohler, Lasco, National Bathing Products, Swan Corporation, Tub-Master, Universal-Rundle, Warm Rain.

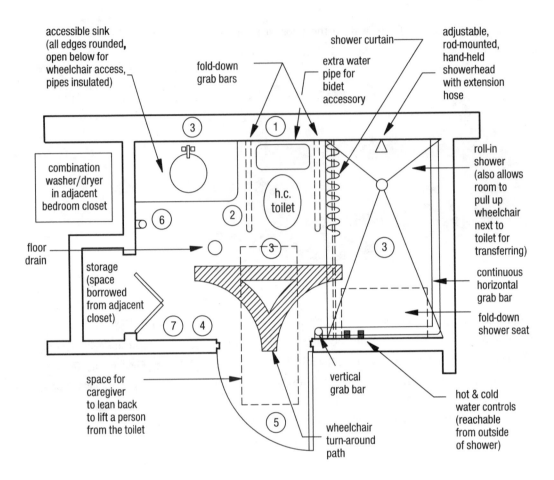

accessible sink (all edges rounded, open below for wheelchair access, pipes insulated)

fold-down grab bars

shower curtain

extra water pipe for bidet accessory

adjustable, rod-mounted, hand-held showerhead with extension hose

combination washer/dryer in adjacent bedroom closet

h.c. toilet

roll-in shower (also allows room to pull up wheelchair next to toilet for transferring)

floor drain

storage (space borrowed from adjacent closet)

continuous horizontal grab bar

fold-down shower seat

space for caregiver to lean back to lift a person from the toilet

vertical grab bar

wheelchair turn-around path

hot & cold water controls (reachable from outside of shower)

(1)   Extra GFI outlet for bidet accessory and/or toilet seat lift.

(2)   Recessed toilet paper holder and telephone jack.

(3)   Lights in the shower, over the sink, and in the center of the bathroom for general illumination.

(4)   Motion-detecting light switch, switches for ceiling heater, lights, and fan. Provide and locate outlets for night lights.

(5)   Toilet visible from open door. Door opens outward. No locks on door. Handicapped door threshold.

(6)   Vertical grab bar on wall next to sink.

(7)   Intercom on constant listening mode.

All bathroom walls constructed with a layer of 3/4" plywood attached directly to wood studs (allowing grab bars, etc., to be located where needed).

Even an average bathroom with a bathtub can be converted into an accessible bathroom by changing the swing of the door and replacing the tub with a roll-in shower. To gain an extra storage area, take some space from the adjacent closet. This design is based on a typical 5' × 8' bathroom excluding adjacent closet and storage space.

bathroom by replacing the tub or shower (next to the toilet) with an open, roll-in shower.

For many older people, lifting themselves from the toilet is awkward and requires more strength and coordination than is available. To assist your loved one provide her with the tools that allow her to take advantage of the strength that remains.

Install grab bars on both sides of the toilet. There is a grab bar for every possible bathroom and need. Locate the grab bar precisely so that it provides the most leverage and assistance for your loved one's height, reach, and special needs. (See chapter 9.)

Elevate the toilet to make the trip up and down shorter and easier. One company manufactures platforms intended to raise the entire toilet 4 inches. (Refer to the photo on page 286.)

There are a few points to keep in mind when elevating a toilet:

- Make sure that your family member's feet can still rest comfortably on the floor, to avoid loss of circulation in the legs, discomfort, or fear from being up too high. Elevating the toilet also increases the possibility of a fall, since it will be both higher and new to your family member.
- Make sure the area around the toilet is soft and forgiving (one advantage of carpeting in the bathroom). Install grab bars on both sides of the toilet and cushioning pads along adjacent counter edges and the bathtub wall. (See chapter 4 for sources.)

Another option might be a motorized or mechanical toilet seat lift that attaches to your toilet and mechanically raises and lowers your family member.

In those cases when this is not enough, provide a means by which someone can call for assistance. Provide a pager, remote doorbell, baby monitor, or bell to jingle next to the toilet. (Refer to chapter 4 for sources.)

Using the Bathtub or Shower

Getting in and out of the shower or bathtub offers its own unique difficulties, especially when the person to be bathed is not so willing. In addition to making the bath and shower safe,

"Mom just doesn't have the strength to lift herself up from the toilet. Last week she was stuck there for half an hour."

Toilet Riser:

MedWay Corp.

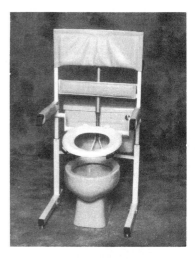

The Toilet Seat Lift mechanically raises or lowers the user. Photo courtesy Stand-Aid of Iowa.

Toilet seat lifts:

Home Care Products LLC, Stand-Aid of Iowa, Transfer Master Products, Ultimate Home Care.

"I can help Alfred get into the tub, but I can't lift him out. Last night he was in there for an hour before my neighbor got home to help me."

recognizing potential difficulties before they occur and making the appropriate modifications will help when bathing becomes a little more difficult. (See also chapters 4 and 9.)

Bathtub and Shower Seats

Two inherent problems with bathtubs are:

- standing up (pulling and lifting oneself up from the bottom of the tub), and
- transferring in and out of the tub (stepping over the tub wall).

Let's first look at how standing can be made easier. The best way is to eliminate the need to stand—at least from the very depths of the tub. Bathtub seats accomplish this by making it possible to bathe while sitting in the tub, elevated on a seat or chair. Granted, your loved one can no longer soak in a tub of warm water, but her fears of drowning may be alleviated.

Bathtub seats (these companies offer a variety of bathtub seats):

Activeaid, AdaptAbility, Aids for Arthritis, AliMed, ASI, Care Catalogue, Carex, Easy Street, ETAC USA, Frohock-Stewart, Graham Field, Guardian Products, Invacare Continuing Care, Judson Enterprises, Lumex, McKesson, North Coast Medical, R. D. Equipment, Sammons Preston, Sears Home HealthCare Catalogue, St. Louis Medical Supply, Wheelchair Warehouse, and home medical supply and home improvement centers.

Bathtub seats help not only the person taking the bath, but also the caregiver. They allow the caregiver access to all parts of your family member's body (since your loved one sits much higher in the tub), minimizing the need to bend and reach. In addition, bathtub seats lessen the distance your loved one needs to be lifted when being helped out of the tub.

There are several types of bathtub seats:

- a bench that fits over and spans the tub,
- a seat that fits in the tub,
- a bathtub transfer seat,
- a bathtub insert, and
- mechanical seats that raise and lower your loved one.

Simple bathtub benches resemble boards spanning across your tub, using the tub walls on both sides for support. Their primary advantage is to allow the user to sit higher and not have to lift himself or be lifted from the bottom of the tub.

The second type of bathtub seat is a waterproof stool or chair (or wall-mounted, fold-down shower seat) that fits in the tub. They too allow a person to bathe seated, higher up, so as to make standing up and sitting down much easier. Fold-down seats offer the added advantage of being able to be folded out of the way when not in use. (See the discussion later in this chapter on shower access for sources.)

One often-overlooked feature of bathtub (and shower) seats is that they are adjustable. If the seat is too low, the legs on most can be extended. Thus the seat can be made higher so the trip back to a standing position is shorter. In combination with arms on the seat and grab bars, the problem of standing or sitting may be much easier.

When using bathtub seats make sure:

- your chair has rubber feet that won't slip or slide,
- you have a non-slip floor mat or slip-resistant floor strips to allow good, dependable footing when standing and sitting,
- you have a hand-held showerhead (see chapter 4), and
- grab bars are available and properly located (for both caregiver and your family member).

Getting in and out of the bathtub or helping someone do so is no simple task. This is especially true when helping a person unstable on his feet, resisting the bath, or afraid of the shower or tub. Furthermore, it requires a series of complex, multi-sequential tasks:

- approaching the tub,
- balancing and stepping over the bathtub wall,
- sitting down,
- getting up, and
- stepping out of the tub (again over the tub wall).

All these tasks require certain skills, balance, timing, weight transfer, strength, and coordination. If your loved one fails at any one, a serious fall could result, injuring both him and caregiver.

One of the easiest ways to safely transfer in or out of a tub (or shower/tub combination) is by means of a transfer seat. A bathtub (or shower) transfer seat helps an individual move in

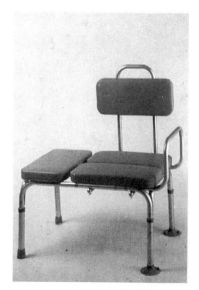

A bathtub transfer seat makes sitting down and standing up in the bathtub much easier and safer. Photo courtesy Sammons Preston, a BISSELL® Healthcare Company. Reprinted with permission.

and out of the bathtub or shower. Some fit in the tub, yet extend outside, beyond the tub wall, while others are similar to a chair mounted on a pole that swings over the tub or into the shower. Both types are safe because the user sits down outside of the tub (or shower) before entering, eliminating the tasks required to step over the tub wall or shower curb.

Transfer seats make it easier to get into the tub or shower without the usual balancing act of lifting one's legs up and over a wall or curb. There are several types, ranging from simple seats that extend outside the tub to a seat on a rail that slides over the tub.

To help your loved one stand up from a transfer seat, you can add a fold-down grab bar, offering something right in front of the bather to grab onto and pull himself up. One of the beauties of a fold-down bar is that it can be pulled down when needed and then raised out of the way when not. (Refer to the section on grab bars in chapter 9.)

If your loved one is afraid of water or if being immersed in the tub presents problems, a bathtub insert may be helpful. A bathtub insert is a shallow, contoured pan that fits over a standard tub. Your loved one sits on the insert, rather than the bottom of the tub. Bathtub inserts are contoured to drain the water down into the tub below. They can be "full length" (spanning your entire tub) or "half length" (spanning only part of your tub, similar to a large bathtub seat). Partial inserts resemble a contoured bathtub seat that you can sit on while bathing and soaking your feet in the tub below. Some bathtub inserts are cushioned for additional safety and comfort.

Again, don't forget to install grab bars. A bathtub insert is not a conventional product, and it may be unfamiliar to both family member and caregiver. Having grab bars to hold may be invaluable.

Mechanical bathtub seats:

Apex Dynamics, Clarke Health Care Products, SafeLift.

Finally, there are also mechanical bathtub seats that will raise and lower your loved one in and out of the tub. Some are designed to allow him to sit down outside the tub, swivel over it, then lower him down into the tub—all the way to the bottom. For those who value their baths, this may be just what is needed!

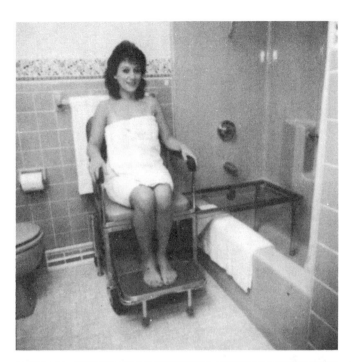

Bathtub transfer seats:

Aids for Arthritis, Frohock-Stewart, Guardian Products, Independent Care Products, Judson Enterprises, Sammons Preston, Shamrock Medical Equipment, home medical supply and home improvement stores.

Sliding bathtub or shower transfer seat:

Clever Solutions, R. D. Equipment.

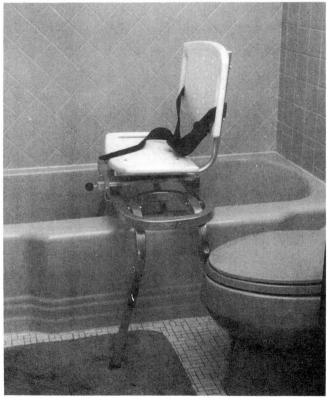

Sliding bathtub seats can differ from each other. The various options include arms to hold on to, seat belts, and locks to keep them from sliding once in place. Top photo courtesy R. D. Equipment; bottom photo courtesy Clever Solutions, Inc.

Pole-mounted bathtub or shower transfer seat:

Independent Care Products.

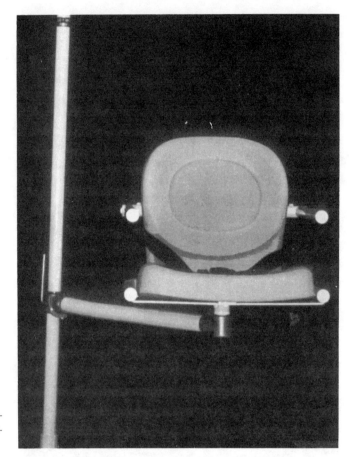

Another type of bathtub transfer seat rotates on a pole. Photo courtesy Independent Care Products, Inc.

Bathtub inserts:

Clarke Healthcare Products,
Diversified Fiberglass Products.

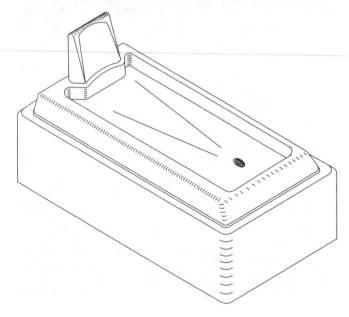

A bathtub insert is useful if standing to get out of the tub is difficult or if your loved one is afraid of being immersed in water.

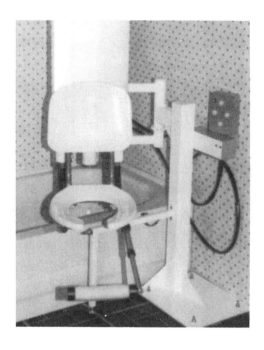

This mechanical bathtub seat transfers the occupant from outside the tub to over the tub, then lowers him into the tub. Photo courtesy SafeLift, Inc.

Bathtubs with Doors

No kidding—there really are bathtubs with doors for both institutions and homes. Some bathtub doors seal with a sensor (which requires electrical service), and others seal manually with a lever. A third type has a roll-up door that seals automatically once in place.

Some bathtubs with doors come with built-in seats. You enter, sit down, and close the door behind you, then fill the

Bathtubs with doors:

American Standard, BathEase, Carderock Limited, Invacare Continuing Care, Kohler, Grand Traverse Technologies, Technically Unique Bathing.

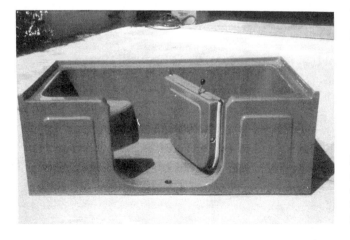

Several companies offer bathtubs with doors. No more balancing act stepping over an awkward tub wall—just open the door and walk right in. Photo courtesy BathEase, Inc.

Wheelchair-friendly bathtubs with doors:

Carderock Limited, Grand Traverse Technologies.

tub with water and take a bath. These are also wheelchair transferrable, allowing your family member to relocate from her wheelchair to a convenient seat inside the tub. Once inside, you close the door, seal it by pulling a lever, and fill it up. Another advantage to these tubs is that you sit on a built-in chair, not at the bottom of the tub at floor level. When you get out, you do not have to lift or pull yourself up, you just open the door, turn, and stand up or transfer to your wheelchair.

Shower Access

First of all, what kind of shower do you have? Is it a bathtub/shower combination, a walk-in shower, or an accessible roll-in shower? Do you have a single shower door, sliding shower doors, or a shower curtain?

Some people use bathtub transfer seats to safely enter the tub, then shower normally, standing up. (For more information on bathtub transfer seats refer to the discussion earlier on bathtub transfer seats.)

Replace your sliding shower doors with a shower curtain. Sliding shower doors, no matter how you arrange them, always block half the opening. This makes transferring in and out of the shower difficult, and if there were an accident in the shower, the doors would make assistance much more difficult. Remove them now, before there is a problem, and replace them with a strong, sturdy shower curtain.

Shower seats allow the bather to sit rather than stand and risk falling. Sitting in the shower is also calmer and more secure. Moreover, a shower seat combined with a hand-held showerhead makes for a much easier and less threatening shower for all involved. Shower seats include simple shower chairs, fold-down padded chairs, and roll-in chairs.

Patio chairs may also work in the shower. Larger than the small stools sold for showers and tubs, patio chairs have arms to grasp and are usually more comfortable (available with soft, waterproof cushions). Make sure yours is heavy, stable, and won't tip over. It would also be a good idea to add slip-resistant fittings to the feet (available at your hardware store or local home improvement center), so it won't slide on the slippery tile floor.

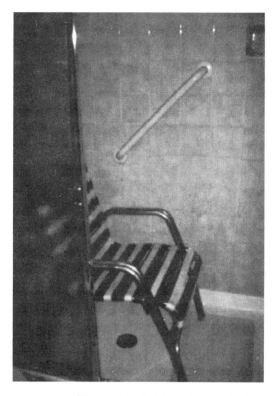

A patio chair can be used in the tub or shower.

Because many older people find it easier to pull themselves up, rather than pushing on the seat to lift themselves, properly located grab bars are very important. Once again, consult your occupational or physical therapist to identify the best location for your grab bars. In this particular case the side wall may not be the best location, but rather the wall in front of the seat. Locating a grab bar in front of your seated loved one, parallel to the floor (not vertical), allows her something visible, close, and comfortable to reach, grasp, and use to pull herself up. (See the photo on page 330.)

The most frequently used shower seat is the common stool or bench, available at your local health care supply store or home improvement center. Many of the companies listed in the back of this book also offer them.

Among the most dependable and convenient seats for the shower is the wall-mounted, fold-down seat. There are many types available, from inexpensive metal models to heavy-duty, enamel-coated seats.

When installing a wall-mounted shower seat, consider what

Fold-down shower seats:

American Health Care Supply, ASI, Bradley, ETAC USA, Graham Field, Häfele America, HEWI, Invacare Continuing Care, Lumex.

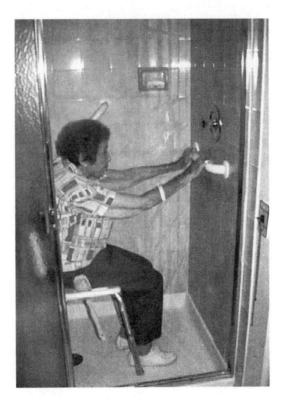

A horizontal grab bar in the shower located in front of your family member allows her to use both hands to sit down and stand up. Photo courtesy Juliet Mason.

height is best for your family member. There is no standard height, perfect for everyone. Make sure your shower seat is located low enough for feet to comfortably reach the floor and high enough to make standing easy. For additional comfort and height, add an outdoor patio chair cushion. They are already waterproof and won't be damaged by a wet environment.

Roll-in shower seats (special waterproof rolling chairs for the shower) are intended for accessible roll-in showers. They allow you to transport and bathe your family member while he remains seated.

Roll-in, wheelchair-accessible shower kits:

Aqua Bath, Clarion, Concept Fibreglass, Fiberglass Systems, Invacare Continuing Care, Kohler, Lasco, National Bathing Products, Swan Corporation, Tub-Master, Universal-Rundle, Warm Rain.

Another possibility might be to replace your tub with a more accessible barrier-free, roll-in shower. A roll-in shower has no curb to prevent your loved one from being rolled into the shower. There are kits to replace your tub with a roll-in shower. Your family member could then use a roll-in shower chair and take her shower while remaining seated, with no need to worry about standing, sitting down or getting up. (Refer to the discussion later in this chapter on wheelchair accessibility.)

Showers are typically designed for one person only, not two. The doors and openings are narrow, usually with a four-inch curb. The shower itself is often only three feet by three feet, hardly enough room for a caregiver to help your family member. If your plans call for building or renovating a bathroom, make room for an oversized shower, one with space not only for the caregiver but also for a shower seat or roll-in shower chair. A general rule here is the bigger, the better. The more room you have, the easier it will be to bathe your loved one, from all angles and with the greatest of ease. (See also the section later in this chapter entitled "Accessibility.")

If you're considering any of these ideas for creating accessible showers, talk with a contractor, interior designer, or an architect who specializes in accessible design or construction. For recommendations, contact your local agencies on aging, professional organizations (for architects, interior designers, or contractors), or organizations for the disabled.

Lifts

Alzheimer's is a progressive disease. Eventually there will come a time when your family member has difficulty standing and walking. Often caregivers are older themselves and lifting their loved one is too much for them. When this becomes a problem, you will need to look into equipment to help you lift and transfer your loved one to and from important locations (the bed, chair, sink, toilet, and tub).

For help getting in and out of the tub your answer may be a bathtub lift. These devices are located next to or over the tub and help lift, transfer, and lower a person in and out of the tub, avoiding painful and dangerous strain on the caregiver. They can be manual or motorized and are operated only by the caregiver.

Patient lifts are rolling mechanical devices that lift, carry, and lower your loved one to and from the shower, bath, toilet, etc. They too can be manual or motorized.

There are also ceiling track lifts. These are motorized seats or hoists that travel on an overhead track. They are commonly used

Bathtub lifts:

Barrier-Free Lifts, Columbus McKinnon, Easy Lift, Ferno-Washington, Graham Field, Invacare, Guardian Products, Handi-Move International, McKesson, Moving Solutions, Porta-Lift, Sammons Preston, Sunrise Medical.

Patient transfer lifts:

AliMed, American Health Care Supply, Apex Dynamics, Barrier-Free Lifts, Care Catalogue Svcs., Columbus McKinnon, Easy Lift, Enrichments, Ferno-Washington, G. E. Miller, Graham Field, Handi-Move International, Invacare, Guardian Products, McKesson, Moving Solutions, Porto-Lift, SafeLift, Sammons Preston, Sears Home HealthCare Catalogue, Sunrise Medical.

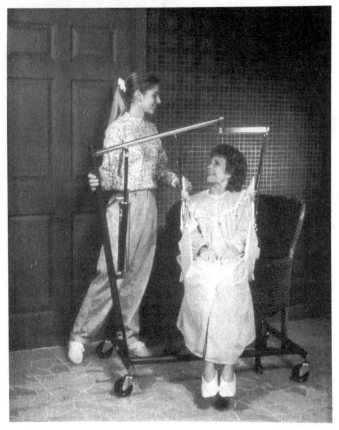

A patient transfer lift is important when lifting and transferring becomes difficult and dangerous. Photo courtesy Porto-Lift Corp.

Ceiling track lifts:

Apex Dynamics, Barrier-Free Lifts, Columbus McKinnon, Easy Lift, Guardian Products, Handi-Move International.

to transfer people to locations that are repeatedly and commonly used, such as from the bed to the toilet, sink, shower or easy chair. Ceiling track lifts can be expensive, and they require time to install. They can also be frightening to someone with dementia. These are good reasons to have them installed early, when workers in your home are less likely to upset your loved one, especially working in his room.

Most ceiling track lifts attach directly to structural members already in your ceiling. If your joists or trusses run the wrong direction or are inadequate, additional support may be needed. Discuss these issues with your architect and the sales representative, in a meeting at *your* home, where you can discover and solve other problems that might arise. In particular, you will want to discuss turns, changes in floor heights, the source and location of electricity for the equipment, and where the device will be stored when not in use.

The final destination for the lift can be a corner, closet, or wall storage cabinet, where the equipment can be kept out of sight when not in use. Discuss this option with your sales representative as well.

Be aware that lifts travel slowly, and that the number of turns as well as the distance greatly affect the time it will take to move from one stop to the next.

If you're constructing a new bathroom and planning to install a ceiling lift, design the bathroom so that the bed, easy chair, bathroom door, toilet, sink, and shower (or bathtub) all line up. This will save you money when installing the lift and time when making the transfer.

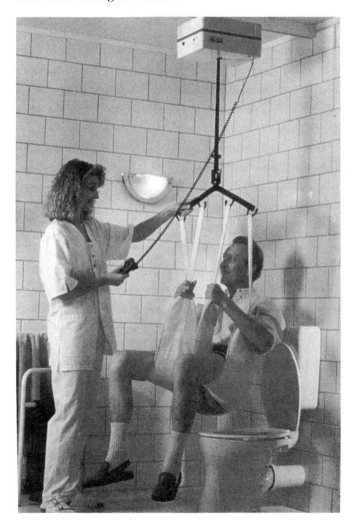

A ceiling track lift transfers the user to and from commonly used locations (a bed, a chair, the toilet, the bathtub). Photo courtesy Barrier-Free Lifts, Inc.

Lifting equipment is not for everyone. This unusual equipment can frighten and overwhelm. Some people with AD become frightened just being moved by hand—imagine suddenly being moved by a motorized hoist. Consider your family member's particular fears and needs, and see what works for you.

Stairs and Stair Lifts

Stairs are a real problem when it comes to caregiving, especially if your family member's room is on the second floor and the caregiver's daily activities are mostly on the first. This is the best reason for converting a first-floor room to the master bedroom for your loved one.

Consider relocating your family member's room to the first floor, thereby eliminating the stairs as an obstacle. Although your loved one may have enjoyed her upstairs bedroom for many years, the time may come when it is in everyone's best interest to avoid those dangerous and tiring trips up and down the stairs.

When this is not an option, making it safer and easier to get up and down the stairs and eliminating unnecessary trips may be your only option.

Stair lifts are motorized seats on wall-mounted tracks that slowly take your family member up or down the stairs. You can "call" the seat from the top or bottom with the push of a button. For straight staircases, these lifts can be relatively inexpensive. The more complicated the stairs, the more expensive the stair lifts. They can, however, be designed to fit almost any staircase, even the most graceful curving one with numerous landings.

When installing a stair lift, consider the height of the seat. If the seat is too low for one to easily stand up, the lift isn't going to be much good—it may even be dangerous, as a fall at the top of the stairs could have disastrous results. Wheelchair users may need a lower height than ambulatory users to make the transfer from a wheelchair to a lift seat. There are also stair lifts that take your loved one up and down—wheelchair and all.

Also, for those with Alzheimer's, we would suggest looking

Stair lifts:

Access Industries, American Stair-Glide, Bruno, Concord, Econol Lift Elevator Co., Flinchbaugh Co., FlorLift of New Jersey, Garaventa, Handicapped & Elderly Life Products, Inclinator Company of America, National Wheel-O-Vator, Stannah, Whitakers.

Mini stair lifts for short staircases:

Access Industries, Whitakers, Wrightway.

Stair lifts (platforms) that accommodate a wheelchair:

Access Industries.

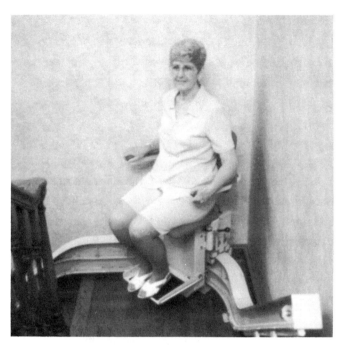

For homes with stairs, a stair lift is a safe and easy way to get up and down. Photo courtesy National Wheel-O-Vator.

for stair lifts with arms to allow your family member to feel at least a little more secure when riding this unfamiliar piece of equipment.

To prevent the possibility of your loved one's falling back down the stairs once at the top, consider installing a gate or fold-down grab bar. Given the difficulty one might have just sitting down in a stair lift (from the top looking down that long flight of stairs) you might want to provide this additional security. Your loved one can sit down, you can raise the bar or open the gate, and the ride down can begin. At the top you can close the gate or lower the bar before allowing your loved one to get out of the seat. Discuss this idea with your stair lift representative and see what other options are available. (Refer also to the discussions of platform lifts and residential elevators later in this chapter.)

Wheelchairs

As your family member forgets how to perform more and more functions, a wheelchair will become a better and safer option than risking the possibility of a fall. Your home will now need to be wheelchair accessible.

Accessibility

This is not a book on wheelchair accessibility or on how to make your home wheelchair accessible. There are many good books available on that subject, or you can contact a contractor in your area that specializes in accessible design and modifications.

The term "wheelchair accessible" has its own meaning when applied to those with Alzheimer's disease (compared to those with other disabilities). Disabled adults do not characteristically suffer from dementia and they often have greater upper-body mobility and strength. Some even play wheelchair basketball and tennis! We will address only those issues that apply to caring for someone with AD. Keep in mind that the person with AD does not usually propel herself in a wheelchair. All too often, the caregiver is elderly, without the stamina of a younger person. Ramps conforming to every requirement of the Americans with Disabilities Act are often still too steep and offer too few places to rest.

Focus attention now on the caregiver and make it as easy as possible for him or her to transport a loved one in a wheelchair to and from key locations. Create clear paths in and out of the home, and to and from the bathroom, dining room, den, porch, and bedroom. Provide and locate chairs or benches for the caregiver to rest after pushing the wheelchair in the hot sun or along difficult pathways.

An accessible home conserves effort and energy. It makes life easier for both the caregiver and your loved one.

Don't forget the special places that you created for your family member. These too need to accommodate your loved one in a wheelchair. Can she get into the kitchen? Will she need a higher table for her wheelchair to help you fold napkins, sort silverware, or supervise your attempts to make her famous apple pie?

Minimize Obstacles

Numerous obstacles around the house suddenly reveal themselves when a wheelchair becomes necessary—thick carpeting, throw rugs, thresholds at doors, changes in flooring materials, steps at doors that you never really noticed. Even walkways made of Chatahoochee stones or brick pavers can create a drag on a wheelchair that quickly tires the person pushing it. The caregiver may not have the strength or energy to overcome some of these obstacles. The more obstacles that can be eliminated, the easier it will be for everyone.

It is difficult to push a wheelchair through thick, plush carpeting. Some families we know have replaced theirs with low-nap, flush carpeting early, before there is a problem. Changes in floor finishes can cause difficulties. Caregivers pushing a wheelchair often unconsciously lean on the chair for support. If the chair suddenly lurches forward on a smooth floor after they have been struggling on thick carpeting, they can easily lose their balance.

Thresholds or transition strips between floor finishes can also present obstacles. Check doorways and changes in flooring materials for obstructions, such as a strip between the carpeting and vinyl flooring. Replace high thresholds with lower, "handicapped" thresholds to create smooth transitions for a wheelchair. This can eliminate unnecessary pushing, tugging, and sudden stops. Consult a local contractor specializing in accessible design and construction.

Identify the most important routes within your home and first remove the obstacles along them. Wheelchairs come with an inflexible set of requirements. They are usually at least 26 inches wide and require pathways three feet or wider for easy navigation.

Check for excess furniture in hallways that might get in the way. Don't overlook protruding wall-mounted shelves or other such objects. It's not unusual for people to clear their halls to make room for their family member in a wheelchair and then themselves walk into a shelf or wall-mounted light fixture they forgot about.

Wherever you can, make it possible to get from point A to point B in a straight line. Can a person get through rooms by going in a straight line, or must he weave through a maze of furniture?

Move tables or other objects that get in the way when trying

Protective wall corner guards:

Arden Architectural Specialties, American Health Care Supply, Crest, IPC, Laurel Designs, Mercer Products, Pawling, Reese, Tepromark International, Tri-Guards, Tubular Specialties.

Kick plates for doors:

Brookstone, Crest, Improvements, IPC, Pawling, Renovator's, hardware stores, and home improvement centers.

to turn the wheelchair. Create areas in the home with enough clear space to allow the caregiver to turn a wheelchair completely around and proceed in the opposite direction. The rule of thumb is a circle five feet in diameter. This may be accomplished simply by removing the coffee table in the living room.

Install corner guards to protect walls. Accidents will happen. Kick plates will make doors easier to open by merely pushing them with the wheelchair.

You may need to replace some of your steps with ramps or install platform lifts. (Refer to the section on platform lifts later in this chapter.) You will also need places to store the wheelchair that are out of the way, yet close to where it is needed. If your home has stairs, you may need a wheelchair (and space to store it) both upstairs and down.

Widen Doorways

Doors need a *minimum* clear opening of 32 inches wide to comfortably allow a standard wheelchair to pass. Wheelchairs are usually about 26 inches wide (measure yours to be sure). The additional width is for clearance and to allow hands to hang down or help propel the wheels through the doorway without getting scraped.

You may find that some doors in your house simply cannot be enlarged, due to a wall, adjacent closet, or other obstruction. In any case, before you invest in a major project of tearing out a door and replacing it with a wider one, think twice and consider all your options.

You don't have to widen all the doorways in the house. Focus on the doorways along the paths that are most important:

- pathways leading out of your home, starting at your loved one's bedroom (for trips to the doctor, outings, or an emergency).
- from the bedroom to the bathroom. (Unfortunately, the bathroom door is usually the narrowest doorway in the house. Nonetheless, you'll be doing yourself and your loved one a favor if you make sure this doorway is not a troublesome barrier.)

- doorways leading to favorite locations, such as the easy chair in the den, the porch, and the dining room.

Here are a few ways that you can widen those important doorways with minimal demolition, construction, and expense:

- Install offset or swing-clear hinges. These are designed to allow your existing door to move completely out of the way when it is opened. (Normally when a door is opened, the thickness of the door narrows the opening.) Offset hinges can widen your door opening by almost two inches (depending on the thickness of your door).

- Remove the trim on both sides of the door from the floor up to 48 inches above the floor. This will give you an extra half inch on each side where the wheelchair passes through yet still allow the upper part of the door to close normally. (See the illustration on page 340.)

- Remove the door and replace it with a curtain or shower curtain. (In addition to allowing access to the full width of the door opening, a good-quality, heavy-duty fabric curtain provides privacy and immediate entry. This alteration is also easily reversible: When you want to re-install the door, just remove the curtain and do so.)

For certain doors in your home you may need an expert opinion. Ask a contractor to examine your doorways and advise you on the most efficient and inexpensive ways to widen them. Look in your phone book, or contact local agencies on aging to find contractors knowledgeable in installing or widening doorways for wheelchair accessibility.

Note that most bathroom doors swing in. Closing or opening a bathroom door with a wheelchair inside is often difficult. This is another good reason to replace that door with a curtain. It will allow you to maintain some privacy and dignity for your loved one while also solving the problem of accessibility.

Finally, pocket doors are certainly an option. However, because they require a pocket to slide into, considerable demolition

Offset or "swing-clear" hinges:

Accent on Living, AdaptAbility, American Health Care Supply, Facilis, LDB Medical, Maxi Aids, Sammons Preston, Sears Home HealthCare Catalogue, Stanley, home improvement centers.

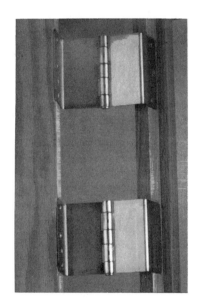

With offset hinges, an open door is completely removed from the doorway. Photo courtesy Sammons Preston, a BISSELL® Healthcare Company. Reprinted with permission.

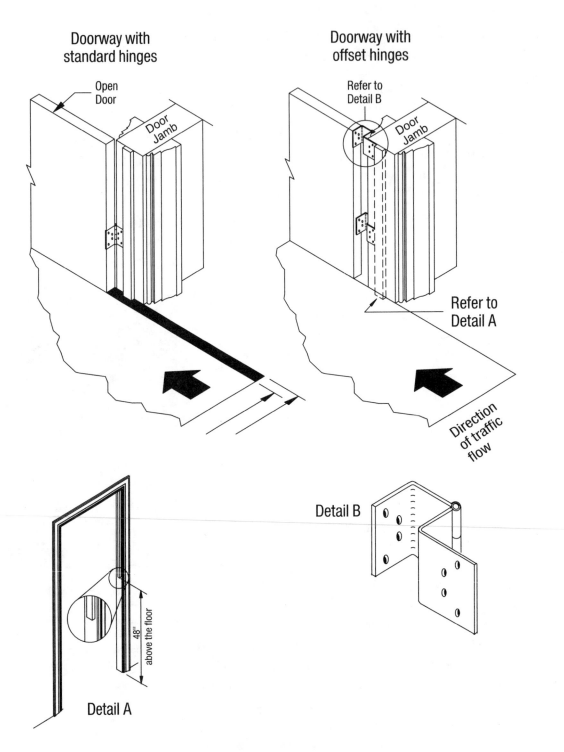

Though your door may be 30" wide, the opening may only be 28", as shown on the top left. On the right, offset hinges have been installed, and door trim has been removed.

and construction is required. This is therefore not a way to widen a doorway with minimal expense and construction.

The Bathroom

The bathroom, as small as it is, is one of the most important rooms in your home. In the course of a day, more happens in that one room than in any other room in your home. It is the one room that is used every day, no matter what the occasion. It is a room that needs to remain usable and accessible for as long as possible.

The threshold at the bathroom door is usually ¾" high. It doesn't have to be. You can replace it with a ½" "handicapped" threshold or a barrier-free threshold, which will be much easier to get past with a wheelchair. Ask your handyman or a contractor about either of these options.

Needless to say, there are three primary destinations in the bathroom: the sink, the toilet, and the shower or tub. Once past the door, how can we make each usable for someone in a wheelchair?

An accessible bathroom sink is open below, providing space for knees, and allowing someone in a wheelchair to get as close as possible. To make your sink accessible, replace your vanity with a pedestal sink, or modify the base cabinet to allow a wheelchair to roll under. You'll need an opening under the sink to 29" above the floor and 30" wide (minimum). In addition, the sink and counter should be lowered to no higher than 33" above the floor, a useable height for a family member sitting in a wheelchair.

That said, don't forget to insulate the pipes and any sharp objects under the sink to prevent scalding or injury to knees and legs. Your loved one may not know how to react or tell you if his knees touch a hot drain pipe or sharp object. (See chapter 9 for suggestions on how to accomplish this inexpensively.)

Install an adjustable, or canted, mirror over the sink that can be angled so that your family member can see herself from a lower, sitting position. Adjustable mirrors make it possible for others in the family to use the same mirror.

In the shower one of the biggest obstacles is that four-inch curb that everybody has to step over. You can install a

Adjustable mirror:

Basco, Bradley, Häfele America, Maddak.

Small wall-mounted adjustable mirror:

AdaptAbility.

Mini-ramps for showers:

Access to Recreation, AdaptAbility, Aqua Bath, HomeCare Products, Prairie View Industries, Swan Corp., Van-Duerr Industries.

Barrier-free shower curbs (water-retention strips):

Aqua Bath, Tub-Master.

Wheelchair-accessible bathtubs with doors:

Carderock Limited, Grand Traverse Technologies.

mini-ramp to get over the curb in your shower or you can remove the curb entirely and replace it with a barrier-free compressible water-retention strip. Talk to a local contractor or handyman.

There are a variety of bathtubs designed to serve people in wheelchairs. (Refer to the discussion on bathtubs and showers earlier in this chapter.)

Entrances and Exits

Your home's front door should be at least 36 inches wide, with a "handicapped" threshold (no more than half an inch high).

Provide space next to out-swinging doors that will allow a wheelchair to get out of the way while the caregiver opens the door.

In case of an emergency, create smooth and direct paths from key locations within your home (your loved one's bedroom, for example) all the way to the street or driveway. Don't think that just getting out the door is sufficient, only to get stuck at the step just beyond it.

If possible, a sliding glass door might provide the quickest and easiest exit from your family member's room. Make sure that you have a ramp there and the transition can be smooth and easy. A continuous sidewalk to the driveway will allow you to get far enough away from the house.

Outside the Home

Don't overlook your home's exterior. Sidewalks need to be smooth, firm, and free of any surprises. Paths made of stepping stones, dirt, sand, gravel, mulch, pavers, or some finishes can be bumpy and difficult for wheelchairs. Sidewalks with sections or broken areas that have risen to different heights need to be repaired. If you live in a development and have these problems, notify the management.

Make sure the outside of your home is well lit. It is important to be able to see obstacles and steps at night as well as during the day.

Ramps

Ramps are not just helpful for those in wheelchairs. Often older people find it easier to walk up a slight incline than to risk a single step that requires them to lift their foot, place it down (finding firm footing again), transfer their weight, and then re-establish their balance. For a person with Alzheimer's disease a single step can be a complicated series of maneuvers.

Use a ramp to bypass steps. Using a ramp will be far easier than trying to negotiate steps with an occupied wheelchair. Pay particular attention to the route leading out of the house and to the car. There will be times when you want to take your family member to the doctor or on an outing.

Ramps need not be a major investment. A single step or a few steps can be easily, inexpensively, and temporarily replaced with a prefabricated ramp. A prefabricated ramp is one that you buy and install over your step(s). They can be either steel or aluminum, with or without railings. Most come with slip-resistant finishes and are very convenient. Many manufacturers offer prefabricated ramps for just this purpose.

Use a small ramp to get past a single step, perhaps the one leading from the garage into the house or along the path from the driveway. Use mini-ramps at sliding glass doors to make it easier to get through them with a wheelchair. Often sliders have a one-inch lip on the inside (and more on the outside).

Prefabricated ramps:

AccessAbility, Access to Recreation, AdaptAbility, AliMed, American Health Care Supply, Care Catalogue Svcs., Easy Street, Enrichments, Facilis, Ltd., Guardian Products, Handi-Ramp, HIG's, HomeCare Products Inc., J. H. Industries, Lumex, McKesson, Portable Entry Systems, Prairie View Industries, Rampit, Sammons Preston, Sears Home HealthCare Catalog, St. Louis Medical Supply.

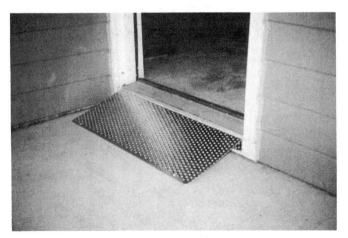

An awkward threshold, such as the one at an exterior door or a sliding door, can be bridged over with a mini-ramp. Photo courtesy Handi-Ramp, Inc.

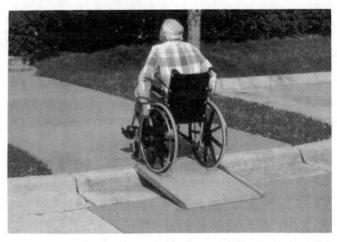

Strong, lightweight prefabricated ramps are available for more difficult barriers. Some can be folded and come with a carrying handle for trips. Photo courtesy Sammons Preston, a BISSELL® Healthcare Company. Reprinted with permission.

Ramp Installation

The formula for determining the minimum appropriate length of a ramp is based on the ratio 1:12; that is, the height of the step in *inches* = the length of the ramp in *feet*. Thus a four-inch step will require a four-foot ramp.

The *minimum* acceptable slope for a ramp is twelve inches horizontally for every inch you need vertically. However, for an older caregiver pushing his loved one in a wheelchair, this may still be too steep. Where possible, we recommend a more gradual slope of 1:20 (for each inch vertically, allow 20 inches horizontally; see the diagram below).

A ramp that is too steep can be more dangerous than no ramp at all. A 1:12 slope is good, but 1:20 is better. (Be sure to install railings on both sides of the ramp and level platforms every ten feet. Your ramp should have a non-slip surface.)

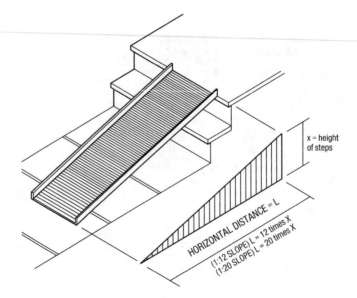

x = height of steps

HORIZONTAL DISTANCE = L

(1:12 SLOPE) L = 12 times X
(1:20 SLOPE) L = 20 times X

Ramps should have a constant, uniform slope—no surprises or sudden changes.

Since ramps are not level surfaces, the likelihood of a fall or loss of balance is far greater there. Railings can supply the necessary support to prevent a fall. They also:

- warn of an approaching change in slope that might otherwise be overlooked;
- give your loved one and the caregiver a chance to rest while holding onto something strong and secure;
- assist when a caregiver loses his balance or tries to prevent your family member from falling;
- allow the person in the wheelchair a way to help pull himself along;
- prevent the wheelchair from going over the edge of the ramp; and
- identify and locate the ramp for anyone looking for an accessible pathway to your home.

Call attention to your ramp. Make it almost impossible not to notice, even for someone who may be paying little attention to where she may be going. Use color, lighting, and railings to help you make your ramp more visible.

Provide sufficient lighting at your ramps. Make sure that the caregiver has every opportunity to see (and prepare for) the change in slope, and to see the railing in case of a fall or stumble, day or night.

Ramps can be slippery, so make sure yours has a non-slip surface. Prefabricated ramps normally come with non-slip surfaces. If you are building a ramp yourself or have one already that's a little slippery, here are a few tips:

- Use special non-slip paints. Certain paint manufacturers offer additives that make their paints slip-resistant. (Call your local paint store to discuss available products.)
- Install non-slip adhesive strips, which come in either individual strips or rolls.

Mini-ramps for small changes in elevation:

Access to Recreation, AdaptAbility, Care Catalogue, Fibreglass Systems, Handi-Ramp, HIG's, Home-Care Products, Pemko, Prairie View Industries, Reese, Sammons Preston, St. Louis Medical Supply, VanDuerr Industries.

Non-slip adhesive-backed outdoor strips:

home improvement centers.

- Install railings. If a slip occurs, a railing might prevent it from turning into a fall.

You can easily create a great non-slip finish on a new concrete ramp by brushing the concrete (before it sets) with a broom (perpendicular to the direction of travel). This will put small ribs in the concrete, resulting in a slip-resistant surface.

Make sure your ramps are wide enough for navigating a wheelchair. The minimum width is 3 feet, but wider is better. Four feet allows 26" for the wheelchair and a little extra space for someone to pass by it. Five feet would allow two wheelchairs to pass.

Ramps can be tiring. Longer ramps may be compared to scaling a small mountain for those who aren't used to them or who are pushing a wheelchair in addition to themselves. Provide a place to sit down at the top, bottom, and at intermediate landings along the way for those who may need a rest. Fold-down shower seats make excellent seats at landings. They are waterproof and can be lowered when needed and folded up and out of the way when not.

If you are going to install railings or build a ramp, do it right. Don't skimp on something so important. If you're not sure you can do this properly yourself, find a builder or contractor who can.

For plans or more information on creating an accessible home, visit your local library or bookstore. If they don't have the books you need, ask to order them from a publisher or through interlibrary loan. (Refer to some of the books mentioned in the list of suggested reading at the end of this book.) You can also contact an architect, interior designer, or contractor in your area that specializes in accessible design and modifications.

Fold-down shower seats:

American Health Care Supply, ASI, Bradley, ETAC USA, Graham Field, Häfele America, HEWI, Invacare Continuing Care, Lumex.

Platform Lifts

As mentioned above, ramps require 12 to 20 inches in length for every vertical inch required. To go from the ground to a porch only four feet up requires a ramp 48 to 80 feet long (plus intermediate landings). You might not have this much room available.

Where changes in elevation are too high for a ramp, a platform lift may be just what you need. This device is much like an outdoor, open, mini-elevator that transfers you and your loved one, standing or in a wheelchair, from the ground to levels as little as a few feet to as high as twelve feet (sufficient for many second-floor apartments). They can be locked with a key, just like a front door.

These platform or porch lifts are weather-resistant and vary quite a bit. Some have seats, allowing the passengers to sit down during their trip, and some come with overhead covers.

Platform lifts are particularly helpful for those who live in mobile homes. Mobile homes typically sit three to four feet above the ground. Climbing this height would require a very long ramp. Platform lifts take up only a few square feet.

Platform lifts:

Access Industries, Barrier-Free Lifts, Columbus McKinnon, Concord, Econol Lift Elevator Co., Flinchbaugh, FlorLift of New Jersey, Giant Lift Equipment, Inclinator of America, LectraAid, Mac's Lift Gate, National Wheel-O-Vator, Wrightway.

Platform lifts that can reach up to the second floor:

Access Industries, FlorLift of New Jersey, Inclinator Company of America.

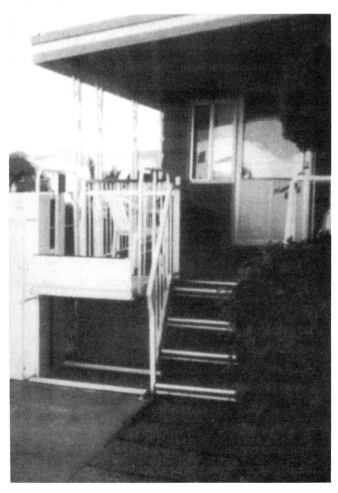

When there's not enough room for a long ramp, a platform lift may be just what you need. Photo courtesy National Wheel-O-Vator.

Platforms lifts are usually a last-resort option, installed only when all others are exhausted.

- Platform lifts can be expensive and may require a good deal of work to install.
- A platform lift will require a concrete foundation pad, usually six feet by eight feet (this varies by manufacturer) and a dedicated electrical circuit. Discuss this with your sales or manufacturer's representative and don't forget to consider these expenses when adding up the total price.
- Platform lifts need periodic maintenance, lubrication, and safety checks. Most manufacturers offer a maintenance program (for an additional charge).

Residential Elevators

Residential elevators:

Access Industries, American Stair-Glide, CEMCO, Concord Elevator, Inc., FlorLift of New Jersey, Handicapped & Elderly Life Products, Inclinator Company of America, National Wheel-O-Vator, Schumacher, Waupaca.

Elevators are not just for hotels and office buildings. There are residential elevators that don't require bulky equipment, elaborate elevator shafts, pits, or special rooms for the motors. They are simple and raise you from the first floor to the second by going through a hole in the first floor ceiling. (Be sure to consult with an architect or structural engineer before cutting any structural members supporting your second floor.)

If you're planning a new home or an addition or doing major remodeling, consider locating closets over one another on each floor, so that at a later date a residential elevator can be installed easily and conveniently. Check with manufacturers to determine how large a space you will need, the electrical requirements, and other considerations that might save you money and inconvenience later (such as installing an easily removable panel between floors).

Becoming Bed-bound

At some point the inability to walk or even stand will require your loved one to spend more time in bed or in an easy chair. Over time, even sitting upright without leaning to one side may become a problem. The only safe and comfortable place for him may be in his bed.

Alzheimer's disease is both progressive and terminal. Over time, the disease gradually robs your loved one of his abilities to perform more and more functions. Eventually, few remain, and he or she will be able to do little more than just lie in bed.

The following discussion is about making the time in bed and the bedroom pleasant, safe, and easier for everyone involved.

Making the Bedroom Safe and Comfortable

The bedroom is now the most important room in the house for your loved one. Families who have not anticipated and planned for this time may end up with a family member isolated in the back of the house or upstairs in a room that is not only remote but uninteresting and uneventful. Please plan ahead so your loved one can enjoy the benefits of a safe, comfortable room downstairs, closer to family activity and the outside world.

Reality tells us that a caregiver cannot spend all of her time in the room with her family member. Other activities (laundry, preparing meals, respite, etc.) will require the caregiver to be in other parts of the home, leaving the person with AD alone in his room. You will want to be able to monitor your loved one wherever you are or listen as you continue to perform your daily activities. At this stage it is unlikely that your family member will be able to operate devices as complicated as a pager or even ring a bell. A monitor, intercom, or surveillance camera may prove to be more helpful, allowing you to supervise or converse from various locations within your home. There are surveillance cameras that come with a small TV that can be carried with you from room to room. (Perhaps you had the foresight to install an intercom system—wired or wireless—in your home.)

Anticipate the needs of someone with a medical condition who is now confined to her bed. Install additional electrical outlets next to the bed to avoid dangerous extension cords stretching from more distant outlets, overloading circuits, and possibly blowing fuses. In addition to the lamp, telephone, and clock radio, you may find yourself needing outlets for an electric bed or various pieces of medical equipment. These outlets

Wireless baby monitor:

Kids Club, Hammacher Schlemmer, Radio Shack, Safety 1st, The Right Start, The Safety Zone, and most stores that sell products for babies.

Wireless intercom:

Radio Shack, The Safety Zone, Solutions. Also check home improvement centers and the phone book, under "Intercom Systems."

Surveillance camera:

Alsto's Handy Helpers, Canwood Products, J. C. Penney Special Needs Catalogue, Radio Shack, The Right Start, The Safety Zone, Vivitar, or home improvement centers.

will need to be located conveniently and safely, near the bed, so that electric items are not dependent on the length of their cords or the locations of your present outlets. Have an electrical contractor take a look at your home early to see if he can add a few outlets where they will be needed. (Don't overlook the possibility that your family member may eventually need to be relocated to a room other than the one he is using today. The room for the contractor to look at may be one downstairs, not upstairs.)

In the bedroom, locate things where they can be seen. Tunnel vision, your loved one's reduced mobility, and the limited number of comfortable positions will govern what she can see. Her view may be limited to only items that are relatively close, large, and straight in front of her. Take note of the most visible directions and wall spaces when she is lying in bed.

"Mom only looks at two things by her bed—the pictures of her family and Jesus."

Consider your family member's values and priorities. For most people, photographs of family are important. Photos are often proudly displayed in hallways or the living room, where they can no longer be enjoyed by a person in bed. Provide pictures of family and grandchildren in locations where they can be enjoyed from the bed. Enlarge some favorite photos of family and friends and hang them on the most visible walls.

Surround your family member with items of interest to him and to stimulate conversation. You might want to include religious pictures and articles that represent your loved one's association with her religion. Which religious pieces are important? Where could you put them to make your family member happiest?

Sun shields for windows:

American Health Care Supply.

Make your loved one's bedroom cheerful and bright—but avoid annoying glare. Glare can be reflected into your family member's room from outside of the window. The glare from your neighbor's white house or newly fallen snow may be particularly annoying. Sheer curtains or sun screens can soften the look and feel of too much sun, yet still admit gently filtered light.

Consider the orientation of the sun throughout the day to make sure that it does not shine directly onto your loved one, which could be irritating or make her hot and uncomfortable.

She might have no escape but to roll over—if she is able. Check the room at different times of the day to make sure this is not a problem. Remember her comfort zone; it is probably very different from yours.

Be aware of what a person on his back looks at all day. Is there a ceiling fan with a bright overhead light? Imagine looking at the spinning blades of an overhead fan hour after hour, day after day. Maybe it would be a good idea to remove it (or just turn it off) and add a more comfortable light on the night table. To operate this light you can easily install a wireless remote switch. (See the photo on page 49.)

Remote wireless electrical switch: Improvements or home improvement centers.

Your family member can still take a bath . . . in bed! (See chapter 4.)

Arrange furniture and locate the bed to provide access from all sides. There will be times, such as bath time, when access from all directions is needed. Making your family member as accessible as possible will be easier for both the caregiver and family member.

Consider everyone, including the caregivers, your loved one's friends, and other members of the family. Make the room as pleasant and cheerful as possible, not only for your loved one but also for guests who may have difficulty dealing with the changes in your family member. Emotions will elevate, and visitors who are not prepared or familiar with Alzheimer's may find their visits difficult. Don't forget pictures and conversation pieces for those difficult and awkward moments of silence. Provide a comfortable chair near the bed for the caregiver and visitors. Taking steps to make their experience more comfortable will allow you some free time and make their visit easier and more enjoyable.

"Windows to the World"

As more time is spent in bed, your loved one's world will be limited to only what surrounds him. In addition to the views and activities in his room, pay attention to what he can see and hear from bed. The bedroom windows and door will become his only "windows to the world," his only sources of stimulation.

Maximize the views and the activity that your loved one can see and hear through his "windows to the world." For example, if you build a sandbox for the grandchildren in the backyard, locate it so that your loved one has a clear view and can listen to and watch the activity from his bed. Create a special place for the whole family in your loved one's bedroom. Have enough chairs to sit and discuss the day's events. It may be difficult for your loved one to contribute to these conversations, but listening is easy.

Look at how the bed is oriented. Can your loved one easily and comfortably see outside? Could the bed or room be rearranged to improve views of the doorway or window(s)? The bedroom may have been set up one way for years, and changing it might cause confusion. But once your loved one is bedbound, travel will occur only with assistance, and getting lost will no longer be an issue.

Maximize the activity taking place outside your windows. Take advantage of your backyard. Anything that changes is worth watching and listening to, including parking lots, street activity, a playground, bird feeders, weather, even the neighbors!

Create an entertainment center with gardening and landscaping. Plant trees, bushes, perennials, and annuals that attract birds, squirrels, insects, and butterflies. Trees and bushes that change color with the seasons and plants that provide colorful flowers at different times of the year are the most interesting. Locate a garden where your loved one can watch and enjoy the companionship of those gardening.

Two helpful gardening magazines:

Fine Gardening (800) 888-8286 or (800) 477-8727, *Birds & Blooms* (800) 344-6913.

Place a birdfeeder or a pot filled with plants to attract birds or butterflies outside the window or in a window box. For more ideas on gardens and plants that will attract butterflies, birds, and other animals, contact your local nurseries or Audubon chapter, or check your local library for books and magazines on the subject.

Remove or trim landscaping that blocks or limits views.

Create more "windows to the world." If funds are available and the walls allow it, consider converting a window to a sliding glass door. (Have an architect or contractor look at your home ahead of time to determine whether this is possible.) Sliding glass doors in the bedroom offer a wonderful, unobstructed, full-height view. From the comfort of bed your loved one can enjoy the sunlight, rainstorms, animals on the ground, and so much more. A sliding glass door also offers a much larger panorama than a window and a greater opportunity for breezes and fresh air.

There are other "windows to the world" that you can take advantage of or add: a television, radio, and telephone. Install a high, wall-mounted television shelf, easier to watch for someone lying in bed. This might be reminiscent of a hospital room, but nonetheless, if your loved one spends most of the time lying down, it will be helpful to be able to see the television without having to look over her knees or sacrifice comfort. Some wall-mounted television shelves can be tilted for a more direct view of the television.

Locating the television directly in front of the bed limits the positions one can lie in and still see it. On the other hand, if the TV is slightly to one side, your family member can watch TV sitting up, lying on his back, or lying on one side.

If your family member has difficulty holding the telephone, install a telephone equipped with a speaker phone, so he can talk while lying in bed or perhaps just listen in on a conversation between you and someone dear to you both.

Mobility is indeed a difficult and complicated issue, especially when it applies to the person with Alzheimer's disease. The age-old riddle of "What animal walks on four legs, two legs and then three legs?" never took these concerns into account, did it?

Preparation and planning ahead remain your best tools and strategies. Make your to-do list, create a plan, assemble those you need to help (your family, contractor, and handyman), and take action. The sooner you get the work done, the easier it will be.

Adjustable wall-mounted television shelves:

American Health Care Supply, Crest, Get Organized, Hammacher Schlemmer, Improvements, Peerless Industries, The Safety Zone, The Woodworker's Store, home improvement centers.

Speaker telephones:

Enrichments, Hello Direct, HITEC, LS & S, Radio Shack, telephone stores.

9

Safety

Keeping a person with Alzheimer's disease at home and safe throughout the entire course of the disease is a challenge that requires extraordinary preparations and foresight. Consider the recommendations in this chapter as examples of a mindset that goes beyond the limits of normal safety-proofing, recognizing and responding to the special needs of a person with a dementing illness.

Safety is a particularly important issue for anyone living with Alzheimer's disease. The word "safety" takes on a whole new meaning when applied to Alzheimer's disease, as it no longer refers just to accident prevention. "Safety" now also means creating environments that are easy to understand, less intimidating, more likely to result in success; it means recognizing the unique demands that accompany Alzheimer's disease.

People with AD may not be able to distinguish right from wrong, appropriate from inappropriate, or safe from unsafe. For someone who is confused, even common, everyday items pose a danger. Lawn tools, for example, require judgment and coordination. Skills no longer as well-tuned as they once were may cause injury when one is trying to use an ax, shears, or a lawnmower, for example. Relying on common sense and good judgment no longer suffices. Your husband may check to see if the lawnmower is operating properly by looking underneath or feeling with his hand without remembering to turn it off.

Accidents can also be reminders that something is wrong. Some people can't accept that they have this disease until the accidents and episodes of forgetfulness become too frequent to ignore or cover up. When they are no longer able to use certain products and tools safely, it is wiser to remove them from sight and out of reach than to risk injury or psychological damage.

Sensory impairments also present safety issues. Olfactory (sense of smell) impairments associated with AD may explain why some people don't realize that they are eating or drinking something inappropriate, such as a bottle of pickle juice or spoiled food. Other age-related conditions, such as visual and hearing impairments (which may or may not be related to Alzheimer's), can also contribute to accidents.

Because Alzheimer's disease has many stages and everyone's situation is different, your decisions regarding safety must be based on your specific situation. Safety steps should be tailored to the cognitive stage and physical skills of your loved one. It certainly is not appropriate to gut your home, removing everything of potential danger, as soon as your loved one demonstrates a few episodes of forgetfulness. On the other hand, when he fails to recognize his home for the first time, it may then be appropriate to take precautions against his wandering away from home.

Keep in mind, too, that creating a safer environment also makes the caregiver's job easier. Removing as many potential dangers as possible means the caregiver has less to worry about and can devote attention to more important matters than worrying about what her loved one will get into next.

Because Alzheimer's is a progressive disease, conditions are constantly changing, sometimes slowly and at other times remarkably fast. Caregivers must stay on their toes, watch for changes, and act accordingly.

The first strategy for safety-proofing a home is to learn as much about Alzheimer's disease as possible. Join a support group, attend lectures, and use your computer if you have one. (There are resources and on-line support groups abounding in information.) Alzheimer's education is an ongoing process with new ideas and information appearing every day.

This chapter focuses on potential dangers and principles of safety-proofing that specifically apply to people with dementia. We'll cover the six most common types of injury that occur around the home, a few Alzheimer's-specific concerns, and offer detailed coverage of grab bars, an important and versatile tool for safety.

Getting Started

Rule Number One: Plan for the Future

Plan for future needs, such as a wheelchair. Keep in mind, too, that in the latter stages of the disease, activity will become limited to the bed and favorite chair. At that time it will probably be safe to reverse some of the modifications that you have made to the rest of the house.

Rule Number Two: Observe and Act in the Appropriate Manner at the Appropriate Time

There are no definitive rules with Alzheimer's disease. Your loved one may experience conditions that others do not, and vice versa. You'll need to react and take action uniquely appropriate to your situation. Each stage of AD is different also. As soon as you adjust to the symptoms of one stage, the disease seems to move on, with new demands and adjustments required. You need to watch and learn, adjusting to each change as it occurs. By keeping your eyes and heart open to the needs of your loved one, you will be able to make the appropriate changes.

Rule Number Three: Make Your Modifications Early

As the disease runs its course, social skills decline and interaction with strangers may become more of a threat than a pleasure. Contractors coming into your home may be seen as intruders, and may not be as understanding of your loved one's behavior as you are. Your family member may remove construction materials, hide their tools, or accuse them of stealing things now missing. The earlier you get these people in and out of your home (and their work completed), the better it will be for everyone.

Rule Number Four: Identify Zones within Your Home

As discussed in chapter 1, there are three types of zones: the Danger Zone, the Respite Zone, and the Safe Zone.

Remove sources of danger and install locks on doors leading into danger zones. If you need more lockable storage space for dangerous items, now is the time to add or create it.

Create a "Forgiving" Home

A "forgiving" home is one that:

- recognizes the potential for accidents;
- reduces potential failures and upsets; and
- minimizes injury or trauma if and when accidents do occur.

Look through this book for tips on simplifying your home, creating clear and open pathways, removing furniture that is easy to trip over, providing soft and stable furniture that can be relied on in a fall and won't cause bruises or cuts. Simplify decisions and look for places and items in your home that repeatedly disturb your family member. These are just a few ideas that contribute to a "forgiving" home. (See chapter 1.)

Child-Proof Your Home

Examine your home, looking at it much the same way you would if you were living with a young child. Be on guard for anything that a young child might explore: small items he might put in his mouth, potentially hazardous electrical appliances, items that represent danger if not used properly or understood. Identify the potential problems, then use your good judgment to determine the appropriate action.

However, don't rely too heavily on child-proofing techniques to protect an adult with dementia. Child-proof products are intended and designed for children, not adults. Your loved one has a lifetime of experience to draw from and the strength of someone much larger and older. In addition, products intended for children may not be ergonomically designed for adults. A child-proof gate, for example, may be just right for a small child, but a taller and stronger person may simply step over it or force her way through.

On the other hand, you may find excellent uses for some of the hundreds of cleverly designed child-proof products that really do take a good deal of creativity and clearheadedness to outsmart—items such as locks that open only with magnetic keys, child-proof doorknobs, medicine cabinet locks, and electric outlet caps. (For more information, visit stores, contact companies that sell child-proofing products, and check your local library for books on making homes safe for children.)

Child-proof products:

Alsto's Handy Helpers, Brainerd, Gerber Products, Kids Club, National Manufacturing, OFNA Baby Products, Perfectly Safe, Rev-A-Shelf, Safety 1st, The Safety Zone, The Right Start, home improvement and baby supply stores.

Additional Safety Strategies

It is often better to safety-proof a room than to declare it off-limits. In the early stages of Alzheimer's, people retain much of their reasoning and cognitive abilities. Furthermore, they have spent their entire adult lives free to do what they want within their homes. Though your family member may trust your good judgment, he may not understand or fully accept being denied access to areas in his home. He may enter forbidden areas when your back is turned or at night while you are asleep, or become agitated at a locked door.

"It's my home and I can go anywhere and do anything I want in it."

Improve lighting. Lighting contributes to safety by:

- helping your family member see what she is doing;
- eliminating shadows that can be misinterpreted or provide places for "strangers" to hide; and
- guiding and making it possible for your loved one to see and identify destinations.

Recognize that while your family member may need more light, too much light can create dangerous glare. Be careful not to overload your lighting fixtures to provide more light. Many fixtures are designed to handle bulbs no brighter than

60 watts. Check the labels on your light fixtures and do not exceed their recommendations.

Hide a spare key outside or leave it with a trusted neighbor in case you get locked out of the house.

Consider installing monitoring equipment. There are several different types available, from clandestine baby monitors to surveillance cameras to intercom systems (wired and wireless). (See chapter 5 for more on monitoring equipment.)

Common Types and Sources of Injuries

Burns

For a person with Alzheimer's, burns and fires can be caused by something as simple as forgetting ordinary safety precautions that most of us take for granted, such as using mitts when removing a hot pan from the oven. In addition to the common and typical burn hazards around the home, such as the stove, many other items can get hot or cause fires—things that the rest of us know to avoid, but that your loved one may not remember.

Many of these hazards might be best moved to a more secure, inaccessible location in a Danger Zone. You may want to rent storage space to move certain items and appliances out of harm's way.

Common Items around Your Home That Get Hot

There is no shortage of appliances around the home that get hot and can cause burns. Here are just a few:

toasters	hair dryers
hot plates	curling irons
laundry irons	bread makers
waffle irons	tea kettles
coffee makers	stoves and ovens
toaster ovens	barbecues

The lid on your patio barbecue can get extremely hot—and when it does, it doesn't look any different from when it was cold. Your loved one may not recall lighting the barbecue or associate it with the scorching temperature, and may get burned. It may be best to remove the barbecue, not only to avoid accidents, but also to avoid agitation. The barbecue may represent a family responsibility that your family member can no longer perform safely, and he may find someone else's taking over his job upsetting.

It is all too easy for your loved one to use the stove or oven and forget to turn it off. Hot items from the microwave, too, can cause burns. Look into child-proof stove and oven locks (available at baby supply stores) and remote switches that make a stove or microwave inoperable. (See chapter 6.)

Any source of heat, including your furnace and water heater, can cause burns. Consider placing secure locks on the doors leading to these pieces of equipment.

Radiators and space heaters are obvious culprits. Use protective radiator covers to prevent burns. In the bathroom, ceiling-mounted heaters or heat lamps may be far better options than floor-mounted space heaters, which can be touched, knocked over, or put in the tub, shower, or toilet while still plugged in the outlet.

Place a "Stop-Hot" label on any item that might burn your family member if touched. These small stop signs are specially designed to be applied to items that get hot. They may not create an impenetrable line of defense, but could call your loved one's attention to something hot and divert a possible accident.

"Stop - Hot" label:
American Thermometer Company.

Don't forget your fireplace. Tending a fire may be another long-standing family responsibility that can no longer be performed safely. Remove firewood, lighter fluid, and matches used to light the fireplace. Store them in a safe, remote location.

Night lights with bulbs can get very hot and are often left on 24 hours a day. You can avoid nasty burns by installing night lights with bulbs that burn cool.

Night lights that burn cool:
The Limelite is one example. Austin Innovations, home improvement centers or hardware stores.

Incandescent light bulbs also get very hot. One caregiver told us about a family member who accidentally knocked over a bedside lamp. The lampshade came off and the lamp came to rest with the bulb wedged between the mattress and the night table. The confused family member went to get the

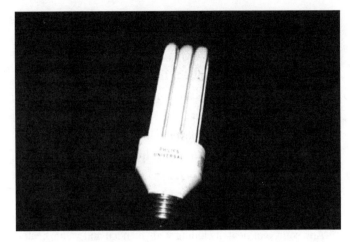

A compact fluorescent bulb screws into your regular light fixture but does not burn as hot as an incandescent bulb.

caregiver, and by the time they came back the mattress was smoldering.

Compact fluorescent, screw-in light bulbs:

Philips Light Company, hardware stores, home improvement centers, or grocery stores.

Replace incandescent bulbs in lamps that may be knocked over or touched with compact fluorescent bulbs. Compact fluorescent bulbs burn cooler. They are far less likely to cause a burn when touched, and they will not cause a fire. These much safer bulbs screw into the same socket as your regular bulbs. They are more expensive, but the cost is offset by the fact that they last much longer than conventional incandescent bulbs.

Safe, cool-to-the-touch torchere lamps with fluorescent bulbs:

Energy Federation Inc.

Halogen lamps are the most dangerous, because they reach much higher temperatures than incandescent bulbs and can easily start a fire. Just touching a metal lampshade on a halogen lamp can be painful. Free-standing halogen floor lamps, which might be grasped or knocked over if your loved one loses his balance, are especially hazardous. Put them away for the time being, where they cannot be used, touched, or knocked over.

Explosives

Microwave ovens can cause explosions if used improperly. Food in glass jars or other sealed containers (even eggs) can build up enough pressure to explode. (See chapter 6.)

Flammable liquids are another explosive and burn danger. Charcoal lighter fluid for the barbecue, paint thinners, even common nail polish removers can ignite or explode if they come in contact with a live flame. Pay particular attention to common flammable products stored around the house, especially those normally located near sources of fire.

Fires

Certain precautions are wise in every home. Locate lightweight hand-held fire extinguishers conveniently and prudently in key areas of your house. Small 2½ pound units are available at your local home improvement center or fire extinguisher dealer and are easy to carry and use. Store them near places where a fire is most likely to occur, but not so close that the fire would make them inaccessible. For example, keep an extinguisher in the kitchen, but not next to the stove, where a fire could prevent you from reaching the extinguisher.

Purchase fire extinguishers labeled "ABC," which are able to put out all kinds of fires. Periodically check your extinguishers to make sure they're still charged with sufficient pressure.

- Class A extinguishers put out fires involving items such as paper, wood, and cloth.
- Class B extinguishers put out fires fueled by flammable liquids such as gasoline, oils, grease, and oil-base paint.
- Class C extinguishers are good for electrical fires.

Contact a local security alarm company to discuss installing a central smoke alarm system. Ask about systems that use your telephone line to notify somebody in the event of an emergency.

Nighttime wandering is a major concern regarding fires in the house. Stoves can be turned on and food left on the burners or cigarettes lit and forgotten, just to name a few possibilities. (See chapter 5 for ideas about how to deal with this.)

Would your loved one know what to do if he did start a fire? In addition to smoke detectors, you might want to consider installing a sprinkler system in your home. A good residential sprinkler system doesn't just alert you, it extinguishes the fire.

With these systems, sprinkler heads are installed in key locations throughout your home. Each head has a tiny glass cylinder that breaks at approximately 135 degrees Fahrenheit, dispersing enough water to put out most small fires. Only those sprinkler heads that sense the fire go off, not all of them simultaneously. Look in your phone book under "Sprinkler Systems" or "Fire Protection" for local companies that install these systems.

To determine your best fire-protection options, contact your local fire department and request a home inspection. In many communities there is no charge for this service. However, a gift of food or whatever you care to offer will be much appreciated at the station. (Most firemen have to pay for their meals while they sit in the firehouse waiting for an alarm.)

Smoking

Smoking should only be allowed under supervision. It creates the potential for serious danger. Cigarettes, pipes, or cigars lit and forgotten or dropped in crevices of furniture can have catastrophic results. In addition, a confused person may go to extremes to light a cigarette, possibly using the fireplace, furnace, or stove burners, if he can't find matches. There is a real danger of jeopardizing the safety of everyone in your home or building, just for something to smoke.

If your loved one smokes, we recommend that you remove items that remind him of his habit and need, including pipes, packages of cigarettes, cigars, matches, and lighters. Store them in a secure location and allow them to be enjoyed only under strict supervision. Ashtrays should be removed only if you have done a thorough job of removing all of the other reminders, otherwise your family member may try to smoke with nothing safe to put the ashes in. Also, without matches, your family member may use other, more dangerous means to light her cigarette, such as the stove.

Smoking can be a difficult problem. We realize that you may feel torn between the obvious fire and health hazards of smoking and the guilt of denying your loved one a pleasure that he enjoys. But consider the potential for serious injury and damage. While this may be a hard decision, remember that your loved one does not want to endanger the lives of those he loves, either.

Miscellaneous Burns

Acids and other caustic chemicals are another burn hazard that may be silently lurking in your home, especially in the kitchen, garage, or near the pool. Cleaning chemicals, including drain cleaners and pool chlorine, are often dangerous if used improperly. Lock 'em up! Get rid of those cans, bottles, and boxes of miscellaneous chemicals in the garage whose labels have worn or fallen off, leaving the containers and their contents unmarked and unknown. If, by any chance, they were mishandled, you wouldn't know what chemical was in the can.

Danger from scalding is often overlooked. Tactile sensation may be dulled and reaction time slowed in older people. Your family member may not realize that he is being burned in time to remove his hand or foot from hot water. He may not realize that he has been scalded or is unable to explain what happened. Once again the result may be agitation or some other means of venting discomfort.

The least expensive and probably most effective strategy is to lower your water heater thermostat to its lowest setting—no higher than 120 degrees. This way the water can never get hot enough to cause discomfort or injury. If you are not sure how to do this, ask your local handyman to take a look at your water heater and turn the thermostat down. Then wait until the next day (giving your water time to cool down), and test it.

Install anti-scalding devices in your faucets and shower-heads. These are inexpensive devices placed on or in your faucets. If the water gets too hot, their internal parts expand and turn off the flow.

For showers, the next step up from an anti-scalding device is replacing your hot and cold mixing valve with a pressure-sensitive and/or temperature-limiting anti-scalding valve. This device senses and compares the pressure in the hot and cold water lines. When there is a sudden change in pressure (for example, if your husband flushes the toilet while you are in the shower), the valve compensates so that you don't get caught in

Anti-scalding devices:

Accent on Living, AdaptAbility, Joan Cook, Independent Living Aids, Keeney, Memry Corporation, or home improvement centers.

Anti-scalding showerheads:

Accent on Living, AdaptAbility, Brookstone, Independent Living Aids, Keeney, Lighthouse Enterprises.

Anti-scalding devices for bath-tub faucets:

Keeney.

These small anti-scalding devices turn off the water flow if it gets too hot.

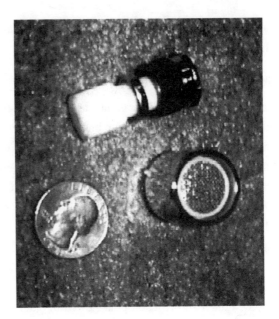

Pressure-sensitive, temperature-limiting anti-scalding bath and shower valves:

Delta, Kohler, Moen, Price Pfister, or a plumbing dealer.

Non-slip, color-changing floor mats:

Joan Cook, Underfoot.

Safety pipe covers for under-the-counter pipes:

Keeney, Plumberex, Truebro.

a stream of scalding water. A temperature-limiting feature allows you to pre-set the valve to ensure that the water will not get too hot. Consult a plumber for more information.

There are also non-slip tub mats that change color to alert you that the water is too hot. These may not work for the person with Alzheimer's, but could be a visual alarm to the caregiver that the water is too hot.

Don't overlook the teapot on the stove or the instant hot water dispenser at your sink. An innocent attempt to make a cup of soup, as your family member may have done for years, may now pose new dangers. Disconnect or unplug your instant hot water dispenser and remove the teapot from the stove.

For those in wheelchairs, insulate exposed pipes under sinks to protect knees from touching hot pipes. Hot water going through the hot water supply pipe or down the drain can make those pipes very hot.

To cover hot water pipes inexpensively, use pipe insulation tubes available at your local home improvement center. These foam tubes are slit lengthwise, come in various diameters, and wrap around your pipes. They cost as little as two dollars per eight-foot length, which is more than enough for several pipes. To hold them in place, wrap them with a few strips of plastic electrical tape.

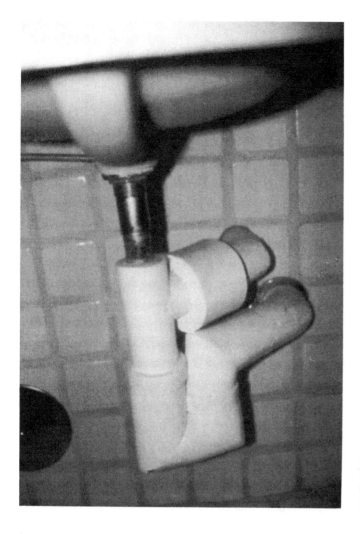

Pipe covers prevent burns and cuts to knees of the wheelchair user when she's pulled up close to the sink. Photo courtesy Truebro, Inc.

Cuts

The kitchen is the first room in the house that comes to mind when thinking about sharp, dangerous objects. Knives, forks, and sharp cooking tools are all-too-readily available in most kitchens. Ceramic plates can be easily dropped and break into sharp pieces. Glasses are especially vulnerable because they are clear and difficult to see. (People with AD often have difficulty seeing clear objects and may only see those items directly in front of them.)

Consider limiting metal tableware to spoons. They have no pointed tips and are easier to use. Avoid plastic utensils, especially forks, which can be bitten and the tiny plastic ends swallowed or choked on. Relocate sharp utensils used for cooking and food preparation to secure locations (locked drawers and cabinets). You might also consider leaving at least one drawer unlocked and filled with safe items to divert attention from drawers that need to remain locked and off-limits.

Ceramic dishes might best be replaced with paper or plastic to avoid the danger, trauma, and concern of breaking them. Replace glasses and flimsy plastic or paper cups with large, stable, heavy-duty plastic mugs that will be easier to handle and less likely to be knocked over. (You may be able to use the excuse that you are providing them for the grandchildren when they come to visit.)

The kitchen is not the only location in your home where sharp implements abide. Pencils, hangers, and hobby and gardening tools can also be dangerous. Survey your home for these potential hazards and for "weapons," especially those that are small enough to throw—and most certainly if your loved one has demonstrated a tendency to react violently.

Don't overlook table or oscillating fans. Make sure yours have protective screens to keep curious fingers from touching the rotating blades, or that they're kept securely out of reach.

Kitchen Appliances

Take precautions with electrical or motorized cutting appliances, such as blenders, food processors, mixers, and electric knives. Although these appliances may represent a lifetime of caring and family responsibility, they may now be dangerous for your loved one, who no longer has the judgment, skills, or knowledge needed to operate them safely.

When you have to deny access to appliances for safety reasons, also consider creating a special place in the kitchen where your family member can perform alternative tasks that make a meaningful contribution to family care. Substitute safe utensils for those that need to be removed. Make it possible for your loved one to continue to assist in meal preparation or be there while other activities are taking place, offering advice, and conversation.

Home utensils and gadgets:

Accent on Living, AdaptAbility, Aids for Arthritis, Easy Living Specialties, Enrichments, ETAC-USA, Improvements, Independent Living Aids, J.C. Penney Special Needs Catalogue, Lifestyle Catalogue, Maddak, Maxi Aids, Rifton, Sammons Preston, and Shamrock Medical.

The Disposal

The garbage disposal is sometimes an irresistible curiosity for those who rummage and hide things. Its switch on the wall can easily be confused with a light switch when more light is needed to search that intriguing hole. The results could be catastrophic.

Some disposals (called batch feed disposals) will only operate when the cover is securely locked in place, making them much safer. Perhaps it might be a good idea to replace your disposal with a safer batch feed disposal. For existing disposals or those not offering this feature, disconnect them. There is often a plug underneath the sink and sometimes a dedicated circuit in your electrical panel. Unplug the disposal or flip the

Disposals that will only operate with the cover on:

In-Sink-Erator, Maytag, appliance dealers.

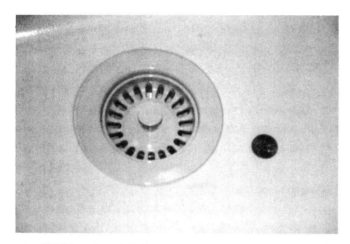

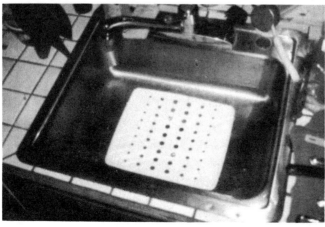

A drain cover (top) or a sink mat (bottom) conceals the garbage disposal.

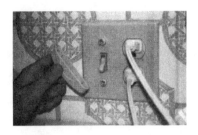

Use switch covers to hide dangerous switches, like the one for the disposal, pictured above.

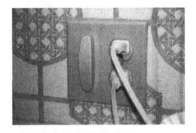

Installation is easy. Once in place, the cap snaps on, and the switch "disappears."

Switch covers:

Improvements.

circuit breaker and place a label on it indicating that this breaker is *not* to be turned back on.

To discourage hiding things in the disposal, camouflage the hole. Install a disposal-size strainer or a perforated mat in the sink that will totally cover and remove the hole from sight. (Do not rely on this alone to protect your loved one from the danger of the disposal. Disconnect it also!)

Sharp Tools and Power Tools

Your family member may have once enjoyed, and still feels that he can perform, tasks such as yard work, pruning, wood-carving, food preparation, or sewing. These activities are normally associated with sharp, pointed tools that require judgment, coordination, and special skills that he may no longer have. Something as apparently harmless as fingernail clippers can be dangerous if the skills to use them are no longer intact. (See also chapter 4.)

Your garage or shed may be full of tools that can cause serious injury. Provide secure locks on doors leading to rooms or sheds containing tools such as power saws, lawn tools, or gas-operated equipment. Devices that cannot be relocated (table saws, grinders, etc.) should be unplugged and the circuit breakers controlling the electrical outlets turned off.

Don't overlook the lawn mower. Your family member may still see mowing the lawn as his responsibility. We have also heard of families who took the keys to the car away, only to find their loved one going down the street on the riding lawnmower!

Glass and Mirrors

Kitchens and bathrooms are filled with all types of glass. Your loved one may have used the same drinking glass for years. Although replacing it with a more stable plastic mug that is easier to see and hold contradicts our suggestion to maintain familiarity, the consequences of dropping a glass and breaking it go way beyond losing a familiar friend. Furthermore, even the slightest accident, especially the trauma of breaking something, may represent failure and a reminder that something is wrong.

Survey your home thoroughly, taking note of everything

made of glass, including windows, sliding glass doors, and shower doors. If any were installed before 1977, they may be made from plate glass, rather than tempered safety glass. Plate glass is dangerous when it breaks, whereas safety glass, as the name implies, is much safer. If you are unsure, contact a local glass contractor to examine your sliding glass and shower doors. (See chapter 1 for more on plate and tempered glass.)

Consider replacing tempered glass sliding tub or shower doors with shower curtains. Sliding doors, at best, allow access to only half the shower when fully open, making it difficult to assist your loved one while he's bathing. Also, if there's an accident in the shower or bath, sliding doors might hinder the caregiver or rescue personnel when helping your loved one out or attending to her in the tub or shower.

Every year hundreds of people accidentally walk into sliding glass doors, thinking they are open. It might help to apply decals to the glass to make it more visible—but for someone with dementia this may not be sufficient. Fake mullions covering the entire glass area may not only eliminate the problem, but also make the door appear to be a window (not an exit), an additional advantage for those who may try to leave home. (These fake mullions are also removable later, when mobility problems—becoming bed-bound or chair-bound—make visibility more important than accessibility.) (See the photo in chapter 1.)

Fake mullions for sliding glass doors and windows:

New Pane Creations.

Mirrors present a variety of challenges. Hand-held mirrors can be dropped, much like drinking glasses. Larger, wall-hung mirrors may reflect the image of an unrecognizable "stranger" who may frighten or threaten your loved one. Mirrors can also contribute to difficulties with wayfinding, especially when there are more than one in a room. Two or more mirrored walls can be confusing and make a room appear to have no exit. Depending on how your loved one reacts to mirrors, you may want to cover or remove them. (See chapter 2 for more suggestions and ideas.)

Furniture with glass inserts (such as end tables, etageres, breakfronts, china cabinets, and coffee tables) can be hazardous. Your loved one might reach for a table or breakfront to

support himself in the midst of a fall, only to have his hand
go through the glass. Other panes of glass can be broken by
thrown objects. They can also reflect images or lights that
your loved one may not understand. Put these dangerous
pieces of furniture in storage now, before an accident happens. Or you could replace the glass with something non-
breakable, such as wood or Plexiglas (check your yellow pages
under "Plastics").

Glass-covered paintings present safety problems from both
glare and reflections, in addition to breakage. Use nonbreakable, nonreflective Plexiglas rather than glass. Visit a local
picture framing company for more information on this type of
plastic for your pictures.

Some people with AD try to remove framed photos, paintings, or lithographs from the wall, causing them to fall and
break. Contact a local framing store and ask about nonremov-
able, wall-mounting brackets that attach the picture directly
and securely to the wall.

Poisoning

Many common household items, if eaten, can cause discomfort, illness, or death. Some are intended to be consumed, but
only in limited quantities (such as spices or toothpaste), and
may cause temporary discomfort if larger amounts are swallowed. Furthermore, if your loved one eats something that
makes him uncomfortable, he may not understand the source
of his discomfort or be able to relate it to you. The result may
be unnecessary suffering, on everyone's part.

Foods

For a person who is confused, food may take on different
meanings. It may be hoarded or hidden in the bedroom for
the person in the mirror, or to prevent running out (maybe
reflecting back to times when food was scarce). The purpose
of toothpaste or shaving cream may escape your family member. Instead he may try to eat it. And foods such as raw meats
might be consumed without being properly cooked. Spices

may be ingested to excess, and products that only resemble food (such as plastic grapes) may be mistakenly swallowed.

As we age, we gradually lose some of our sense of smell and taste. The problem is often compounded by AD and may offer some explanation for the otherwise inexplicable ingestion of inappropriate products found while rummaging in the refrigerator or of hidden food that has long since spoiled. (See chapter 2.)

A weekly refrigerator check, throwing out spoiled foods, is a good practice. Consider installing a child-proof lock on the refrigerator to prevent your family member from eating inappropriate or spoiled foods. You might also consider buying a mini-refrigerator and locating it in a remote, secure location to keep certain items (like medications) out of harm's way.

Remove alcoholic beverages or lock them in a liquor cabinet. Your family member doesn't have to be an alcoholic to get into trouble here. Certain beers and wines can be replaced with non-alcoholic versions, thus satiating the need but eliminating the danger. One family we heard about went to the trouble of refilling bottles containing their family member's favorite brand of beer with a non-alcoholic brand.

Make sure you remove pet foods and pet products from easy access. Family members who grew up during the Depression may not think twice about consuming pet food. Often pet products (shampoos and insecticides) are brightly colored and could possibly be mishandled or swallowed. Litter boxes should be put in locations accessible only to the cat. Install a pet door or a chain that only allows the door to remain open wide enough for Fluffy.

Small, compact refrigerators:
American Health Care Supply, Koolatron,* Igloo Products,* Intirion, Marvel, U-Line, or appliance dealers. (*Make sure you ask for the converter that allows you to plug the unit into a wall outlet.)

Common Household Products

Dangerous chemicals, household cleaners, and other products that combine potential toxicity with attractive packaging should be stored in remote, secure locations. For people who are confused and are looking for cues that might indicate a correct decision, a tempting color or a smiling face on a package may be all that is needed to encourage a taste. Products that are scented and colored to resemble food, like lemon-scented furniture cleaners or detergents, offer an additional temptation.

Medications

Your loved one might take the wrong medications, the incorrect dosages, or forget she took her pills and take them again. Don't forget the dangers of over-the-counter, nonprescription medications, such as aspirin, or vitamins. (Refer also to the section in chapter 4 entitled "Medication Administration.")

Locking medicine cabinets:

American Health Care Supply.

Consider all the locations in your home where you might be storing medication. Certainly remove them and other dangerous products from your family member's bathroom, and install locks on your own medicine cabinet.

Check the refrigerator, where you may be storing medications that require refrigeration. You can install a child-proof lock on the refrigerator or place a small refrigerator in one of your inaccessible Danger Zone rooms to keep your medications.

Also make sure you don't have anything lying around the house that resembles pills or medications, such as small decorative beads, which that could be mistaken for pills. On the other hand, be aware that many medications look like candy, another misleading signal.

Plants

Many household plants are toxic. (Refer to the list of poisonous plants in chapter 1.) Read the instructions that accompany your new household plants. If you have questions, check with your local poison control office. Don't overlook your front, back and side yards, as well.

Choking

Do not have small items around the house that can be placed in the mouth and cause your loved one to choke. Sometimes people in the later stages of Alzheimer's forget how to swallow or how to chew. Swallowing alone is a complex series of timed and coordinated actions, multi-sequential tasks that your loved one may no longer be able to perform. Even items intended to be placed in the mouth can be dangerous if the person does not know what to do with them. Then harmless foods such as hard candy, popcorn, or nuts can easily cause choking.

Like a young child who knows no better, your loved one may no longer recognize the appropriate purpose of items discovered around the house. Survey your home and remove small objects that, if placed in the mouth, could cause choking. Although the list is virtually endless, here are a few items to give you a good idea of what to look for:

buttons	cotton balls
pebbles in planters	dry pet food pellets
paper clips	gum balls
pins and needles	popcorn
hard candy	pills
marbles	bowls of nuts
jewelry (rings, earrings)	decorative bits of soap
small toys (and toy parts)	fruit seeds or pits
loose keys	coffee beans
nails and screws	mothballs
bottle caps	loose change

Electric Shock

Common knowledge is no longer "common" with Alzheimer's disease. For someone with AD, electrical outlets may become interesting holes. You don't want to find your family member exploring these curiosities with a paper clip, screwdriver, metal coat hanger, or kitchen knife.

Install child-proof safety caps in all accessible electrical outlets.

Install GFI (ground fault interrupted) outlets where appropriate. GFI outlets or breakers in your electrical panel sense an electrical short in only a fraction of a second and turn off the power, preventing accidental shock or electrocution. They won't protect your loved one from shock if she inserts something metallic in the outlet, but they will offer some protection if she drops an electrical appliance in water while it is still plugged in the outlet. Your family member may not understand the potential danger of an electrical appliance and the water in the sink, shower, toilet, or bathtub nearby.

Child-proof caps for electrical outlets:

Gerber Products, Perfectly Safe, The Right Start, The Safety Zone, Safety 1st, baby supply stores, home improvement centers.

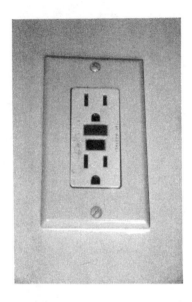

A GFI outlet senses a short circuit and turns off the power, reducing the likelihood of shock or electrocution. It can also be used as a secret switch to turn off the outlet.

If you already have GFI outlets in these locations, test them and make sure they work. One family we know had GFI outlets in their home, but over the years, paint had gotten into them and they no longer worked. To test yours, all you have to do is push the test button that is located on all GFI outlets or breakers. It should make a popping sound and then need to be reset (by pushing the reset button). If nothing happens, the outlet offers no protection. If you are not sure, don't take any chances. Ask your local electrician to check it for you and to install GFI outlets where they may be needed. (You may wish to leave the GFI outlet off, without resetting it, making it inoperable and therefore safer, even if something is plugged into it.)

Survey your home for extension cords and hazards hindering the route to interesting views or places. Check and make sure that you do not have any frayed electrical cords, overloaded extension cords, and cords going under furniture or carpeting or hanging from tables, where they might be snagged.

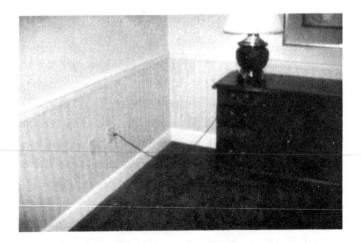

Check all electrical cords in your home—many accidents can be avoided. It is just a matter of time before this cord is snagged and the lamp broken.

Remove portable fans and heaters. Place safety covers on radiators.

Identify and remove potential hazards—including that lovely aquarium in the corner with the electric light, pump, and filter ... and water. If you just can't live without your aquarium, how about giving the exotic fish to a nice home and replacing them with some that do not require the air pump, filter, and light, like guppies or goldfish? (Or perhaps even artificial fish!)

Repair any faulty appliances. Remove and put away small, portable electrical appliances normally kept on the kitchen or bathroom counter that could fall into the sink or be carried to a wet location. (Refer to chapter 1 for a brief list.)

Take multiple steps to protect against shock or electrocution. It's good to have GFI outlets or breakers. It's even safer to supplement them with child-proof outlet caps.

Drowning

It is said that a person can drown in as little as two inches of water. I think a person can drown in less than two inches, especially if he falls face down into water, as in a bathtub. Remember that people with dementia may no longer have swift reaction times to help them adjust to a loss of balance.

Pools can be both beautiful and deadly. Swimming pools, decorative pools, Jacuzzis, and spas are potentially dangerous areas, not only because of electrical shock, but because of slips and falls that could lead to a drowning.

Make sure your loved one does not have access to dangerous bodies of water. Install a protective railing or fence, allowing a view, but denying access and protecting him from a fall. Provide gates, locks, and alarms on the doors leading to the pool area. You can also install child-proof alarms that will sound if the water in the pool is disturbed. Consult a local pool supply dealer to discover what products are available, which work best, and who can install them for you.

Pool guard alarms:

Improvements, Perfectly Safe, pool supply and home improvement stores.

Pool alarm with remote alarm: Improvements.

Bathtubs are easily overlooked, though they are the cause of numerous deaths every year. We strongly recommend that you install grab bars and make bathroom, bathtub and shower floors slip-resistant. This can be done easily and inexpensively with slip-resistant strips, appliqués, or bath mats.

Consider your neighborhood. If you live near a river, pond, lake, canal, or other body of water, you need to be extra diligent in preventing your loved one from wandering out of the home. (See chapter 5.)

Trips and Falls

Many older people, especially those with Alzheimer's disease, have difficulty with stability, equilibrium, and reacting to a loss of balance. They are no longer able to quickly reach in front of them to cushion their fall or protect their face. (Refer also to chapter 8.)

Survey your home and yard for things that are broken and need to be repaired. Look for obvious dangers: rotting planks, cracked stair treads, wobbly handrails, lights that don't work, worn carpeting, uneven sidewalks, protruding deck nails, etc. Repair them now, before an accident occurs.

Remove pieces of furniture that are hard to see and easy to trip over, including small ottomans, magazine racks, standing floor lamps, coffee tables, end tables, and miscellaneous floor decorations.

Declining strength, hearing, or vision can also cause problems with balance, as can side effects from medications. If your loved one is taking sedatives or medications to induce sleep, or has difficulty hearing, his equilibrium may also be affected. Alzheimer's disease also creates unusual phenomena, such as visual cliffing and hallucinations. Your loved one may lose her balance or trip and fall while trying to avoid imagined obstacles. In addition, your home's lighting may cause shadows that can be misinterpreted.

Strategies that can help prevent falls include improved lighting, and sturdy, dependable furniture for support. Remove unreliable tables and chairs on wheels, furniture that wobbles or rocks or has only three legs. Install continuous railings along commonly used paths, especially along routes to and from the bathroom. (See chapter 8.)

Since people with Alzheimer's disease frequently do not sleep well at night, your loved one may tire easily and quickly. There may be times when she needs to sit down but cannot get to or find a chair. Provide comfortable chairs in convenient locations and create a soft, safe environment, just in case a fall does occur.

Clear pathways inside and outside your home. Often people with AD have a form of tunnel vision and don't see obstacles unless they are directly in front of them and at eye level. Remove low decorative furniture and pieces that blend into their background. Hard-to-see tables or chairs may be walked into or tripped over.

Installing grab bars and railings is among the best and least expensive ways to prevent falls. Put them anywhere and everywhere they may be needed. They are not just for the bathroom. (See the discussion on grab bars in this chapter.)

Stairs and steps are some of the most dangerous features of any home, but particularly for someone with Alzheimer's disease. So many skills and abilities are needed to negotiate a single step or go up and down stairs successfully—coordination and judgment, good vision and depth perception, timing, and adjustments to unanticipated changes, etc. We may take stairs for granted, but for a person who may no longer be able to operate two cabinet latches simultaneously, steps and stairs may be an impossible challenge. (See chapter 1 for more discussion on steps and stairs.)

Limit access to stairs or make them unnecessary. If you convert a first-floor room to a bedroom for your family member, he (and the caregiver) may no longer need to go upstairs. Stairs in multi-level homes are often a primary reason for converting a first-floor room to a master bedroom.

"Dad goes up the stairs fine, but he comes down backwards and very carefully."

For all the stairs and steps in your home, make sure that you have strong railings that continue for the full length of the stairs and around landings. Install railings on both sides of the stairs, so your family member can use them with her strongest arm both going up and coming down.

Often caregivers install gates only at the top or the bottom of stairs. This alone is a great precaution—but stairs and steps can be accessed from both the top and the bottom. If your loved one climbs the stairs and finds a closed gate at the top, his only alternative may be to turn around and come back down the stairs, a task that he may not be able to complete successfully. You can prevent this situation by installing strong, lockable gates at both the top *and* the bottom. (See also chapter 6.)

Provide multiple cues to alert both you and your loved one

when he has reached the top and bottom steps. All too often the next-to-the-last step is mistaken for the last, or the traveler gets to the top and expects one more step, resulting in a fall. Install full slip-resistant treads on the first and last step to make them different from the other steps. (You can provide front-edge, slip-resistant strips on all the others). A tactile warning strip (perhaps a piece of adhesive-backed Velcro) attached to the railing is also a good idea.

Slip-resistant safety stair treads:

American Health Care Supply, Consolidated Plastics, Mercer, Musson, R.C.A. Rubber Co., Reese.

First and last step alerts for stair railings:

Mature Mart, Step Ahead Product Innovations.

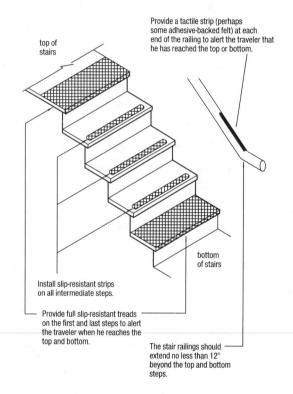

Provide a tactile strip (perhaps some adhesive-backed felt) at each end of the railing to alert the traveler that he has reached the top or bottom.

top of stairs

bottom of stairs

Install slip-resistant strips on all intermediate steps.

Provide full slip-resistant treads on the first and last steps to alert the traveler when he reaches the top and bottom.

The stair railings should extend no less than 12" beyond the top and bottom steps.

Full-size non-slip treads on the first and last steps offer subtle warnings that you have reached the top or bottom of a stairway. Intermediate steps can be equipped with smaller safety strips.

If you live on an upper floor, be particularly aware of doors leading to a balcony. Your family member may not realize that she does not live on a ground floor. If this represents a possible problem, install multiple locks and an alarm on the door leading to the balcony. (See chapter 6.)

Slippery winter ice on outdoor paths is dangerous. This hazard may be difficult to see or anticipate, even for those who are not confused. Take particular notice of areas where water and ice collect regularly. These would be good locations for a secure railing, whether there is a step there or not. Use locks or alarms on doors leading outside, even to yards that have been carefully safety-proofed for warmer seasons of the year.

Falls do not happen only when people are standing. Those with equilibrium problems can lean and fall when sitting on the toilet and hit their heads on the side of the tub or counter. Use fold-down grab bars on both sides of the toilet, not only to prevent such an incident but also to hold onto while sitting and getting up. (Refer to the discussion on grab bars later in this chapter.) Seat belts are also available to help keep your loved one from leaning and falling. However, the restraining factor may be frightening and will need to be dealt with carefully. An additional preventive measure is to cushion the edge of the sink and bathtub wall.

The sink counter can be padded with child-proof products specifically designed for this purpose. Inexpensive foam rubber pipe insulation can also be applied with adhesive-backed Velcro. These are both available at many home improvement centers. Specially designed bathtub wall cushions will make the tub much safer in the event of a fall. (See also chapter 1.)

"Irene can't sit up straight. She leans to one side. Last night she leaned over and fell right off the toilet, hitting her head on the side of the sink counter."

Seat belts to support and prevent leaning in chairs:

Posey Healthcare.

Toilet seat belts:

Posey Healthcare, Sammons Preston.

Child-proof table and counter edge cushions:

KidKusions, Perfectly Safe, Safety 1st, or baby supply stores.

Adhesive-backed Velcro:

Consumer Care Products, Sammons Preston, Smith & Nephew.

Bathtub wall cushions:

KidKusions.

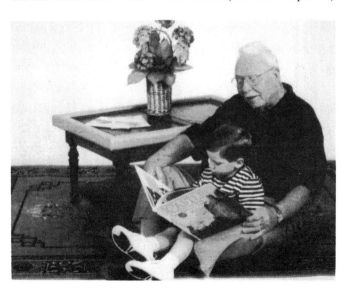

Edge cushions can be used to soften the edges of sharp tables and countertops. Photo courtesy KidKusions, Inc.

Remove outdoor furniture with flexible slats that allow a person's foot to go through them. Your loved one may try to stand on it or use it as a step to go over a fence and then become entangled in the slats.

Alzheimer's-Specific Dangers

In addition to common causes of injury, there are other dangers of which caregivers need to be aware. These hazards may only exist for those who are confused, such as trying to avoid imagined obstacles, protecting oneself from a perceived stranger, or defending personal space. Your best precautionary steps are observing your loved one and removing the conditions that seem to be causing the problems, real or imagined. For example, if a colored strip on the floor appears to be a hole, then cover it or paint it so that the "hole" is no longer there.

Uninterrupted Supervision

If your loved one has reached a stage where he is unable to care for himself, you certainly will want to ensure that he is never without quality care and supervision. This means considering the health and well-being of both the caregiver and the person with AD. If anything happened to the caregiver, such as a serious accident or sudden illness, what would happen to your family member? Would the paramedics realize that there was anything wrong with him, or would he be left alone to fend for himself? (Refer to the section entitled "Just In Case" in chapter 5 for precautions that you can take to help ensure that your loved one is not left alone in an emergency.)

Planning ahead is also important when you need to maintain uninterrupted supervision. Maximize storage throughout your home and provide extra storage in important areas, like the bathroom. You should never have to leave your loved one alone to get something as foreseeable as another roll of toilet paper or a towel.

Weapons in the Home

Without exception, either remove all weapons from your home or securely lock them away. It is not sufficient just to unload guns and rifles or place a trigger lock on them.

Imagine the following scenario: your family member accidentally happens upon an unloaded gun. He realizes that he should give it to you immediately. Off he goes looking for you, carrying the gun and walking down the corridor of your condominium or apartment complex. What would the neighbors think? What would the police do, maybe not realizing that your family member has Alzheimer's disease?

The same scenario could happen with knives or other weapon collections, even if they are far from the ammunition that would make them operable. Also consider toy guns that look real enough to be convincing, even to the police, or real pistols with locks that can still be picked up and carried.

Remove both weapons *and* ammunition. Even without a gun, ammunition is still dangerous if subjected to the right conditions—a fireplace, stove, furnace, oven, microwave oven, disposal, hammer, etc.

Wandering Away from Home

"Elopement," or wandering away from home, is one of the biggest concerns for those caring for a person with dementia, and rightly so. Beyond your front door are countless dangers over which you have no control: winter weather, rivers and canals, highways, woods, and people who prey on those less fortunate. It may be all too easy for your family member to wander outside and not be able to find his way back home. (See chapter 5.)

Driving

People with dementia and cars don't mix. This goes beyond getting lost. They can easily forget, for example, which pedal is the brake and which is the gas. They can hurt both themselves and others. Carefully observe your loved one. You will have to use your better judgment to determine when it is in everyone's best interest to take away driving privileges.

If your family member makes repeated attempts to drive, install a secret "kill" switch in your car that must be turned on before the car will start. This can be done by any store that installs car alarms or, of course, your mechanic; suddenly the car may "just need to be repaired."

Be sure to consider anything in your home that can be driven, including motorcycles, bicycles, and even a riding lawnmower.

And finally, remove reminders of driving, including keys to the car, suitcases, hats on hat racks, and briefcases, which may suggest driving to work, the store, etc.

Nocturnal Wandering

Nighttime wandering and sleep disturbances are common to those with AD, occurring usually when everyone else is asleep. Safety-proof your home to create the safest possible home to wander in. Minimize the possibility of accidents that may occur when your loved one is tired and it is dark, times when disorientation is most likely to occur. Do whatever you can to avoid accidents that might happen when no one is supervising and helping your loved one. (See chapter 5.)

Personal Space

Recognize that personal space is important to your family member, who may need definable and "defendable" space around her easy chair or seat on the porch. Your family member may feel she needs to take desperate actions to defend and protect herself, possibly reacting aggressively to perceived violations of her personal space. If this is a problem, clearly define the boundaries of her space, so that visitors, repairmen, and family members, as well as your loved one, know which lines of demarcation should not be violated. This can be achieved with furniture arrangements, tape, color, or any other creative means you can devise.

In addition to being a buffer zone, this space will allow your loved one to safely observe her surroundings, offering assurance that nothing is happening without her knowledge and that she is not being abandoned by the caregiver. Often the corners of rooms provide security on all sides, safe distance, and good opportunities for observation.

For times when your family member feels threatened, create a special place that represents safety and comfort. This should be a calming, favorite spot, with pleasant activities and diversions to take your loved one's mind off the concerns that are upsetting her. This could be a bench on the back porch or a favorite chair in a quiet room.

Diversions

Diversions are one of your best tools to defuse agitation, upsets, and catastrophic reactions. Here your family member's poor short-term memory can actually work to good advantage if you can divert his attention from what is bothering him long enough for him to forget.

"Look, Dad, that pesky squirrel is eating the bird seed again!"

Anything of interest can be a diversion: a bird feeder with a fake bird or a ceramic squirrel in the garden. Colorful flowers, pets, and chairs located in front of windows for viewing outside activity can all be used for diversion. Use your own creativity and knowledge of what catches your family member's attention. Provide opportunities for diversions throughout your home, particularly in places where agitation seems to repeatedly occur. Where your creativity fails, install a secret button that you can push at times of trouble, causing a doorbell or telephone to miraculously ring and require you both to refocus your attention on the "caller." (Refer to chapter 3 for more on diversions.)

Catastrophic Reactions

Catastrophic reactions are extreme reactions to seemingly normal or imagined events. Their cause can be rational, obscure, or only in the mind of your loved one. They can lead to violent behavior sufficient to cause accidents or injury.

Creating a therapeutic, forgiving environment and recognizing the special needs of a person with Alzheimer's may make it possible to avoid catastrophic reactions and the injury that may accompany them. Your goal is to create a home that is both safe and calming; one that encourages the successful completion of tasks and avoids opportunities for failures and upsets.

"Sometimes my husband gets so angry that he becomes violent, throwing anything he can get his hands on."

Recognize that catastrophic reactions can have serious consequences. For example, if someone (caregiver, family, or friend) gets seriously hurt and the police become involved, they might not realize that your loved one suffers from Alzheimer's. They have a protocol in assault situations, and without this information your loved one could wind up in jail. (Refer to the section entitled "Just in Case" in chapter 5.)

If your loved one is prone to catastrophic reactions, don't wait for a serious accident. People with dementia sometimes throw things or use common household items as weapons. Anything within reach may be fair game. These unusual behaviors may justify extraordinary precautions. Replace anything that can be used as a weapon or projectile with softer, safer items that are less likely to cause injury or damage.

Avoiding Unpleasant Reminders

Avoid reminders of the disease. Any failure or inability to complete a task is a reminder that something is wrong—and a possible trigger for a catastrophic reaction. Accidents, trips or falls, forgotten events, and misplaced items are potential reminders of the disease. Even forgetfulness or absentmindedness, common to us all, takes on a disproportional meaning to a person with Alzheimer's disease and the person caring for them.

Bear in mind that your home may contain reminders of a departed loved one: photographs, portraits on the wall, letters, and personal possessions. Do they trigger sadness and discomfort from mourning a loss over and over, each time your family member is reminded of a loved one's passing?

If this is a problem, consider editing photo albums and displays of memorabilia to limit their contents to people that are still alive. If, on the other hand, these reminders are not sources of discomfort, but rather pleasurable reminders that bring back good feelings, then by all means encourage these activities. Observe your loved one and act accordingly.

Anything can be a source of discomfort or loss. One woman we know had a sundial in her backyard, but to her it looked like a cemetery stone. She would go there and sob as if she had just lost her sister (who had died a few years before)— every day, over and over and over. The sundial was eventually removed, and the problem was eliminated.

Grab Bars and Railings

Alzheimer's disease is an extraordinary disease with its own unique problems. Many common tools and devices can be used in creative ways to address these problems. Grab bars are an excellent example. They can be used not only to assist one in getting up from the toilet and preventing falls in the bathtub or shower, but also in other ways.

Grab bars benefit everyone, not only the person with Alzheimer's but also the caregiver, guests, and other members of the family. They are great helps when the caregiver needs something to lean on when lifting or transferring a loved one, and of course they are great aids for a family member wherever extra help is needed . . . *anywhere* in the home.

Grab Bars as Diversions

In the shower install a set of grab bars on the far wall, opposite the door.

When Ernie turns, he'll face away from both the caregiver and the exit from the shower. In this instance the grab bar is not only a safety device but also a diversion, redirecting Ernie's attention from likely sources of agitation—the escape from the shower and the "stranger" bathing him.

"Ernie, turn around and hold on to the grab bar with both hands to make sure you are safe and don't fall in the shower."

The grab bar also enables Ernie to contribute to his own caregiving by assuming a small though significant responsibility. Using the grab bar this way makes an otherwise undignified task (being bathed by a "stranger") a little more dignified. It may make Ernie calmer about bathing and less likely to become upset or resist bathing.

Grab Bars as Guides

Imagine walking to the end of a hallway and you have a choice of going right or left. You look down the corridor to your right and see that it is dimly lit and has no grab bars or railings. The corridor to your left is well lit and has continuous railings and grab bars on both sides all the way to the end. Which way would you go?

Alzheimer's sufferers tend to seek the paths of least resistance, those that appear safe and most likely to result in success. Railings and grab bars represent safety and minimize the likelihood of a fall. They are a guide for your loved one and an invitation to travel the routes that they line. Railings can also be used to direct your loved one away from dangers by making the safer route more attractive.

Add railings wherever they might be useful—in long hallways, on walls along the path from the bed to the bathroom, and in other areas where your loved one may have difficulty. Continue railings around corners to act as directional cues. Railings offer a sense of security that may make otherwise intimidating or confusing paths a little safer and reassuring.

Railings should be continuous wherever possible. Interruptions due to doors can be fixed by installing short railings or grab bars on them, thus maintaining continuity. (Install railings only on doors that are kept locked. If the door were opened while your family member was holding the railing, it could throw him off balance or startle him.)

Have railings and grab bars, especially those on doors, installed by a good handyman or contractor. For example, a hollow core door may need extra reinforcement. A good handyman or contractor will have the proper tools and know how to do this. (For more discussion on installing grab bars refer to the section on installation later in this chapter.)

Grab Bars as Camouflage

Imagine that halfway down a corridor your family member comes to that three-foot gap in the railing caused by a locked closet door. Installing a grab bar on the door will not only continue the railing and eliminate the gap, but also camouflage the door so your family member will be less likely to recognize or try to open it. After all, doors don't have grab bars on them!

Grab Bars as Warnings

Wherever you have a single step or a few steps, provide a grab bar on the adjacent wall. For dangers created by areas like sunken living rooms, a pair of railings will offer much-appreciated support; otherwise they will be avoided or remain hazardous. Railings in these locations will not only provide necessary support to avoid an accident, but also call attention to a danger that might otherwise be overlooked.

Continuous railings on staircases change from sloping to level at landings. They provide both continuous support and subtle warnings of the approaching platform and last step.

Preventing Falls

Quite often paramedics are called to a scene where an older person has fallen off the toilet. Leaning to one side or not maintaining balance is a common problem for those with AD. Many lean, fall, and hit their heads against the tub wall or the edge of the sink counter.

Floor/wall-mounted or fold-down grab bars on either side of the toilet can prevent leaning and falling to either side. Fold-down grab bars offer an added advantage in that they can be lifted up and out of the way when the toilet is used by other family members, or for transferring to the toilet from a wheelchair. (Refer to the discussion of toileting in chapter 4.)

A fold-down grab bar mounted at the top of the stairs can be lowered to prevent your loved one from falling back down the stairs, maybe while getting up from a stair lift, or just to help him regain his stability once at the top. Once balance is regained and your family member is no longer near the stairs, the bar can be raised out of the way.

Fold-down grab bars:
American Health Care Supply, ASI, Barclay, Basco, Bobrick, Carex, DSI, Elcoma, ETAC USA, Frohock-Stewart, Häfele America, HEWI, Invacare Continuing Care, Lumex, McKesson, Otto Bock, Sammons Preston, Tubular Specialties Mfg., or home improvement centers.

Fold-down grab bars that store almost flush with the wall: Lumex.

Miscellaneous Uses

One long railing in the hallway or in the backyard can be a way your loved one can judge his physical strength and provide valuable, safe exercise that can also be supervised from a distance. Freddy was proud of his ability to go up and down that bar, often telling me (with great pride), "Today I made it up there and back *three times*." Exercise is a part of peoples' lives and can continue to be important as long as there are safe means provided. Your home offers plenty of opportunities for you to provide exercise, whether it is with a wandering

"For as long as he could, Freddy would take me down the hallway to his favorite railing and show me how many times he could walk up and down without help, all by himself."

path, long railing, or exercise equipment. (See chapter 4 for more suggestions.)

We have described only a few creative uses for grab bars and railings. This type of imaginative thought is part of any difficult challenge, especially when caring for a loved one with Alzheimer's disease at home. Though we mentioned only a few, I am sure you will discover new locations where grab bars will serve you and your loved one well.

Locations for Grab Bars

Different uses and specific requirements should be carefully considered when selecting locations for grab bars. The general rule is: Provide a grab bar anywhere and everywhere you or your loved one might need one.

Locate grab bars where your family member or the caregiver may need a little extra support—next to the bathroom scale, at a step going into the house, at the kitchen or bathroom sink, where your family member stands to get dressed or to dry off after a bath or shower. Many grab bars are reasonably priced, making it possible to put them wherever they may be needed throughout the home. Grab bars that are designed for wet environments (the bathroom) are also good for outdoor locations.

Locate grab bars also where the caregiver may need a little extra help. Caregivers often have to lift the person they are caring for out of bed, assist them in the shower or tub, or get them up from a favorite chair or the toilet. They may have to take the full weight of your loved one with nothing else to rely on. Grab bars for these purposes have to be selected and located carefully. A few simple steps taken now can be a big help and prevent back pain later, especially when the caregiver is not very strong or is substantially smaller than the care-receiver.

Even the ways people approach and sit down on the toilet may differ. Those needing assistance often approach the toilet head on, turn around, and sit down, holding onto the grab bars on both sides of the toilet for stability. When a caregiver is involved, he or she might stand behind the person approaching the toilet, turn him around, and help by holding his hand (or under his arm), supporting his weight and lowering him in place. For this purpose, an additional set of grab bars might be located higher and closer to where the caregiver will need them. Someone moving to the toilet from a wheelchair will have different uses for grab bars, and they need to be selected and located accordingly.

Every situation is unique, requiring attention to the exact location, angle, height, distance from the user, and type of grab bar. Grab bars need to be selected according to how they will be used, pushed on, pulled on, leaned on, or just held for steadiness. They need to be located according to your loved one's condition, characteristics, strengths, and weaknesses. For example, your family member may be especially dependent on one side of his body, because of right- or left-handedness or the effects of a stroke. If so, grab bars must be located to make use of his stronger side and to offer support coming and going—both getting into the tub or shower and getting out. There is no one rule or standard location for installing grab bars.

A physical or occupational therapist is the best person to help you locate your grab bars for their particular purpose and use. A properly located grab bar can prevent injury and even save lives. It can make the difference between a grab bar that is helpful and one that is useless.

Locate grab bars to assist in *all* tasks associated with each area. One size does not fit all, and one grab bar does not serve all purposes. For example, install grab bars to help a person:

- *get into* the tub
- *sit down* in the tub
- *get up* from the tub
- *step out* of the tub.

Types of Grab Bars

Grab bars come in various shapes, angles, colors, textures, lengths, and combinations. There are grab bars designed for almost any location and conceivable use:

Grab bars:

Access with Ease, Aids for Arthritis, American Health Care Supply, ASI, Basco, Bobrick, Bradley, Carex, Crest, Cwego, DSI, Easy Street, Facilis, Franklin Brass, Frohock-Stewart, Guardian Products, Häfele America, Home Health Care Products, J. C. Penney Special Needs Catalogue, Keeney, Lumex, Maddak, Maxi Aids, McKesson, Olsonite, Sammons Preston, Tubular Specialties Mfg., Winco, home improvement centers.

Plastic-coated grab bars:

Häfele America.

- wall-mounted grab bars
- floor-mounted grab bars
- multiple-handled grab bars
- fold-down grab bars
- grab bars in decorator colors
- single-handled grab bars
- grab bars in modular sections
- grab bar poles with handles or rings
- seat-mounted grab bars (for toilet seats)
- portable grab bars (such as walkers or clamp-on bathtub handles)
- textured grab bars for better grasping in slippery, wet, or soapy locations
- plastic-coated grab bars that do not conduct heat like those with a metal surface. (If the water is too hot in the shower, the grab bar won't absorb that heat and become too hot to touch.)

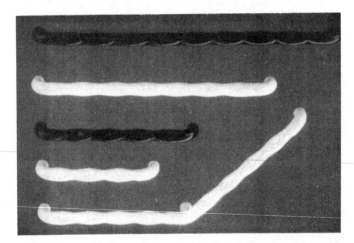

Grab bars come in a number of shapes and sizes for various locations in your home. Photo courtesy DSI.

Some companies offer grab bars to fit custom showers and configurations. These come in lengths that you can special order to line up with your exact wall stud locations or in angles and combinations to wrap around or follow the most complicated shower or bath.

Sturdy poles with grab bar handles can come in handy at the tub, next to the bed, or next to your family member's favorite easy chair.

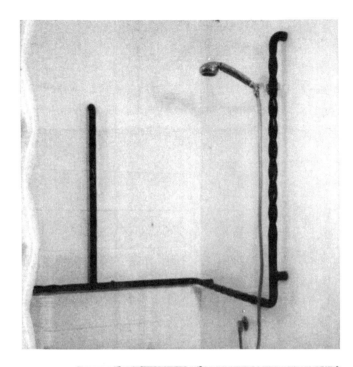

Custom grab bars:

DSI, Häfele America.

Continuous grab bars can be custo-
mized to fit the shape of any shower
or bathtub. Photo courtesy DSI.

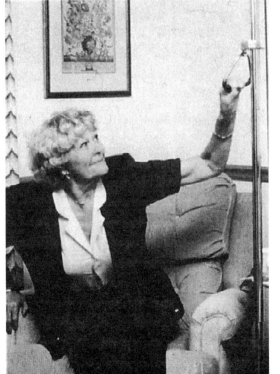

**Poles with handles that attach to
the floor and ceiling:**

HealthCraft Products, Independent
Living Products, M.O.M.S., North
Coast Medical, Sears Home
HealthCare Catalogue.

For locations where there is no wall to
attach a grab bar, provide a pole with
handles.

Textured grab bars:

Basco, Crest, DSI, Frohock-Stewart, Guardian Products, Lumex, Maxi Aids.

Single grab bar handles:

Access with Ease, AdaptAbility, Aids for Arthritis, AliMed, LS & S Maddak, North Coast Medical, Sammons Preston.

WaveGrip grab bars:
DSI.

Grab bars in decorator colors:

Franklin Brass, Häfele America, GAMCO, Keeney.

At the shower or tub, or wherever soapy hands need something to hold, install bars with textured surfaces.

Long grab bars are not always necessary. Simple, shorter grab bars are useful in various locations for a little support and stability. Small handles installed vertically can be secured to a single wall stud, making their installation easier and stronger.

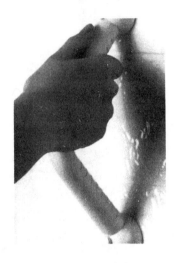 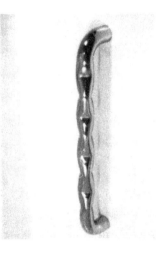

Small, inexpensive grab bars offer valuable support when a larger grab bar is unnecessary. Photo courtesy Sammons Preston, a BISSELL® Healthcare Company. Reprinted with permission.

The WaveGrip grab bar is contoured to fit the shape of your hand. Photo courtesy DSI.

Grab bars do not have to look institutional. There are grab bars in decorator colors, brass and gold-colored grab bars, and grab bars with interesting spiraling textures that ergonomically conform to the shape of a hand. This also makes it possible to install grab bars that contrast to the wall behind, making them easy to spot in a hurry.

And, of course, there are fold-down grab bars that can be mounted to the wall behind a toilet or those that come with their own free-standing columns. (See the photo in chapter 4.)

There are also "residential" and "commercial" grab bars. Residential grab bars vary considerably in quality and often lack the consistency and safety of commercial grab bars, which comply with the standards set by the American Disabilities Act. Whether you buy commercial or residential grab bars, there are certain standards to consider.

Grab bars should be 1¼ to 1½ inches in diameter. Smaller, weaker hands may have an easier time grasping the smaller diameter bar (1¼ inches).

The gap between the grab bar and the wall should be exactly 1½"—no more, no less. If the grab bar is any further from the wall, your family member's arm may slip through the gap and get caught between the grab bar and the wall. If she then falls, her arm could be broken or shoulder dislocated. If the grab bar is any closer to the wall, it may be difficult for her to get her hand around the bar to properly grasp it, or her fingers could get pinched.

These recommendations are in accordance with the Americans with Disabilities Act. Some manufacturers of residential grab bars argue that these standards are for commercial installations only. They offer grab bars for home use that are ⅞" to 1" in diameter and that extend as much as 3 inches away from the wall. They tell us that a 3-inch projection allows users to lean on the bars more fully.

We nonetheless recommend that all grab bars extend no more or less than 1½ inches from the wall for safety. Both commercial and residential grab bars are available for purchase and use in the home. Refer to the following section of shopping tips for grab bars before going shopping.

Towel bars (soap dishes, toilet paper holders, etc.) are not designed or installed to support a person's weight. The well-being of both the caregiver and the person with AD may depend on a grab bar. Don't gamble on a towel bar that can unexpectedly detach from the wall.

Towel bars are not grab bars!

Shopping Tips

- Look for small, single grab bar handles for extra support in special locations.
- Make sure the back plates used to attach the bars to a wall are not plastic. (Plastic back plates can

crack or break if the screw is the wrong type or if it is tightened too much, making the plate and grab bar unreliable.)

- Look for back plates that have multiple holes allowing installation at an angle if needed. You'll need a choice of holes to line the screws up with the vertical wall studs.
- Make sure the grab bars cannot rotate in their own supports. This is more likely to be true for certain residential grab bars or towel bars resembling grab bars.
- The space between the grab bar and wall should be 1½ inches.
- Make sure your grab bars conform to the requirements set forth by the Americans with Disabilities Act (ADA) and are so labeled.

Installation

"Do we have to use those big long screws to attach grab bars?"

"Can we attach our grab bars to the tile?"

Grab bars must be attached properly to do any good—and too often, they're not. An improperly attached grab bar may be more dangerous than no grab bar at all.

Grab bars must be securely attached to strong, structural components inside your wall not the wall finish material (tile, drywall, etc.). The two most common types of walls are stud walls (wood or metal) and masonry walls. Wood studs are the most reliable; walls with steel studs may require a plate on the other side and bolts going all the way through. Each type requires different fasteners, and it is important that you use the right ones. You are depending on strong, secure attachments to support you and your loved one in an emergency.

Grab bars should be installed only by someone who knows what he or she is doing. It is important that your installer knows the construction of your wall and where the studs are located, and has the right tools. He or she should know how many and what kind of screws or bolts to use, how long they should be, whether additional backing (internal wall supports) will be necessary—and how to repair your wall afterward.

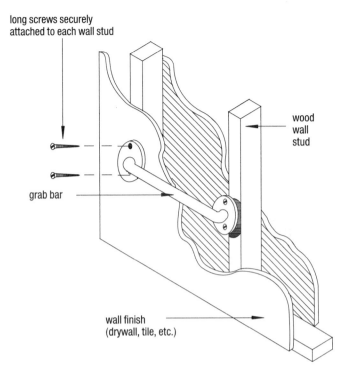

long screws securely
attached to each wall stud

wood
wall
stud

grab bar

wall finish
(drywall, tile, etc.)

Grab bar installation in a wood-stud wall, cutaway view. Remember to consult your physical or occupational therapist to determine the best locations for grab bars. For new construction, you can add a sheet of ¾" plywood behind the wall finish material so that location is not limited by the wall studs.

Your wall studs are supposed to be exactly 16" or 24" on center, depending on the type of wall. Sometimes, though, studs wind up being just a little (or a lot) off. For those situations, there are modular grab bars, which come in sections and can be ordered at specific lengths to fit your exact stud locations perfectly.

Molded fiberglass showers are especially difficult to install grab bars in. Their curved shapes create gaps between the walls and the studs behind them. Any attempt to tighten the screws for a secure fit only deforms the wall, and it ultimately cracks. However, one company offers the Solid Mount, a spacer and mounting bracket specifically designed to fill that gap and allow you to install grab bars in fiberglass showers. It may sound difficult, but all you have to do is locate the studs (with a stud finder), drill a hole, and measure the distance to the stud. Then, by trimming the spacer to your measurement, you'll have the exact fitting to allow you to attach the grab bar and get a nice, strong installation, no matter how complex your curved shower may be.

Modular grab bars:

DSI, Häfele America, Keeney.

The Solid Mount, a spacer for installing grab bars in curved fiberglass showers:

Back to Basics Innovative Design.

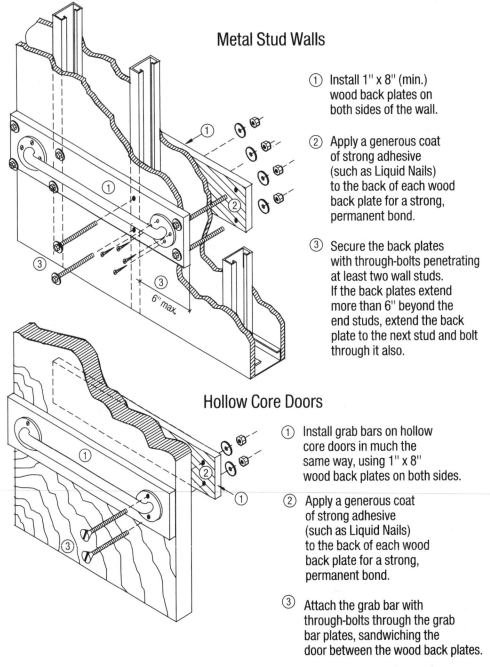

Metal Stud Walls

① Install 1" x 8" (min.) wood back plates on both sides of the wall.

② Apply a generous coat of strong adhesive (such as Liquid Nails) to the back of each wood back plate for a strong, permanent bond.

③ Secure the back plates with through-bolts penetrating at least two wall studs. If the back plates extend more than 6" beyond the end studs, extend the back plate to the next stud and bolt through it also.

6" max.

Hollow Core Doors

① Install grab bars on hollow core doors in much the same way, using 1" x 8" wood back plates on both sides.

② Apply a generous coat of strong adhesive (such as Liquid Nails) to the back of each wood back plate for a strong, permanent bond.

③ Attach the grab bar with through-bolts through the grab bar plates, sandwiching the door between the wood back plates.

(The inside back plate will have to be slightly shorter on both the right and left sides to get past the door trim when closing the door.)

Installing grab bars in difficult locations.

Safety-proofing your home is no matter to be taken lightly. Along with it comes the responsibility of being thorough, discovering every little thing your loved one might get into, and recognizing dangers in your home, given your family member's unique and changing condition. Do the best you can. No one is perfect and the task you are taking on is immense.

Safety-proofing is an ongoing process. No home will ever become completely safe. Continue to observe and adjust. As the disease progresses, you will discover new hazards, and ordinary situations will develop into problems—act on them. Once again, join a support group. These people will help you through each difficult period and help you discover what may or may not be dangerous and some things that you might have forgotten or overlooked.

And finally, don't be too hard on yourself. Alzheimer's disease is a challenge. No one is expected to anticipate or foresee every danger or be able to remove it in time. The best that you can ever provide is the best that you can provide. And no one appreciates that more than your loved one (whether or not he or she is able to tell you).

Products & Manufacturers

Buying through catalogues and mail order houses can be a real lifesaver, especially if getting out and going shopping for hard-to-find products is a luxury. The following is a list of manufacturers offering products of all kinds that are referred to in this book.

These are not the only companies that manufacture these products, nor were we able to mention all of the applicable products that each of these companies offers. We are not endorsing these companies or making any statements about the quality of their products. We are just making the information available to you so that you can call, get the information, and do your homework.

Many of these manufacturers have toll free telephone numbers, making it that much easier for you to call them, ask for their catalogues, local representatives, or where you can buy the products locally. I am sure they will be happy to hear from you.

Different companies offer the same products, and several are representatives of the same manufacturers. They may differ, however, in their prices. So we offer their names in as many places as they may apply. Call, get their catalogues, and compare prices.

Finally, don't forget the additional charges for taxes (if applicable) and shipping and handling. The quoted costs for the individual products normally do not include these additional charges.

There are countless other companies that offer other creative products that would benefit our readers. We may be unaware of some products because they are not marketed widely. And some of the products listed here, though beneficial, have been discontinued because it became too costly to continue manufacturing them. We hope this doesn't continue to happen to even one more product.

I apologize for any inadvertent omissions or out-of-date information. I invite companies to provide us with information on them and their products so that they might be included in future editions of this book and in other books that we publish. Please forward that information to: Ageless Design, 12633 159th Court North, Jupiter, FL 33478.

Companies marked with a single asterisk (*) are mail order companies offering a wide range of products. However, upon review of their catalogues, it was noted that some of their products were applicable and may be of interest to our readers.

Some of these companies may not sell directly to the public. In these cases, call the listed phone number and ask for the name of your local representative. If the company is a large, well-known company and the product is relatively standard, such as a door hinge or thermostat, stores in your local area may carry the product. Or ask your local hardware store or home improvement center if they can order it for you.

Disclaimer—Neither Ageless Design, Inc., nor the author has necessarily examined, reviewed, or tested any product, device, or company referred to in this book. Neither Ageless Design, Inc., nor the author makes any endorsement, representation, or warranty, either expressed or implied, regarding any company or product mentioned. We are not responsible for the actions, products, services, quality, effectiveness, or accidents that might be associated with or caused by products referred to or offered by manufacturers listed in this publication.

Readers should also be aware that requesting catalogues from any company might result in their names getting on mailing lists. You may wish to specifically request that your name not be given to other companies or placed on that company's mailing list if you wish not to receive other unsolicited literature.

COMPANY NAME	TELEPHONE NUMBER	PRODUCT
Abbey Enterprises 235 W. First Street Bayonne, NJ 07002	(800) 552-5629 (201) 823-3690	The Sofa Saver pressure-sensitive pad and alarm
Absolute Environmentals 3504 S. University Drive Davie, FL 33328	(800) 329-3773 (954) 472-3773	Air cleaning and air purification machines
Accent on Living P.O. Box 700 Bloomington, IL 61702-0700	(800) 787-8444 (309) 378-2961	Products for those with special problems and disabilities; the magazine Accent on Living
Access Industries 4001 East 138 Street Grandview, MO 64030-2840	(800) 925-3100 (816) 763-3100	Porch lifts, stair lifts, & residential elevators
Access One 25679 Gramford Avenue North Wyoming, MN 55092	(800) 561-2223 (612) 462-3444	Beyond Barriers catalogue of products for daily living

Access to Recreation 8 Sandra Court Newbury Park, CA 91320	(800) 634-4351 (805) 498-7535	Recreational and accessibility products for those in wheelchairs
Access with Ease P.O. Box 1150 Chino Valley, AZ 86323	(800) 531-9479 (520) 636-9469	Gardening supplies and miscellaneous aids for daily living; "After Therapy" catalogue
Acorn Industries 21400 Tudor Drive Boca Raton, FL 33486-1411	(561) 750-8276	Genijet, a bidet attachment for residential toilets
Activeaid, Inc. 101 Activeaid Road P.O. Box 359 Redwood Falls, MN 56283	(800) 533-5330 (507) 644-2951	Bathroom and bathing aids, bed rails
AdaptAbility (S & S Worldwide) P.O. Box 515 Colchester, CT 06415-0515	(800) 288-9941 (800) 243-9232	Miscellaneous products for daily living
ADD Interior Systems, Inc. (Kruger International) 1330 Belleview Road Green Bay, WI 54302	(920) 468-8100	Chairs designed for seniors
Adden Furniture, Inc. 26 Jackson Street Lowell, MA 01852	(800) 625-3876 (978) 454-7848	Chairs designed for seniors
ADI 213 E. Luzerne Ave. Larksville, PA 18704	(800) 839-9025 (717) 288-5561	The Enhan-Sit motorized platform, which converts an easy chair to a motorized lifting chair
Adjustable Fixture Co. 3726 N. Booth Street Milwaukee, WI 53212	(800) 558-2628	Safe, durable table lamps that can be secured to the table, preventing them from being knocked over
Aids for Arthritis, Inc. 3 Little Knoll Court Medford, NJ 08055	(800) 654-0707 (609) 654-6918	Unique products for the home and for those with special problems or disabilities.

The Air Sponge Filter Co. 11905 N.W. 35 Street Coral Springs, FL 33065	(800) 757-1836 (954) 752-1836	Activated carbon air conditioning filters
Alert Care 591 Redwood Highway Suite 2125 Mill Valley, CA 94941	(800) 826-7444 (415) 381-9009	Wander-alerting and fall-prevention devices
AliMed, Inc. 297 High Street Dedham, MA 02026	(800) 225-2610 (617) 329-2900	Products for daily living
Alsons Corporation 3010 West Mechanic Street Hillsdale, MI 49242	(800) 421-0001 (517) 439-1411	Hand-held shower head assemblies
Alsto's Handy Helpers P.O. Box 1267 Galesburg, IL 61401	(800) 447-0048 (309) 343-6181	Assistive products for outdoor enthusiasts and miscellaneous daily living aids
American Health Care Supply 100 South Milwaukee Vernon Hills, IL 60061	(800) 677-7180 (847) 743-1000	Products from personal care to room accessories
American Health Systems P.O. Box 26688 Greenville, SC 29616-1688	(800) 234-6655 (864) 234-0496	Mattresses with supportive edges
American Medical Alert Corp. 3265 Lawson Blvd. Oceanside, NY 11572	(800) 645-3244	Personal Emergency Response System (PERS)
American Stair-Glide (Access Industries) 4001 E. 138th Street Grandview, MO 64030	(800) 925-3100 (800) 825-1220	Residential elevators, inclined stair lifts
American Technology Network (ATN) 20 South Linden Avenue Suite 1B South San Francisco, CA 94080	(650) 875-0130	Clock radio with hidden surveillance camera that sends picture to television in caregiver's room
American Thermometer Company 6212 Executive Boulevard Huber Heights, OH 45424-1420	(800) 826-9709 (513) 233-5080	Temperature indicators, safety products, and "Stop - Hot" labels

Ameriphone 12082 Western Ave. Garden Grove, CA 92841	(800) 874-3005 TTY (800) 772-2889 (714) 897-0808	Amplified telephone ringers and telephone handsets, lamp flashers, vibrating telephone ringers, remote answering systems, and other telephone devices
Apex Dynamics, Inc. 332 Reece Road Dawsonville, GA 30534	(800) 742-0453 (706) 265-4024	The Concept 2000 mechanical bath seat
Aqua Bath 921 Cherokee Avenue Nashville, TN 37207	(800) ADA-BATH (615) 227-0017	Shower ramp, prefabricated shower modules, bathtubs with built-in seats
Arden Architectural Specialties 151 5th Ave., NW, Suite J St. Paul, MN 55112-3268	(800) 521-1826 (651) 631-1607	Wall and corner protection products
Aremco Grove House Lenham, Kent ME17 2PX England	(44) 1 622-858502	Fall prevention pad alarms and devices that insert under one leg of the bed or chair to alert caregiver that loved one has gotten up.
ASI American Specialties, Inc. 441 Saw Mill River Road Yonkers, N.Y. 10701-9986	(914) 476-9000	Bathroom equipment
Assist Equip, Inc. P.O. Box 1558 1916 West Avenue Levelland, TX 79336	(800) 654-9664 (806) 894-5700	Assistive bed post
Austin Air 500 Elk Street Buffalo, NY 14210	(800) 724-8403 (716) 856-3704	Air cleaning and air purification machines
Austin Innovations P.O. Box 202530 Austin, TX 78720	(800) 669-6766 (512) 339-6765	The LimeLight, a safe night light that is always cool to the touch
Back to Basics Innovative Design 9672 Colchester Drive Anaheim, CA 92804	(714) 533-3636	Special spacers for mounting grab bars to fiberglass showers

Bailey Manufacturing Company 118 Lee Street Lodi, OH 44254	(800) 321-8372 (234) 948-1080	Exercise equipment, wheelchair transfer boards, etc.
Barbara Jacobs Productions, Inc. P.O. Box 6906 San Rafael, CA 94903	(415) 479-2630	Sing-along video respite tapes, complete with lyric book
Barclay Products, Ltd. 400 Porett Drive Gurnee, IL 60031	(847) 244-1234 (800) 446-9700	Shower seats with arms, Sinks that raise and lower, grab bars, relocatable shower water temperature valves, folding shower seat, fold-down grab bar.
Barr Mobility (Transfer Master Products) 368 West Stoneman P.O. Box 917 Postville, IA 52162	(800) 475-8122 (319) 864-7364	Electric adjustable beds
Barrier-Free Lifts, Inc. 9230 Prince William St. Manassas, VA 20110	(800) 582-8732 (703) 361-6531	Lifting and transferring equipment
Basco 40 Aero Road P.O. Box 237 Bohemia, NY 11716	(800) 835-4445 (516) 567-4404	Adjustable and sloping medicine cabinet mirrors
BathEase, Inc. 3815 Darston Street Palm Harbour, FL 34685-3119	(888) 747-7845 (727) 786-2604	Wheelchair-accessible bathtubs and showers
Bed-Check Corp. 307 East Brady Street Tulsa, OK 74120	(800) 523-7956 (918) 592-3338	Pressure-release bed monitoring alarm
Bed Handles, Inc. 4825 S. Tierney Drive Independence, MO 64055	(800) 725-6903 (816) 220-7725	Bed handles & rails
Bendix of North America 2807 Antigua Drive Burbank, CA 91504	(888) 423-6349 (818) 843-1845	Front-loading washer/dryer combination that requires no venting

Better Living 411 Waverly Oaks Road P.O. Box 9199 Waltham, MA 02454-9199	(800) 424-6848	Electric lift that attaches to any easy chair, converting it to a lift chair (item #UL100), gold medical bracelets and "dog" tags (add your own message)
Better Living Products 201 Chrislea Road Vaughan, Ontario L4L 8N6 Canada	(800) 487-3300 (905) 264-7100	Wall-mounted soap & shampoo dispenser for shower
Bissell Inc. 2345 Walker Road Grand Rapids, MI 49544	(800) 237-7691	Small portable wet/dry vacuum cleaner (the Green Machine)
Black & Decker, Inc. 6 Armstrong Road Shelton, CT 06484-4797	(800) 231-9786	Products and aids for daily living, emergency lights and flashlights
Bossert Specialties, Inc. P.O. Box 15441 Phoenix, AZ 85060	(800) 776-5885 (602) 956-6637	Products for the visually impaired, talking clocks and calculators
Bradley Corporation Div. of Washroom Accessories 7020 West Parkland Court Milwaukee, WI 53223	(800) 272-3539 (414) 354-0100	Fold-down shower seats, grab bars, canted mirrors
Brainerd Mfg. Corp. 314 Chimney Rock Road Greensboro, NC 27409	(800) 652-7277	Safety and childproof products
Briggs Corporation P.O. Box 1698 Des Moines, IA 50306-1698	(800) 247-2343	Stop signs, directional arrows, signage, and other products
BRK Brands, Inc. 3901 Liberty Street Road Aurora, IL 60504	(800) 392-1395 (630) 851-7330	First Alert safety products for fire protection
Broda Enterprises 385 Phillip Street West Waterloo, Ontario N2L 5R8 Canada	(800) 668-0637 (519) 746-8080	Rocker Gliders

Brookstone 1655 Bassford Drive Mexico, MO 65265-1382	(800) 926-7000	Miscellaneous products for daily living
Brown Engineering Corporation 289 Chesterfield Road Westhampton, MA 01027	(800) 726-4233 (413) 527-1800	The Bed Bar bed handle
Bruno Independent Living 1780 Executive Drive P.O. Box 84 Oconomowoc, WI 53066-0084	(800) 882-8183 (262) 567-4990	Stair lifts
The Cable Connection, Inc. 5224 Highway 50 East Carson City, NV 89701	(800) 851-2961	Steel cables to add additional cables rails to balcony railings
Canwood Products P.O. Box 585 Beaumont, CA 92223	(909) 769-1449	Automatic telephone recorders, surveillance cameras, and security products
Care Catalogue Services 1877 NE Seventh Avenue Portland, OR 97212	(800) 443-7091 (503) 288-8174	Portable ramps, bathroom equipment, lifting easy chairs
Care Electronics 4700 Sterling Drive Suite D Boulder, CO 80301	(888) 444-8284 (303) 444-2273	Wander-tracking devices
Care Trak Route 1 Box 427A Carbondale, IL 62901-9745	(800) 842-4537	Wander alerting systems with tracking capabilities
Carex Health Care Products (Rubbermaid) 3124 Valley Ave. Winchester, VA 22601	(800) 526-8051 (540) 667-8700	Health care products
Carroll Healthcare 1881 Huron Street London, Ontario N5V 3A5 Canada	(888) 466-7656 (519) 659-1395	Bed that can be raised and lowered

CEMCO P.O. Box 500 2801 Township Line Road Hatfield, PA 19440	(800) 726-7380 (215) 703-0358	Residential elevators
Champion Mfg. Corp. 2601 Industrial Parkway Elkhart, IN 46516	(800) 998-5018 (219) 295-6893	Heavy-duty recliner
Charles-Bar Lok Corp. 111 West 154th Street South Holland, IL 60473	(708) 333-0071	The Charley Bar, a lock for sliding glass doors
Chatham Brass Co. 5 Olsen Avenue Edison, NJ 08820	(800) 526-7553 (732) 494-7107	Lockable thermostat guards and covers
Chicago Clock & Gifts Co. 431 Ogden Avenue Clarendon Hills, IL 60514	(630) 986-9210	Clocks with the day of the week and date
Clarion Fiberglass Mfg. 205 Amsler Ave. Shippenville, PA 16254	(800) 576-9228 (814) 226-5374	Prefabricated fiberglass shower units
Clarke Healthcare Products 1003 International Drive Oakdale, PA 15071-9226	(412) 809-0185	The Aquatec bathtub lift
Clever Solutions, Inc. 2122 Agin Court Ann Arbor, MI 48103	(800) 743-6165 (734) 668-2524	Sliding shower/bath transfer seat with rotating seat, chest and lap belt
Clock's Medical Supply P.O. Box 620 901 Industrial Road Winfield, KS 67156	(800) 362-1314 (316) 221-0550	The Stopper Kit, stop signs that go across door openings, "STOP" and "DO NOT ENTER" signs
Collectors' Choice Music P.O. Box 838 Itasca, IL 60143-0938	(800) 923-1122	Music from the good ol' days
Collins & Aikman Floor Coverings P.O. Box 1447 Dalton, GA 30722-1447	(800) 241-4902 (706) 259-9711	Non-absorbent, anti-microbial carpeting

Colonial Medical Alert 14 Celina Avenue, Unit #15 Nashua, NH 03063	(800) 323-6794 (603) 881-8351	Personal Emergency Response System (PERS) and door alarms
Columbia Medical Mfg. Corp. P.O. Box 633 Palisades, CA 90272	(800) 454-6612 (310) 454-6612	Toilet seats for leaning that offer back support, arms, seat belt, and foot supports.
Columbus McKinnon 140 John James Audubon Pkwy. Amherst, NY 14228-1197	(800) 888-0985 (716) 689-5400	Lifts and transfer equipment
Comfortex P.O. Box 850 Winona, MN 55987	(800) 445-4007 (507) 454-6579	Mattresses with firm, tapered edges for passive restraint and fall prevention.
The Company Store 500 Company Store Road La Crosse, WI 54601	(800) 285-3696	STOP sign floor mat
Comtrad Industries 2820 Waterford Lake Drive Midlothia, VA 23113	(800) 992-2966	Device that plugs into and converts an electrical outlet into a telephone outlet
Concept Fibreglass, Inc. 611 Willow Street P.O. Box 518 Grand Island, NE 68802	(800) 262-3559 (308) 381-1965	Accessible shower kits
Concord Elevator Inc. 107 Alfred Kuehne Blvd. Brampton, Ontario L6T 4K3 Canada	(800) 661-5112 (905) 791-5555	Stair lifts & residential elevators
Consolidated Plastics Co. 8181 Darrow Road Twinsburg, OH 44087	(800) 362-1000 (330) 425-3900	Floor mats and matting products
Consumer Care Products P.O. Box 684 810 N. Water Street Sheboygan, WI 53082-0684	(800) 977-2256 (920) 459-8353	Adhesive-backed Velcro fastener strips
Consumer Engineering, Inc. 2730 Kirby Avenue, NE Unit 6 Palm Bay, FL 32905	(407) 984-8550	911 flashing light adapter

Control Products, Inc. 1724 Lake Drive West Chanhassen, MN 55317	(800) 947-9098 (612) 448-2217	FreezeAlarm Voice Dialer, which automatically dials pre-set numbers (alerting distant caregiver) if loved one's home gets too cold or hot
Crest, Inc. Simon at Third P.O. Box 727 Dassel, MN 55325-0727	(800) 328-8908 (320) 275-3382	Home to hospital related equipment and parts, including wheelchairs, lights, and more
Crestwood Co. 6625 N. Sidney Place Milwaukee, WI 53209-3259	(414) 352-5678	Communication aids for children & adults
Cross Creek Recreational Products P.O. Box 289 Millbrook, NY 12545	(800) 645-5816	Recreational and activity products for those with Alzheimer's disease; video respite tapes.
Curbell 7 Cobham Drive Orchard Park, NY 14127	(800) 235-7500 (716) 667-2520	Pressure-release alarms for wandering
Cwego P.O. Box 2456 Gardena, CA 90247	(800) 292-9326 (310) 538-9440	Grab bars
DAC Technologies of America, Inc. 1601 Westpark Drive, #4C Little Rock, AR 72204	(800) 216-1515 (501) 661-9100	Door and window alarms
D & D Technologies 17835 Sky Park Circle, Unit H Irvine, CA 92614	(800) 716-0888	Attractive outdoor gate locks and latches that are key lockable.
Deaf Products P.O. Box 2185 Placerville, CA 95667	(530) 642-0337 (V/TTY)	Assistive listening and signalling devices for the hearing impaired
Delta Faucet Company 55 East 111th Street Indianapolis, IN 46280	(800) 345-3358 (317) 848-1812	Pressure- and temperature-balanced shower valve

Distinct Medical Supplies 8 Commercial Plaza Elkton, MD 21921	(888) 532-0555	Fall-EZ mat, which goes next to the bed to prevent or minimize injury due to falls out of bed.
Diversified Fiberglass Products P.O. Box 670, Hwy 150 West Cherryville, NC 28021	(704) 435-9586	Bathtub inserts and cushioned bathing tables
DSI 16141 Runnymede St. Van Nuys, CA 91406-2913	(818) 782-6793	Wavegrip grab bars
DTE Edison America 2000 2nd Avenue Detroit, MI 48233-5072	(800) 573-6232	Miscellaneous products for daily living
DuPont Flooring Systems 125 Townpark Drive Suite 400 Kennesaw, GA 30144	(800) 4DuPont (770) 420-7700	Stainmaster Carpeting and SpillBlock carpet backing
Dynamic Living P.O. Box 370249 West Hartford, CT 06137-0249	(888) 940-0605	Miscellaneous products for daily living
Easy Lift P.O. Box 272025 Tampa, FL 33688-2025	(800) 793-5438 (813) 963-5438	Patient transfer equipment and lifting devices
Easy Living Specialties 905 West Grand Avenue Hot Springs, AR 71913	(800) 406-1338 (501) 321-1338	Miscellaneous products for daily living
Easy Street 202 6th Street Providence, RI 02906	(800) 959-3279 (401) 454-7791	Easy Street Products Catalogue—products for daily living
Econol Lift Elevator Co. P.O. Box 854 2513 Center Street Cedar Falls, IA 50613	(319) 277-4777	Wheelchair lifts, residential elevators, stair lifts
The Edge Company P.O. Box 826 Brattleboro, VT 05302	(800) 732-9976	Clock radio (that works) with hidden surveillance camera

Elcoma 1929 36th Street NE Canton, OH 44705	(800) 352-6625 (330) 588-8844	Fold-down grab bars
Elcombe Systems Limited P.O. Box 72088 Kanata, Ontario K2K 2P4 Canada	(800) 563-5564 (613) 591-5678	The MainStreet Messenger automatic telephone dialer
Elder Books P.O. Box 490 Forest Knolls, CA 94933	(800) 909-2673 (415) 488-9002	Books and music for seniors
ElderSong Publications, Inc. P.O. Box 74 Mt. Airy, MD 21771	(800) 397-0533	Sing-a-long music from the good ol' days
Electropedic 907 Hollywood Way Burbank, CA 91505	(800) 233-7382 (818) 845-7488	Electric adjustable beds, inclined stairlifts, recliners
Energy Federation Inc. (EFI) 14 Tech Circle Natick, MA 01760-1086	(800) 876-0660 (508) 653-4299	Safe, cool-to-the-touch fluorescent torchere lamps
Enrichments Catalogue (Sammons Preston) P.O. Box 5071 Bolingbrook, IL 60440	(800) 323-5547 (630) 226-1300	Aids for daily living for those with disabilities
Enviracaire (Honeywell Environmental Air Control) 250 Turnpike Road Southborough, MA 01772	(800) 554-4558 (800) 998-1919 (800) 332-1110	Air cleaning equipment
Envirotrol Company, Inc. 6575 Burger Dr., SE Grand Rapids, MI 49546	(616) 940-0122	Telephone aids for those with hand, motion, & speech impairments.
Equator Corporation 10067 Timber Oak Dr. Houston, TX 77080	(800) 935-1955 (713) 464-3422	Front-loading washer/dryer combination that requires no venting

ETAC-USA P.O. Box 1739 Matthews, NC 28106	(800) 336-7684 (414) 796-4600	Walkers, bath/safety aids, misc. aids for daily living
Eureka Company 1201 East Bell Street Bloomington, IL 61701-6902	(800) 282-2886	The Dream Machine, a residential carpet vacuum that injects water into carpeting and vacuums it up.
Exposures 1 Memory Lane P.O. Box 3615 Oshkosh, WI 54903-3615	(800) 222-4947 (800) 572-5750	Frames, photo albums, and photo displays
Extend Inc. 303 21st North Moorhead, MN 56560	(800) 425-3837 (218) 236-9686	Devices that attach to and convert round door knobs into lever door knobs
EZ 2C Signs P.O. Box 27444 Lansing, MI 48909	(517) 393-9922	Colorful, easy-to-see mailbox numbers that attach to the mailbox post
Facilis, Ltd. P.O. Box 7832 Romeoville, IL 60446-0832	(815) 886-4892	Ramps and daily living aids
Farr Company 2201 Park Place El Segundo, CA 90245	(800) 333-7320 (310) 727-6300	Activated carbon filters for air conditioners
Feeney Wire Rope P.O. Box 23805 Oakland, CA 94623	(800) 888-2418 (510) 893-9473	Screen or porch reinforcing cables
Ferno-Washington 70 Weil Way Wilmington, OH 45177-9371	(800) 733-3766 (937) 382-1451	Patient transfer equipment
Fiberglass Systems, Inc. 4545 Enterprise Boise, ID 83705	(800) 727-9907 (208) 342-6823	Accessible shower kits
Fidelity TeleAlarm Corporation 2501 Kutztown Road Reading, PA 19605-2961	(800) 483-0888 (610) 929-4200	Personal Emergency Response Systems (PERS)

The Fire Extinguisher Company (Kidde Safety Products) 1394 S. Third Street Mebane, NC 27302-9199	(800) 654-9677 (800) 222-4013 in NC (919) 563-5911	Hand-held, lightweight fire extinguishers
Fisher-Price 636 Girard Avenue East Aurora, NY 14052	(800) 432-5437 (716) 687-3000	Child-proof products
Flinchbaugh Company 390 Eberts Lane York, PA 17403	(800) 326-2418 (717) 848-2418	Wheelchair lifts, dumbwaiter products, elevators
Florlift of New Jersey 41 Lawrence Street East Orange, NJ 07017	(800) 752-5438 (973) 429-2200	Residential elevators and inclined stairway lifts
Franklin Brass Mfg. Co. 19914 Via Baron Rancho Dominquez, CA 90220	(800) 421-3375 (310) 885-3200	Grab bars
Frohock-Stewart, Inc. (Invacare) 39400 Taylor Parkway North Ridgeville, OH 44039	(800) 343-6059 (440) 329-6532	Bathroom safety products, grab bars, bathtub transfer seats
G. E. Miller 45 Sawmill River Road Yonkers, NY 10701	(800) 431-2924	Patient transfer lifts
GAMCO One Gamco Place Durant, OK 74701	(800) 451-5766 (580) 924-8066	Bathroom products
Garaventa LTD P.O. Box 1769 Blaine, WA 98231-1769	(800) 663-6556	Equipment and accessories allowing wheelchairs to traverse stairways, inclined stairway lifts
General Electric GE Appliances Headquarters AP6-129 Louisville, KY 40225	(800) 626-2000 (option 4)	Refrigerators with face panels

General Technologies 7417 Winding Way Fair Oaks, CA 95628-6701	(800) 328-6684 (V/TDD) (916) 962-9225	Listening devices and products for the hearing impaired
Gerber Products Co. 445 State Street Fremont, MI 49413	(800) 443-7237	Safety and child-proofing products
Get Organized 600 Cedar Hollow Road Paoli, PA 19301	(800) 803-9400	Products to maximize home storage, clocks with day, date, and time
Giant Lift Equipment Company P.O. Box 626 North Hampton, NH 03862	(800) 524-4268 (603) 964-5127	Platform and porch lifts
Gifts for Grandkids P.O. Box 1601 Secaucus, NJ 07096-1601	(888) 472-6354	Personalized door sign kits
Golden Technologies 401 Bridge Street Old Forge, PA 18518	(800) 624-6374 (570) 451-7477	Adjustable chairs & bed, electric lifting easy chairs
Graham Field, Inc. 81 Spence Street Bayshore, NY 11706	(800) 645-8176	Supplies for doctors, nurses, and health care professionals and daily living products
Grainger Electrical Supply Co. 100 Grainger Parkway Lake Forest, IL 60045	(847) 535-1000	Electrical supplies, timers, and related products
Grand Traverse Technologies (Arjo, Inc.) 50 North Gary Ave., Unit A Roselle, IL 60172	(800) 323-1245 (630) 307-2756	Bathtubs with doors
Guardian Electronics 1001 West Glen Oaks Lane Suite 201 Mequon, WI 53092	(414) 241-4850	Wander-alerting system
Guardian Medical Monitoring 18000 West Eight Mile Road Southfield, MI 48075	(888) 349-2400	Personal Emergency Response Systems (PERS)

Guardian Products (Sunrise Medical) 745 Design Court, Suite 602 Chula Vista, CA 91911	(800) 423-8034 (800) 255-5022	Home health care products
Häfele America Company 3901 Cheyenne Drive Archdale, NC 27263	(800) 423-3531 (910) 889-2322	Fold-down shower seats, grab bars, mirrors, & other bathroom accessories
Hammacher Schlemmer* 9180 LeSaint Drive Fairfield, OH 45014-5475	(800) 543-3366	Miscellaneous items & accessories, easy-to-read scales
Hammatt Senior Products (Flaghouse, Inc.) 601 Flaghouse Drive Hasbrouck Heights, NJ 07604	(800) 428-5127 (800) 428-5128 (201) 288-7600	Recreational and exercise products for older adults
Handicapped & Elderly Life Products (HELP) (Elevators, Etc.) 1773 Blount Road Pompano Beach, FL 33069	(800) 785-8585 (954) 970-0767	Stair lifts, residential elevators, door openers
Handi-Move International (SureHands Lift & Care System) 982 Route 1 Pine Island, NY 10969	(800) 724-5305 (914) 258-6500	Ceiling track lifts
Handi-Ramp 1414 Armour Boulevard Mundelein, IL 60060	(800) 876-7267 (847) 816-7525	Prefabricated & portable ramps
Harriet Carter* Dept. 39 North Wales, PA 19455	(800) 377-7878 (215) 361-5122	Miscellaneous items and accessories
Harris Communications 15159 Technologies Dr. Eden Prairie, MN 55344-2277	(800) 825-6758	Products and aids for the hearing impaired, notification systems, vibrating alert signals, etc.
Hayn Enterprises 51 Inwood Road Rocky Hill, CT 06067	(800) 346-4296	Steel cables to add additional cables rails to balcony railings

HealthCraft Products, Inc. Unit 4, 2750 Stevenage Drive Gloucester, Ontario K1G 5N2 Canada	(888) 619-9992 (613) 738-7222	Super Pole—floor-to-ceiling mounted pole with accessories
Health Enterprises 90 George Leven Drive N. Attleboro, MA 02760	(800) 633-4243 (508) 695-0727	Medical ID bracelets
Health Sense International 657 Newmark Avenue P.O. Box 293 Coos Bay, OR 97420	(800) 422-3858 (888) 379-8463 (541) 267-4459	Drytime Bedwetting Alarm
Hear-More Products P.O. Box 3413 42 Executive Boulevard Farmingdale, NY 11735	(800) 881-4327 (V/TTY) (516) 752-0738 (V/TTY)	Products and aids for the hearing impaired
HeartWarmers 6N 534 Glendale Road Medinah, IL 60157	(888) 256-7322 + (PIN code 0437) (630) 893-5383	Activity videos and sing-alongs
Hello Direct 5893 Rue Ferrari Drive San Jose, CA 95138-1858	(800) 444-3556 (408) 972-1990	Telephones and related products
Hertz Supply Company, Inc. 4670 Schantz Road Allentown, PA 18104	(800) 321-4240 (610) 366-1812	Manufacturers of Volker Beds, which raise and lower and do not look institutional
HEWI, Inc. 2851 Old Tree Drive Lancaster, PA 17603	(877) 439-4462 (717) 293-1313	Makers of grab bars, bathroom accessories, hand rails, etc.
HIG's Mfg. Co. 2917 Anthony Lane North Minneapolis, MN 55418	(800) 733-6220 (612) 788-1183	Prefabricated ramps and miniramps
HITEC 8160 Madison Burr Ridge, IL 60521	(800) 288-8303 (630) 654-9200	Amplified telephones, telephone ringers, Personal Emergency Response Systems (PERS), alerting & signal systems, horn signals, flashing smoke detectors, mattress vibrators

HNE Healthcare 227 Route 33 East Manalapan, NJ 07726	(800) 223-1218 (732) 446-2500	Wheelchair and seat cushions
Hold Everything 10000 Covington Cross Las Vegas, NV 89144	(800) 421-2264	Storage accessories, stand-alone shelving units, closet organizing accessories
Holmes Products Corporation P.O. Box 769 Milford, MA 01757	(800) 546-5637 (508) 634-8050	Home air purification machines
HomeCare Products, Co. 15824 SE 296th Street Kent, WA 98042	(800) 451-1903 (253) 631-4633	Portable ramps, thresholds, the E-Z Bathe and E-Z shower, which allow bathing in bed
Home Care Products LLC 4787 Trail View Drive West Bloomfield, MI 48322	(800) 727-8483	Lifting device that attaches to the toilet and lifts the user to a standing position
Home Health Care Products 5701-D Gen. Washington Dr. Alexandria, VA 22312	(800) 253-9993 (703) 642-3141	Grab bars & bathroom accessories
Home Remedies 13730 State Road 84 Suite 137 Davie, FL 33325	(800) 908-0907 (954) 385-0815	The Careousel automatic medication dispenser
Home Trends* 1450 Lyell Avenue Rochester, NY 14606-2184	(800) 810-2340 (716) 254-6520	Miscellaneous daily living products
Honeywell, Inc. Honeywell Plaza-CAC P.O. Box 524, MN 27-2164 Minneapolis, MN 55440-0524	(800) 468-1502	Thermostats with large numbers and lockable thermostat covers
Hoover Company 101 East Maple Street North Canton, OH 44720	(330) 499-9200	The Steam-Vac wet/dry vacuum cleaner
HumanCare 14930 Main Street Gardena, CA 90248	(800) 767-4001 (310) 767-4040	Furnishings for seniors

Hygiene Specialties (Division of Andermac) 2626 Live Oak Highway P.O. Box 1594 Yuba City, CA 95991-8810	(800) 824-0214 (530) 674-8450	Toilet bidet inserts & toilet hygienic equipment
Identi-Find 5465 Dutch Cove Road P.O. Box 567 Canton, NC 28716	(704) 648-6768	Iron-on name and telephone labels for clothes
Igloo Products Corporation 1001 W. Sam Houston Pkwy. N. Houston, TX 77043	(800) 324-2653 (713) 465-2571	Mini-refrigerator
Improvements Hanover, PA 17333	(800) 642-2112	Miscellaneous daily living products
Inclinator Co. of America 2200 Paxton Street P.O. Box 1557 Harrisburg, PA 17105-1557	(717) 234-8065	Residential elevators, lifts, & inclined stair lifts
Incline Technologies, Inc. 3267 Research Way Suite 212 Carson City, NV 89706	(800) 538-0205 (775) 882-8200	The BagBath in-bed bathing system
Independent Care Products P.O. Box 6258 Abilene, TX 79608	(800) 695-8151 (915) 698-8151	Rotating bathtub/shower seat mounted on a floor-to-ceiling pole
Independent Living Aids 27 East Mall Plainview, NY 11803	(800) 537-2118	The "Can-Do" Products Catalogue—visitors chimes, large-face clocks, photocell night lights, telephone assistive devices, miscellaneous products & gifts
Independent Needs Centre 100 Amber Street, Unit #1 Markham, Ontario L3R 3A2 Canada	(905) 479-1448	Lifestyle Essential Catalogue

Innovative Caregiving Resources P.O. Box 17809 Salt Lake City, UT 84117-0809	(800) 272-9806 (800) 249-5600	Video tapes and products that entertain those with dementia
In-Sink-Erator 4700 21st Street Racine, WI 53406	(800) 558-5700	Batch feed garbage disposals that only operate with the cover on
International Cushion Co. 9505 Haldane Road Kelowna, BC V4V 2K5 Canada	(800) 882-7638	Soft-sided bathtubs
International Environmental Solutions 2830 Scherer Drive, #310 St. Petersburg, FL 33716	(800) 972-8348 (727) 573-1676	The Easy Flow automatic faucet control
Intirion Corporation 10 Walpole Park South Walpole, MA 02081	(800) 994-0165 (508) 660-9200	Mini-refrigerator and microwave combination
Invacare Continuing Care 739 Goddard Ave. Chesterfield, MO 63005	(800) 678-7100 (636) 519-0055	Bathtubs with doors, barrier-free showers
Invacare Corporation 899 Cleveland Street Elyria, OH 44036	(800) 333-6900 (800) 668-5324 (Canada)	Wheelchair accessories, power assisted recliner, pressure relief bedding products, adjustable beds
IPC (InPro Corp.) S80 W18766 Apollo Dr. Muskego, WI 53150	(800) 222-5556 (414) 679-9010	Door and wall protection products
Jaclo, Inc. 1115 Globe Ave. Mountainside, NJ 07092-1252	(800) 852-3906 (908) 789-2880	Hand-held shower head assemblies
Jay Products (A Division of Sunrise Medical) 7477-A East Drycreek Pkwy. Longmont, CO 80503	(800) 648-8282 (303) 218-4435	Cushions and backs for wheelchairs, seats, and scooters

J.C. Mfg. Co. P.O. Box 25455 Cleveland, OH 44125	(216) 663-7385	Device that converts standard toilet to a bidet, miscellaneous bath & shower aids
J.C. Penney Special Needs Catalogue P.O. Box 2021 Milwaukee, WI 53201-2021	(800) 222-6161	"Special Needs" catalogue
J.H. Industries 1981 East Aurora Road Twinsburg, OH 44087	(800) 321-4968 (330) 963-4105	Portable and prefabricated ramps
Joan Cook* 2500 Arrowhead Drive Carson City, NV 89706	(800) 935-0971	Miscellaneous daily living products
Judson Enterprises 23830 WCR 48 LaSalle, CO 80645	(800) 587-5212 (970) 284-6618	Shower chairs and bathtub seats
Keeney Mfg. Co. 1170 Main Street Newington, CT 06111-3098	(800) 243-0526 (860) 666-3342	Colored and modular grab bars, anti-scalding devices, protective pipe insulation
KidKusions, Inc. P.O. Box 1686 129 Midtown Lane Washington, NC 27889	(800) 845-9236 (252) 946-7162	Table corner protective cushions
Kids Club 7835 Freedom Ave. NW North Canton, OH 44720	(888) 373-4031 (800) 363-0500	Safety and child-proof products
Knobbles 7235 S. Steele Circle Littleton, CO 80122-1940	(800) 346-5662	Great Grips, a flexible rubber sleeve that fits over knobs & water faucet handles, making them easier to grasp
Kohler Company 444 Highland Drive Kohler, WI 53044	(920) 457-4441	Bathroom products for those with disabilities

Koolatron 27 Catherine Avenue Brantford, Ontario N3T 1X5 Canada	(800) 265-8456	Very small portable electric refrigerator
Larkotex 1002 Olive Street Texarkana, TX 75501	(800) 972-3037 (903) 793-4647	Bed railings
Lasco Bathware 3255 East Miraloma Avenue Anaheim, CA 92806	(800) 877-0464 (800) 877-2005 (714) 993-1220	Prefabricated accessible shower inserts
Laurel Designs P.O. Box 888 Tiburon, CA 94920	(415) 435-1891	Wheelchair supplies and products
La-Z-Boy Healthcare 1284 N. Telegraph Road Monroe, MI 48162	(734) 241-2435	Reclining chairs
LCM Distributing Company 2506 Southern Avenue Brandon, Manitoba R7B 0S4 Canada	(888) 726-4646 (204) 726-4646	ArcoRail assistive bed rail and handle for next to the bed
LDB Medical, Inc. 2909 Langford Rd., #500 B Norcross, GA 30071	(800) 243-2554 (770) 446-2554	Aids for independent living, offset door hinges
LectraAid 1801 E. Medlock Drive Phoenix, AZ 85016	(888) 224-1425 (602) 265-7370	Platform lifts & chair lifts
Leisure Lifts 1800 Merriam Lane Kansas City, KS 66106	(800) 255-0285 (913) 722-5658	Electric lifting easy chairs
Lifeline Systems, Inc. 111 Lawrence Street Framingham, MA 01702	(800) 543-3546 (800) 642-0045 (508) 988-1000	Personal Emergency Response System (PERS)
Lifestyle Catalogue 110 Lehigh Avenue Lakewood, NJ 08701-8123	(800) 669-0987 (732) 364-5777	Innovative products for daily living; photo telephone

Lighthouse International Consumer Products Division 111 East 59th Street, 12th Floor New York, NY 10022-1202	(800) 829-0500 (800) 334-5497	Products for the visually impaired
Lighthouse of Houston Attn: Sales Store 3602 W. Dallas Houston, TX 77019	(713) 527-9561 ext. 466	Talking clocks, products for visually impaired
Linden 1425 Cranston Street Cranston, RI 02920	(401) 943-2100	Clocks with day, date, and time
Lindustries P.O. Box 66295 Auburndale, MA 02466	(781) 237-8177	Devices that convert round door knobs into levers
Link to Life P.O. Box 1661 Pittsfield, MA 01201	(800) 338-4176 (413) 442-9000	Personal Emergency Response System (PERS)
Locknetics 575 Birch Street Forestville, CT 06010	(860) 584-9158	Electric door locks
Logan Powell Company (Omni Interactive) 861 Market Street Lemoyne, PA 17043	(717) 730-2671	Time-activated and heat-activated disconnect switches for stove and oven
Lowe's Carpet Corporation P.O. Box 1186 Chatsworth, GA 30705	(800) 333-2468 (706) 695-4678	Anti-microbial carpeting for incontinence
LS & S Group P.O. Box 673 Northbrook, IL 60065	(800) 468-4789 TTY (800) 317-8533	Products for the visually & hearing impaired
Lubidet USA, Inc. 1980 South Quebec St., Ste. 4 Denver, CO 80231-3234	(800) 582-4338 (303) 368-4555	Attachment for a standard toilet converting it to a bidet

Lumex Medical Products, Inc. (Graham Field, Inc.) 81 Spence Street Bay Shore, NY 11706	(800) 645-5272	Wheelchairs, recliners, & miscellaneous daily living products
Mac's Lift Gate, Inc. 2715 Seaboard Lane Long Beach, CA 90805	(800) 795-6227 (562) 634-5962	Platform lifts
Maddak, Inc. 6 Industrial Road Pequannock, NJ 07440	(800) 443-4926 (973) 628-7600	"Homecare" Ableware Catalogue of aids for independent living
Magnavox SecureAlert 109 David Lane Knoxville, TN 37922	(800) 584-4176 (800) 647-7454	Personal Emergency Response System (PERS)
Mailbox Factory 7857 Chardon Road Kirtland, OH 44094	(888) 740-6245	Unique decorated mailboxes
Marvel Industries P.O. Box 997 Richmond, IN 47375-0997	(800) 428-6644 (765) 962-2521	Small refrigerators
Mature Mart 1788 Cherny Street Jesup, GA 31545	(800) 720-6278 (912) 427-0553	Miscellaneous products for daily living
Maxi Aids P.O. Box 3209 Farmingdale, NY 11735	(800) 522- 6294 (516) 742-0521	Aids for independent living
Maytag Customer Service 240 Edward Street Cleveland, TN 37311	(800) 688-9900	Frontloading and stacking washer/dryers
McKesson Home Health Care 1 Post Street San Francisco, CA 94104	(800) 482-3784 (415) 983-8300	Health care and daily living products
Medic Aid* 3681 Kempt Road, Suite 201 Halifax, NS B3K 4X6 Canada *not related to Medicaid	(800) 565-9135 (902) 454-8877	Personal Emergency Response System (PERS)

Medic Alert Foundation 2323 Colorado Avenue Turlock, CA 95382	(800) 432-5378 (209) 668-3333	Medic Alert ID bracelets
Med-Lift & Mobility Inc. P.O. Box 1249 Calhoun City, MS 38916	(800) 748-9438 (601) 628-8196	Electric lifting chairs
Medreco Inc. 757 State Road 101 South P.O. Box 100 Liberty, IN 47353	(800) 552-7774 (765) 458-7444	Electric beds and bed rails
MedWay Corporation 103 Graybark Lane Amherst, OH 44001	(800) 817-3118	The Toilet Riser, a platform that raises the toilet
Memry Corporation 57 Commerce Drive Brookfield, CT 06804	(800) 582-5454 (203) 740-7311	Anti-scalding devices for faucets, shower, sinks, and tub
Mercer Products Company (Burker Mercer Industries) P.O. Box 1240 Eustice, FL 32727-1240	(800) 447-8442 (352) 357-4119	Slip-resistant stair treads and protective wall corner guards
Micro-Tech Medical, Inc. 17 Rose Avenue West Hartford, CT 06110	(800) 380-8883 (860) 953-6662	The Bed-Mate and Chair-Mate alarms
Miles Kimball Co.* 41 West Eighth Ave. Oshkosh, WI 54906-0002	(800) 546-2255 (920) 231-1992	Throw rug non-slip backing, photocells for lights, miscellaneous products and gifts
MNO Sales 4329 W. Bluefield Rd. Glendale, AZ 85308	(602) 938-3990	Attachment converting standard toilet to a bidet
Mobility Transfer Systems 7 Pleasant Street Randolph, MA 02368	(800) 854-4687 (617) 963-4564	Bed handrails
Moen, Inc. Consumer Services 25300 Al Moen Drive North Olmsted, OH 44070-8022	(800) 553-6636	Faucets, sinks, & accessories for kitchen & bath; anti-scalding balancing shower valves

M.O.M.S. (Mail Order Medical Supply) 24700 Avenue Rockefeller Valencia, CA 91355	(800) 232-7443	Incontinence products, miscellaneous daily living products
Mondial Industries (Playtex Products) 75 Commerce Drive Allendale, NJ 07401-1600	(800) 843-6430 (201) 785-8000	Confidante adult brief disposal container
Monroe Specialties 3200 13th Street P.O. Box 740 Monroe, WI 53566	(800) 628-0165	ID bracelets
Moving Solutions, Inc. 7980 Alabama Avenue Clarendon Hills, IL 60514-2412	(800) 228-7980 (608) 328-8381	Patient transfer equipment and bathtubs with doors
Musson Rubber Co. 1320 E. Archwood Ave. P.O. Box 7038 Akron, OH 44306-0038	(800) 321-2381 (330) 773-7651	Non-slip stair treads with warning stripes
Name Makers, Inc. P.O. Box 43821 Atlanta, GA 30336-0821	(800) 241-2890 (404) 691-2237	Sew-on or iron-on name and telephone labels for clothes
Nasco Activity Therapy 901 Janesville Avenue Ft. Atkinson, WI 53538	(800) 558-9595 (920) 563-2446	Products for reminiscence, activities and exercise for seniors, music, simple puzzles, and more
National Bathing Products 5 Greenwood Avenue Romeoville, IL 60446	(800) 479-2311 (815) 886-5900	Accessible shower units
National Federation for the Blind 1800 Johnson Street Baltimore, MD 21230	(410) 659-9314	Products and information for the visually impaired
National Flashing Signal Systems (NFSS Communications) 8120 Fenton Street Silver Springs, MD 20910	(888) 589-6670 (V/TTY) (301) 589-6670 (301) 589-6671 (TTY)	Visual alerting systems, telephone amplifiers, fire & smoke alarms, vibrating signalers, TTY machines, etc.

National Manufacturing P.O. Box 577 Sterling, IL 61081	(800) 346-9445 (815) 625-1320	Safety and child-proof products
National Wheel-O-Vator 509 W. Front Street Roanoke, IL 61561-0348	(800) 551-9095 (309) 923-2611	Indoor and outdoor stairlifts and elevators, platform lifts, and private residential elevators
Natural Hardware Store Healthy Home Center 1403-A Cleveland Street Clearwater, FL 33755	(727) 447-4454	Activated carbon filters for air conditioners
Neuropedic 10 New King Street White Plains, NY 10604	(800) 327-6759 (914) 684-2665	Waterproof seat and mattress cushions, queen size rehabilitation bed
New Pane Creations 44799 Fern Circle Temecula, CA 92592	(800) 382-7263	Fake mullions for sliding glass doors and windows
NOA Medical Industries 801 Terry Lane Washington, MO 63090	(888) 662-6699	The NOA Riser Bed that rises and lowers
North Coast Medical Consumer Products Division 18305 Sutter Boulevard Morgan Hill, CA 95037-2845	(800) 821-9319 (408) 776-5000	Functional Solutions Catalogue of products for independent living
OFNA Baby Products 22692 Granite Way, Suite B Laguna Hills, CA 92653	(949) 586-2910	Padded corner and edge protectors and other safety-related child-proofing products
Olsonite Corp. 25 Dart Road Newnan, GA 30265	(800) 521-8266 (770) 253-3930	Grab bars, toilet lift seats, & miscellaneous bathroom safety equipment
One Step Ahead P.O. Box 517 Lake Bluff, IL 60044	(800) 477-2189	Leaps and Bounds catalogue: outdoor equipment for children, non-staining tints for bathtub water, safety products, etc.

Optimum Technologies, Inc. P.O. Box 1537 570 Joe Frank Harris Parkway Cartersville, GA 30120	(800) 562-5574 (770) 386-3470	Lok-Lift non-slip carpet backing for throw rugs
Ortho-Kinetics, Inc. Lark of America P.O. Box 1647 Waukesha, WI 53187-1647	(800) 824-1068 (262) 542-6060	Electric lifting easy chairs
Otto Bock 3000 Xenium Lane North Minneapolis, MN 55441	(800) 328-4058 (612) 553-9464	The Linido Ergogrip system, a line of bathroom accessories. The entire line is designed to be aesthetically pleasing, with a unified style and several color schemes.
Outside the Ordinary 20630 Plummer Street Chatsworth, CA 91311	(888) 251-1051	Outdoor rocker glider
Pawling Corporation Borden Lane P.O. Box 200 Wassaic, NY 12592	(800) 431-3456 (914) 373-9300	Corner protectors, door kick plates
PCP-Champion 300 Congress Street Ripley, OH 45167	(800) 888-0867 (513) 392-4301	Home health care products
Peerless Industries, Inc. 1980 Hawthorne Avenue Melrose Park, IL 60160	(800) 865-2112 (708) 865-8870	Wall-mounted television stands
PEMKO Manufacturing Co. P.O. Box 3780 Ventura, CA 93006	(800) 283-9988 (805) 642-2600	Accessible miniramps for sliding glass doors and thresholds
Perfectly Safe 7835 Freedom Avenue NW Suite 3 North Canton, OH 44720-6907	(800) 837-5437	Child-proof locks and safety products

PERSYS Amcest Nationwide Emergency Monitoring 1017 Walnut Street Roselle, NJ 07203	(800) 631-7370	Personal Emergency Response System (PERS)
Philips Light Co. 200 Franklin Square Drive Sommerset, NJ 08875	(800) 555-0050 (732) 563-3000	Compact fluorescent light bulbs
Phillips Enterprises 10 N. Foote Street Cambridge City, IN 47327	(765) 478-9055	Toilet seat lift
Phonex Corporation 6952 High Tech Drive Midvale, UT 84047-3756	(800) 437-0101 (801) 566-0100	Remote telephone jacks
Pioneer Medical Systems 3408 Howell Street, Suite D Duluth, GA 30096	(800) 234-0683 (770) 476-0837	"Companion Call Light" Personal Emergency Response System (PERS) with optional window call light
Plow & Hearth P.O. Box 5000 Madison, VA 22727-1500	(800) 627-1712	Miscellaneous products for around the home
Plumberex Specialty Products, Inc. 72096 Dunham Way Thousand Palms, CA 92276	(800) 475-8629 (760) 343-7363	Pipe insulation for under-counter hot water and drain pipes
Polyconcept USA, Inc. 69 Jefferson Street Stanford, CT 06902	(203) 358-8100	The Photo Dial Phone
Portable Entry Systems P.O. Box 100 Camden, MI 49232	(800) 286-1181 (517) 368-5583	Portable ramps
Porto-Lift Corp. P.O. Box 5 Higgins Lake, MI 48627	(800) 321-1454 (517) 821-6688	Transfer lifts

Posey Healthcare 5635 Peck Road Arcadia, CA 91006	(800) 447-6739 (626) 443-3143	Medical and healthcare products
Potentials Development, Inc. 779 Cayuga Street, Unit 1 Lewiston, NY 14092	(800) 691-6602 (716) 754-9476	Products, music, and books for seniors
Potomac Technology, Inc. One Church St., Suite 101 Rockville, MD 20850-4158	(800) 433-2838 (V/TTY) (301) 762-4005 (V/TTY)	Telephone amplifiers, doorbells, & phone signalers, products & aids for the hearing impaired
Prairie View Industries, Inc. P.O. Box 575 714 5th Street Fairbury, NE 68352-0575	(800) 554-RAMP (402) 729-4055	Portable and mini-ramps
Price Pfister 13500 Paxton Street Pacoma, CA 91331	(800) 732-8238 (818) 896-1141	Plumbing fixtures
Pride Health Care, Inc. (Mobility Products) 182 Susquehanna Avenue Exeter, PA 18643-2694	(800) 800-8586 (570) 655-5574	Electric lifting easy chairs
Princeton Products, Inc. 717 Lakeview Road Clearwater, FL 33756	(800) 497-4655	The Truman Bed Buddy, a device that converts a regular bed into a mechanical lifting bed
Pyro Control, Inc. 2721 White Settlement Road Fort Worth, TX 76107	(817) 335-5981	The Range Queen automatic fire-extinguishing system for over the stove
Radio Shack Corp. 100 Throckmorton St., Suite 600 Fort Worth, TX 76102	(800) THE SHACK (817) 415-3011	Miscellaneous electrical equipment and devices (ask also for their Special Needs Catalogue)
Rampit 337 Bidwell Road Coldwater, MI 49036	(800) 876-9498	Ramp systems

R.C. Steele Company 1989 Transit Way, Box 910 Brockport, New York 14420-0910	(800) 872-4506 (800) 872-3773	Pet supplies, the SofaSaver, a pressure-sensitive pad that sounds an alarm when stepped on
R.C.A. Rubber Company 1833 East Market Street P.O. Box 9240 Akron, OH 44305-0240	(800) 321-2340 (330) 784-1291	Rubber button flooring, slip-resistant stair treads; tactile warning strips, and abrasive safety floor strips
R.D. Equipment, Inc. 230 Percival Drive West Barnstable, MA 02668-1233	(508) 362-7498	Sliding bathtub/shower seat
Reese Enterprises, Inc. P.O. Box 459 Rosemount, MN 55068-0459	(800) 328-0953 (651) 423-1126	Mini-ramps, thresholds, and corner protectors
Renovator's P.O. Box 2525 Conway, NH 03818-2515	(800) 659-2211 (603) 447-8500	Old-fashioned hardware products
ResponseLink Medical Alert Systems 6101 Lake Ellenor Drive Orlando, FL 32809	(800) 894-1428	Personal Emergency Response System (PERS) that allows trained operators to "listen" to determine if there really is an emergency; offers two-way speaker phone communication
Rev-A-Shelf 2409 Plantside Drive P.O. Box 99585 Jeffersontown, KY 40299	(800) 762-9030 (502) 499-5835	Storage and organizing accessories
R.F. Technologies, Inc. 3125 North 126th Street Brookfield, WI 53005	(800) 669-9946 (262) 790-1771	The Code Alert wander-alerting system
Rifton P.O. Box 255 Farmington, PA 15437	(800) 374-3866	Aids for daily living
Right Start Catalogue 5334 Sterling Center Drive, Unit C Westlake Village, CA 91361	(800) 548-8531 (888) 548-8531	Baby safety products and monitoring equipment

Rubbermaid, Inc. 1147 Akron Road Wooster, OH 44691-6000	(330) 264-6464 ext. 2619	Space-saving and storage products
SafeLift, Inc. 305 Park Drive Chardon, OH 44024	(888) 287-1814 (440) 286-1814	Mechanical bathtub lifts and transfer seats
Safe Return Program Alzheimer's Association 919 N. Michigan Ave., Ste. 1000 Chicago, IL 60611-1676	(800) 272-3900	The Safe Return Program to help find lost people with Alzheimer's disease
Safety 1st, Inc. 45 Dan Road Canton, MA 02021	(800) 962-7233 (781) 364-3100	Safety products
Safety Zone, Inc. 340 Poplar Street, Bldg. 20 Hanover, PA 17333-0019	(800) 999-3030	Safety products
Sammons Preston P.O. Box 5071 Bolingbrook, IL 60440-5071	(800) 323-5547	Orthopedic and products for independent living
S & S Opportunities P.O. Box 513 Colchester, CT 06415-0513	(800) 266-8856 (860) 537-3451	Activity products for seniors
Santa Barbara Promotions 133 West De La Guerra Street Santa Barbara, CA 93101	(800) 333-3201	The Save-A-Sofa seat cushion reinforcer
Sauder Manufacturing Company 930 W. Barre Road Archbold, OH 43502-0230	(800) 537-1530 (419) 446-9384	The Design Care series of chairs and furniture for seniors
Schumacher Elevator Co. 1 Schumacher Way P.O. Box 363 Denver, IA 50622	(800) 779-5438 (319) 984-5676	Residential elevators
Science Products Box 888 Southeastern, PA 19399	(800) 888-7400 (610) 296-2111	Aids for those with visual impairments

Sears Home Healthcare Catalogue (800) 326-1750   Home health care products
3737 Grader St., Suite 110   TDD/TTY (800) 733-7249
Garland, TX 75041

Secure Care Products, Inc.   (800) 451-7917   Wander Alert Systems
39 Chenell Drive   (603) 223-0745
Concord, NH 03301-8501

SecurityLink   (800) 926-7583   Personal Emergency Response
32100 US 19 North   (800) 873-7940   System (PERS)
Palm Harbour, FL 34684

Senior Products   (800) 428-5128   Products and music for seniors
(Flaghouse, Inc.)   (800) 428-5127
601 Flaghouse Drive   (201) 288-7600
Hasbrouck Heights, NJ 07604

Senior Style   (503) 246-8231   Furniture for seniors
P.O. Box 2007
Portland, OR 97208-2007

Senior Technologies   (800) 235-8085   Manufacturers of the TABS
1620 North 20th Circle   (800) 824-4490   and WanderGuard wander
P.O. Box 80238   (402) 475-4002   alerting systems
Lincoln, NE 68501

Shamrock Medical Inc.   (800) 231-2225   Products for use in the home
3620 SE Powell Blvd.   (503) 233-5055   and daily living
Portland, OR 97202

The Sharper Image   (800) 344-4444   Unique products, including the
650 Davis Street   Photo Dial Phone
San Francisco, CA 94111

Skil-Care Corporation   (800) 431-2971   Wander alert pressure release
29 Wells Avenue   (914) 963-2040   and pull-tab alarms, soft floor
Yonkers, NY 10701   mats for next to the bed

Smith & Hawken   (800) 776-3336   Garden benches and outdoor
2 Arbor Lane   furniture
P.O. Box 6900
Florence, KY 41022

Smith & Nephew One Quality Drive P.O. Box 1005 Germantown, WI 53022	(800) 558-8633	Miscellaneous products for those with disabilities, rehabilitation products
Snyder Electronics 2082 North Lincoln Avenue Altadena, CA 91001	(626) 794-7139	Motion detectors that send a signal to a remote chime, pressure-sensitive floor pads and alarms
Solutions P.O. Box 6878 Portland, OR 97228-6878	(800) 342-9988	Miscellaneous products
SOS Wireless Communications 18022 Cowan Avenue, Suite 101 Irvine, CA 92614	(800) 767-3141	Personal Emergency Response System (PERS)-cordless telephone
Sound Choice 14100 South Lakes Dr. Charlotte, NC 28273	(800) 788-4487 (704) 583-1616	Karaoke and sing-along music from the "good 'ol days"
Sparkle Plenty, Inc. 130 East Elm Street, Suite 301 Roselle, IL 60172	(800) 621-6460 (708) 894-0220	Illuminated address signs
Speakman P.O. Box 191 Wilmington, DE 19899-0191	(800) 537-2107 (302) 764-9100	Electronic motion sensor water faucets
The Spinoza Company 1876 Minnehaha Avenue West St. Paul, MN 55104	(800) 282-2327	The Spinoza Bear
Stand-Aid of Iowa 1009 2nd Avenue P.O. Box 386 Sheldon, IA 51201	(800) 831-8580 (712) 324-2153	Mechanical toilet seat lift
Stannah Stairlifts 233A South Street Hopkinton, MA 01748	(800) 877-8247, ext. 100 (508) 435-0416	Inclined stair lifts
Starchild Labs P.O. Box 404 Aptos, CA 95001-0404	(800) 346-7283 (408) 662-2659	SleepDry Bedwetting Alarm

Steinel America, Inc. 9051 Lyndale Avenue S. Bloomington, MN 55420	(800) 852-4343 (612) 888-5950	Motion detectors for floodlights, electrical outlets, and remote chimes
Step Ahead Product Innovations, LLC 60 Ora Way San Francisoc, CA 94131	(415) 285-3512	Last Step Alert for stair railings
St. Louis Medical Supply 10821 Manchester Road St. Louis, MO 63122-1298	(800) 950-6020 (314) 821-7355	Miscellaneous medical and health care products
Sub-Zero Freezer Co. P.O. Box 44030 Madison, WI 53744-4130	(800) 222-7820	Refrigerators that resemble cabinets, dressers and night tables
Sunrise Medical 100 Devilbiss Drive P.O. Box 635 Sommerset, PA 15501-0635 or 7477 B. East Drycreek Pkwy. Longmont, CO 80503	(800) 333-4000	Medical equipment and products for daily living
Swan Corporation 1 City Centre St. Louis, MO 63101	(800) 325-7008 (314) 231-8148	Accessible shower kits
The Take Care Store 12400 East Marginal Way South Seattle, WA 98168	(800) 447-2839 (888) 379-8463 (206) 883-5995	SleepDry Bedwetting Alarm
Tamarac Development Group 23542 Lyons Avenue #207 Santa Clarita, CA 91321	(877) 255-0907 (661) 255-0907	Door murals
Technically Unique Bathing Systems 7 Monroe Street Troy, NY 12180	(518) 274-2284	Bathtub with doors
Telko, Inc. 26651 Cabot Road Laguna Hills, CA 92653	(800) 888-3556 (949) 367-1234	Battery-operated motion-detecting chime/alarm

Tepromark International 99 West Hawthorne, Ste. 408 Valley Stream, NY 11581	(800) 645-2622 (516) 825-7707	Corner guards, chair rails, hand rails, and wall protectors
TFI Engineering 529 Main Street Boston, MA 02129	(617) 242-7007	Products & equipment for the visually impaired; talking clocks, scales, watches, calculators, etc.
3M Company Customer Service 225-4S-08 St. Paul, MN 55144-1000	(800) 364-3577	Scotchshield intrusion-resistant window glazing, Scotchgard carpet treatment
Toto Kiki USA, Inc. 1155 Southern Road Morrow, GA 30260	(800) 938-1541	Bidet that can be added to an existing toilet, automatic toilet and faucet valves
Trail Side Mail Box (Cutler Manufacturing) 3240 Flightline Drive Lakeland, FL 33811-2844	(800) 237-2312 (863) 644-3573	Locking mail boxes
Transcience 11 Ryan Street P.O. Box 4917 Stamford, CT 06907-0917	(800) 243-3494 (203) 595-0432	Personal Emergency Response System (PERS)
Transfer Master Products 103 West Greene Street Postville, IA 52162	(800) 475-8122 (319) 864-7364	The Hi-lo bed
Tri-Guards, Inc. 490 Hintz Road Wheeling, IL 60090	(800) 783-8445 (847) 537-8444	Battery-operated strobe light smoke alarm, wall corner guards
Truebro, Inc. P.O. Box 440 Ellington, CT 06029-9985	(800) 340-5969 (860) 875-2868	Pipe insulation for under-counter hot water and drain pipes
Tub-Master L.C. 413 Virginia Drive Orlando, FL 32803-1892	(407) 898-2881	Accessible showers, shower doors, shower seats, and other accessible products

Tubular Specialties Mfg., Inc. 13011 S. Spring Street Los Angeles, CA 90061-1685	(800) 225-5876 (310) 515-4801	Grab bars, shower seats, corner guards, shower soap dispensers, and other bathroom products
U-Line 8900 North 55th Street P.O. Box 23220 Milwaukee, WI 53223	(800) 779-2547 (414) 354-0300	Small refrigerators
Underfoot, Inc. Route 8, Box 691 Micaville, NC 28755	(888) 248-8999 (828) 675-4345	Safety bathtub mats that indicate water temperature
Unison Metal Products 1300 Valleyfield Avenue St. Vincent De Paul, Laval Quebec H7C 2K6 Canada	(514) 871-1295	Free-standing rack for towels or clothes
Universal Medical Products 4100 First Avenue Brooklyn, NY 11232-3321	(732) 583-0077 (718) 499-0020	Fall prevention alarms for bed or chair
Universal-Rundle Corporation (Crane Plumbing Co.) 41 Cairns Road Mansfield, OH 44903	(800) 955-0316 (800) 955-1218	Accessible shower unit
Vann-Duerr Industries 820 W. 7th Street Chico, CA 95928	(800) 497-2003 (530) 893-1596	Mini-ramps for sliding glass doors and small changes in elevations, plus other products for a barrier-free environment
Vivitar Monitoring Systems 1280 Rancho Conejo Blvd. Newbury Park, CA 91320	(800) 421-2381 (805) 498-7008	Surveillance and monitoring equipment
Vornado Air Circulation Systems 415 East 13th Street Andover, KS 67002	(800) 234-0604 (316) 733-0035	Air-cleaning equipment

WanderGuard (Senior Technologies) 1620 North 20th Circle P.O. Box 80238 Lincoln, NE 68503	(800) 235-8085 (402) 475-4002	Wander alerting systems
Wander Watch (Response USA) 3 Executive Campus 2nd Floor South Cherry Hill, NJ 08002	(800) 333-9845 (856) 661-0700	Wander alerting systems
Warm Rain P.O. Box 600 Houghton County Airpark Hancock, MI 49930	(800) 236-3754 (906) 482-3750	Accessible shower kits
Waupaca Elevator Co. P.O. Box 246 1050 South Grider Street Appleton, WI 54914-4858	(800) 238-8739 (920) 991-9082	Dumbwaiters, small residential elevators
Weibrecht Communications 2716 Ocean Park Boulevard Suite 1007 Santa Monica, CA 90405	(800) 233-9130 (V/TTY) (310) 452-8613 (V) (310) 452-5460 (TTY)	Large-faced LED clocks, alerting systems, amplified telephones, products and aids for the hearing impaired
Westek 9295 Farnham Street San Diego, CA 92123-1201	(800) 331-3366 (858) 268-3422	Lighting systems & assistive devices
Westinghouse (Tappan & Frigidaire) Consumer Assistance Program 6000 Perimeter Drive Dublin, OH 43017	(614) 792-2153	Stacking washer/dryers and other appliances
Wheelchair Warehouse 100 East Sierra, Suite 3309 Fresno, CA 93710	(800) 829-0202 (209) 436-6147	Electric lifting easy chairs, bathroom aids, wheelchair accessories, and numerous other products
WhisperGlide 10051 Kerry Court Hugo, MN 55038	(800) 944-7737 (651) 439-0979	WhisperGlide outdoor swing

Whitakers 1 Odell Plaza Yonkers, NY 10703	(800) 445-4387	Elevators and inclined stairway lifts
Winco 5516 SW First Lane Ocala, FL 34474-9307	(800) 237-3377 (352) 854-2929	Grab bars, bathroom accessories, geriatric furniture
Wireless Minnesota Public Radio P.O. Box 64422 St. Paul, MN 55164-0422	(800) 669-9999	Products for fans and friends of public radio
The Woodworker's Store 4365 Willow Drive Medina, MN 55340	(800) 279-4441	Offset hinges, magnetically keyed locks, and old-fashioned hardware
Wrightway, Inc. 175 Interstate 30 Garland, TX 75043	(800) 241-8839 (972) 240-8839	Porch and stair lifts, ramps, automatic doors, kitchen & bath equipment

Appendix
Stages of Decline with Alzheimer's Disease

Level 1

No cognitive decline. No subjective complaints of memory deficit. No memory deficit evident on clinical interviews.

Level 2

Very mild cognitive decline (forgetfulness). Subjective complaints of memory deficit, most frequently in the following areas: (a) forgetting where one has placed familiar objects; (b) forgetting names one formerly knew well. No objective evidence of memory deficit on clinical interview. No objective deficits in employment or social situations. Appropriate concern regarding symptoms.

Level 3

Mild cognitive decline (early confusional). Earliest clear-cut deficits. Manifestations in more than one of the following areas: (a) patient may have gotten lost when traveling to an unfamiliar location; (b) co-workers become aware of patient's relatively low performance; (c) word and name finding deficit becomes evident to intimates; (d) patient may read a passage of a book and retain relatively little material; (e) patient may demonstrate decreased facility in remembering names upon introduction to new people; (f) patient may have lost or misplaced an object of value; (g) concentration deficit may be evident on clinical testing. Objective evidence of memory deficit obtained only with an intensive interview. Denial begins to become manifest in patient. Mild to moderate anxiety accompanies symptoms.

Level 4

Moderate cognitive decline (Late Confusional). Clear-cut deficit on careful clinical interview. Deficit manifest in following areas: (a) decreased knowledge of current and recent events; (b) may exhibit some deficit in memory of one's personal history; (c) concentration deficit elicited on serial subtractions; (d) decreased ability to travel, handle finances, etc. Frequently no deficit in the following areas: (a) orientation to time and person; (b) recognition of familiar persons and faces; (c) ability to travel to familiar locations. Inability to perform complex tasks. Denial is dominant defense mechanism. Flattening of affect and withdrawal from challenging situations occur.

Level 5

Moderately severe cognitive decline (Early Dementia). Patient can no longer survive without some assistance. Patient is unable during interview to recall a major relevant aspect of their current lives, e.g., an address or telephone number of many years, the names of close family members (such as grandchildren), the name of the high school or college from which they graduated. Frequently some disorientation to time (date, day of week, season, etc.) or to place. An educated person may have difficulty counting back from 40 by 4's or from 20 by 2's. Persons at this stage retain knowledge of many major facts regarding themselves and others. They invariably know their own names and generally know their spouse's and children's names. They require no assistance with toileting and eating, but may have some difficulty choosing the proper clothing to wear.

Level 6

Severe cognitive decline (Middle Dementia). May occasionally forget the name of the spouse upon whom they are entirely dependent for survival. Will be largely unaware of all recent events and experiences in their lives. Retain some knowledge of their past lives but this is very sketchy. Generally unaware of their surroundings, the year, the season, etc. May have difficulty counting from 10, both backward and sometimes forward. Will require some assistance with activities of daily living, e.g., may become incontinent, will require travel assistance but occasionally will display ability to familiar locations. Diurnal rhythm frequently disturbed. Almost always recall their own name. Frequently continue to be able to distinguish familiar from unfamiliar persons in their environment. Personality and emotional changes occur. These are quite variable and include (a) delusional behavior, e.g., patients may accuse their spouse of being an impostor, may talk to imaginary figures in the environment, or to their own reflection in the mirror; (b) obsessive symptoms, e.g., person may continually repeat simple cleaning activities; (c) anxiety symptoms, agitation, and even previously nonexistent violent behavior may occur; (d) cognitive abulia, i.e., loss of willpower because an individual cannot carry a thought long enough to determine a purposeful course of action.

Level 7

Very severe cognitive decline (Late Dementia). All verbal abilities are lost. Frequently there is no speech at all—only grunting. Incontinent of urine, requires assistance toileting and feeding.

Lose basic psychomotor skills, e.g., ability to walk, sitting and head control. The brain appears to no longer be able to tell the body what to do. Generalized and cortical neurologic signs and symptoms are frequently present.

Reprinted with permission from B. Reisberg, S. H. Ferris, M. J. de Leon, and T. Crook, "The Global Deterioration Scale for the Assessment of Primary Degenerative Dementia," *American Journal of Psychiatry* 139 (Sept. 1982): 1136-39.

Glossary

Certain words throughout this book are enclosed in quotation marks and have special meanings pertaining to Alzheimer's disease. For example, reading "mail" may refer more to reading anything perceived as mail, including magazines, junk mail, etc. "Strangers" may not be actual strangers, but rather those no longer recognized by a person with Alzheimer's disease and therefore perceived as strangers.

Access denial. Creating barriers; making cabinets or doors leading to danger unavailable by installing locks, alarms or gates; hiding or camouflaging cabinets or doors; removing dangerous products, chemicals, tools and appliances in order to prevent a confused person from mishandling them.

Accessible. Within reach, convenient, and usable by everyone, particularly those with disabilities. An accessible home is one that also recognizes the needs and requirements of those using such devices as walkers, canes, and wheelchairs. Making a home accessible includes widening doorways and installing ramps, grab bars, railings, etc.

Accessible design. A relatively new concept in architecture and interior design that recognizes the needs of those with disabilities.

"Accident." An episode of soiling one's clothing, bed, chair, floor, etc., resulting from incontinence.

Activities of daily living (ADL's). Basic daily tasks, functions, and responsibilities required to maintain one's health, sustenance, and independence. The primary activities of daily living include toileting, bathing, dressing, eating, ambulation, and continence.

AD. Alzheimer's Disease.

Aging in place. The desire and practice of seniors to remain living in their own home, despite difficulties associated with growing older, providing or receiving care, if necessary, and avoiding geriatric residences and institutions; remaining in one's own home and neighborhood, in familiar and comfortable environments, surrounded by family, friends, possessions, and pets.

Agitation. The state of being irritated, upset, or annoyed. Agitation in those with AD can be

444

caused by any one of a number of reasons, including environmental factors and perceptions occurring only in the mind.

Agnosia. The inability to recognize or comprehend sensory information and input. It is also referred to as "mind blindness" or the inability of the mind to recognize and identify what the eyes see.

Alois Alzheimer. A German pathologist and psychiatrist who discovered Alzheimer's disease in 1907.

Alzheimer's disease. A progressive disease of the brain that destroys cells within the brain, interfering with one's ability to process information and recognize otherwise familiar people, places, and objects. Alzheimer's disease (AD) manifests itself in forgetfulness, inexplicable and abnormal behavior, and mood and personality changes. Alzheimer's disease is a terminal disease taking from 2 to 30 years to run its full course. It is the most common form of dementia.

Ambulatory, Ambulation. The ability to walk unassisted. Those dependent upon a cane or walker are still considered to be ambulatory.

Anomia. A cognitive disorder whereby a person is unable to associate, or has difficulty associating, words with objects (word/object association: knowing what something is, for example, yet unable to affix the right word to it).

Aphasia. The inability to recognize, comprehend, and understand words. It affects language skills and one's ability to read, understand signage, communicate, follow instructions, participate in conversations, and express desires or needs.

Apraxia. The inability to execute complex, coordinated movements or a series of movements. Apraxia inhibits the successful completion of multi-sequential tasks (an undertaking requiring more than one step to complete—for example, getting dressed, regaining one's balance in a fall, or operating multiple locks simultaneously).

Assessment. The evaluation of an individual and/or his living conditions in order to render advice or evaluate his ability to live independently.

Atrophy. The degeneration of a body part or tissue, including muscles. Often muscles become smaller and weaker from lack of use. This usually results in instability, lack of endurance, and potential falls caused by the absence or loss of strength in the muscles needed to perform certain tasks.

Autonomy. The state of being capable of living independently and making decisions, without assistance.

Behavioral difficulties. Difficulties associated with conduct, including catastrophic reactions, rummaging, hiding, hoarding, agitation, combativeness, aggression, resistance to caregiving, sundowning, shadowing, inappropriate sexual behavior, cursing, spitting, flailing, etc.; acts not in compliance with normal social standards.

Caregiver. Anyone providing supervision or care for another. It may be a friend, spouse, sibling, child, or professional caregiver. We consider caregivers modern-day heroes.

Caregiver's disorder, caregiver stress. A term referring to the consequences resulting from the stress involved with caregiving; psychological disorders or difficulties resulting from the burdens of caring for another.

Catastrophic reaction. An extreme emotional response. A catastrophic reaction can be a change in mood or personality, stubbornness, hostile and violent reactions, cursing and abusive behavior, etc.

Clinging. Following a caregiver or loved one, wherever she goes, whatever she does. Clinging burdens the caregiver, often giving her no relief or privacy. It is also referred to as tailgating and shadowing.

Cognitive. Relating to thought.

Cognitive abilities. Skills associated with the mind, including thought, perception, recognition, association, information processing, problem solving, and memory.

Cognitive impairment. Mental obstacles, weaknesses, or difficulties involving the mind, interfering with cognitive abilities.

Combativeness, combative behavior. Violent or aggressive behavior. Combativeness sometimes results from such things as attempting to defend personal space, resisting a task (bathing), or inexplicable reasons. Combative behavior is often a means of self-protection rooted in delusions that the targeted person is in some way trying to cause harm.

Compact fluorescent light bulb. A screw-in fluorescent bulb that can replace an incandescent bulb. It lasts considerably longer, burns cool to the touch, and takes a full minute to reach its maximum brightness, allowing older eyes time to adjust.

Contracture. A condition resulting in the contortion and rigid positioning of part of the body, often the arm and hand, though not necessarily so.

Contrast. The differentiation of two or more objects in color (blue vs. red), tone (light vs. dark), texture (smooth vs. rough), and pattern (solid vs. plaid). Furniture and floor finishes, for example, should contrast to each other, allowing one to differentiate one from the other easily and quickly. As we get older and become more prone to visual impairments, greater contrast helps us to distinguish objects from one another.

Cue. See Environmental cue.

Day care. Community social services providing daily activities and entertainment at a day-care center for those with physical, mental, or age-related difficulties. Day care is a valuable resource for support and respite for the caregiver. We strongly recommend that you include day care as a part of your caregiving plan.

Dead-end corridor. A hallway or corridor with no exit or apparent destination. Arriving at the end of a dead-end corridor can be a problem for many with AD who are unable to figure out how to turn around and find their way back.

Deceptive therapy. A tongue-in-cheek label applied to white lies or misleading techniques used by caregivers in the best interest of those they are caring for. Examples might include diversions to distract agitated family members (the telephone ringing), providing fake keys to the car to discourage driving, or telling a loved one that his departed wife is at the store rather than having him unnecessarily and repeatedly mourn his loss.

Delusion. A story based on an inaccurate, but solidly adhered to, belief. People with AD often feel strongly that others are stealing from them, talking about them, or out to get them, with no apparent basis or logical explanation. Their actions and behavior may be based on these delusions.

Dementia. A condition characterized by the loss of memory or impairment of cognitive functions and abilities to such a degree that it interferes with daily life.

Depression. The condition of chronic sadness. Depression is a diverse ailment, but it is treatable. If depression is suspected, it is wise to seek appropriate medical advice.

Disorientation. The loss of one's position in time or place. Disorientation may be manifested in your loved one's forgetting where she is (home, city, or neighborhood) or her inability to recognize people, including family members, spouses, or friends. Disorientation can also refer to episodes of becoming lost in one's own home, neighborhood, or just outside of the home, even though he may be standing right in front of his own door.

Dutch door. A single door, cut horizontally in or about the middle, resulting in independent top and bottom sections. You can use hardware to join the two halves, allowing the door to open or close as one, or you can close (and lock) the bottom, leaving the top open. This allows communication with, and views of, all that is happening outside, yet humanely and safely confines one to an area, such as the bedroom.

Dysphagia. The inability to chew and/or swallow food. Swallowing is a complex series of coordinated, timed movements and functions. Often AD hinders certain bodily functions, including chewing and swallowing.

Elopement. Wandering away from home.

Environment. The cumulative sum of objects, sounds, smells, tactile sensations, and occurrences that surround us.

Environmental cue. A feature of the environment that provides information or triggers behavior. Cues direct or help your loved one to understand, decipher, or recognize something. A sign is an example of an environmental cue that we all use. A stop sign triggers you to stop, a highway sign cues you to go in the right direction, while the sign on the grocery store identifies it as a place to buy food.

Environmental incontinence. Incontinence caused or affected by an environmental factor. For example, a chair that is too difficult to get up from may prevent a person from getting to the bathroom when needed. The result may be an "accident" perceived as incontinence.

Environmental modification. The incorporation of a strategy or product that results in a change in one's surroundings.

Family member, loved one. Affectionate terms used in this book to refer to the person with Alzheimer's disease.

Forgiving environment. Surroundings that minimize trauma and injury in the event of an accident. An example of a forgiving environment would be a room with soft, stable furniture, minimizing the injury that could occur from a fall.

Ground fault interrupted (GFI) outlets or circuit. A special electrical outlet or circuit breaker that senses an electrical short and disables itself in a fraction of a second, thereby preventing injury to the user. A GFI outlet or breaker is recognizable by a test and/or reset button. They are particularly useful in rooms containing sources of water (the bathroom, kitchen, and laundry room), where an appliance can be dropped into the water (or touched by wet hands) while still plugged into the electrical outlet.

Gait. The characteristics or functions making up the act of walking or taking individual steps. Gait is a composite of the speed, height, and length of one's steps, plus all of the coordinated tasks composing them (balance, coordination, etc.).

Gait disturbance. An impairment or dysfunction inhibiting one's ability to walk or take steps.

Hallucination. Hearing, seeing, feeling, tasting, or smelling something that does not really exist, other than in the mind of the person experiencing it. Hallucinations are very real to the person having them but invisible to everyone else.

Hearing impairment. Any difficulty hearing, whether due to a medical condition or a noisy environment.

HEPA. High Efficiency Particulate Air. HEPA refers to a more efficient type of filter for air cleaning equipment that is able to remove very small particles, resulting in cleaner air. HEPA filters are helpful in filtering out odors and improving the air quality in homes dealing with incontinence.

Hoarding. The tendency to collect items, often to the extreme. Items of choice may be logical or not, including coat hangers, rubber bands, napkins, cardboard boxes, or anything found around the house or outside.

"Home." 1) the present abode, 2) the image of where your family member remembers once living, or 3) in some remote cases, going "home" can also refer to dying.

Hospice. A philosophy of special care for those who are terminally ill that focuses on relief of suffering, pain control, and comfort. Hospice advocates that no one should die alone and provides personal, emotional, and spiritual support in the latter stages and days of life.

Hyperthermia. Abnormally high body temperature.

Hypothermia. Abnormally low body temperature.

Illusion. A misinterpretation of an object or occurrence (that is seen, heard, or felt). Voices coming from the television are commonplace. However, if they are misinterpreted as people in the room, they are illusions.

Incontinence. A medical condition resulting in failure or inability to control one's bladder (urinary incontinence) or bowels (fecal incontinence). The result is often an "accident" or soiled clothing. This book suggests that there may be environmental factors that contribute to certain cases of incontinence. (*See* Environmental incontinence.)

Induction cooktop. A type of stove that uses electro-magnetic fields to heat only special metallic cooking containers, allowing the actual cooktop to remain relatively cool. Early induction cooktop units have been accompanied with warnings that advise against someone with a heart pacemaker using them.

Instrumental activities of daily living (IADL's). A secondary level of activities of daily living that require the use of accessories, tools or appliances. They include housekeeping, meal preparation, traveling, shopping, using the telephone, laundry, transportation, medication administration, and money management.

Landmark. A conspicuous, recognizable environmental feature that helps to locate, guide, or orient a person. A good example of a landmark is a lighthouse, which guides ships in the night and signals the presence of land for seagoing wayfarers. Landmarks are especially important for persons with Alzheimer's seeking to navigate in an increasingly baffling environment.

Life review. The activity of privately and internally reflecting upon the events of one's life. Life review is often healthy and pleasurable.

Long-term memory. Experiences, learned information, and memories that occurred and accumulated over the years. In comparison to short-term memory, long-term memory usually refers to occurences that happened in more distant years rather than more recent minutes, hours, or days. Events of one's childhood, for example, are a part of his long-term memory, whereas today's lunch would be a part of his short-term memory.

Memory book. A specially prepared scrap book or photo album containing items selected to stimulate interest, conversation, and stories about your family member's life. A memory book is especially helpful with visiting friends who may face awkward periods of silence or for visiting caregivers, who may not know your family member, his skills, interests, or accomplishments.

"Mind blindness." See Agnosia.

"Miraculous Moment." A rare, wonderful and inexplicable occurrence in which the person with AD momentarily seems to emerge from his confusion to have a brief lucid conversation or perhaps recognize you after having been unable to do so for a long time. Sometimes a miraculous moment appears as simply a phrase uttered with special meaning or maybe a well-timed smile. Others are, in fact, brief, but meaningful occurrences that have no other explanation than being "miraculous moments."

Misinterpretations. See Illusions.

Mullions. The slender vertical and horizontal members in a door or window that contain panes of glass or panels.

Non-ambulatory. The inability to walk without assistance; dependent upon a wheelchair or bed-bound, for example.

Olfactory. Dealing with or relating to the sense of smell.

Olfactory impairment. Difficulties smelling and tasting that may contribute to improper hygiene, ingestion of spoiled or inappropriate foods, and the ability to smell smoke in the event of a fire.

Orientation theory or therapy. See Reality orientation.

Paranoia. A reaction (often to a delusion) characterized by irrational suspicion and feelings of persecution or mistreatment.

Passage lock. A doorknob having no locking mechanism on either side, allowing free access by simply turning the knob.

Passive barrier. An environmental feature that affects behavior or limits accessibility. An example of a passive barrier may be a dark strip on the floor that your family member is afraid to cross or the cat's bed next to a door (which causes him to stop and pet the cat, forgetting his original mission of walking out of the door).

Perimeter. A defined boundary within your home outlining areas that are safe for your loved one to move about or wander in.

Peripheral vision. The outer fields of one's area of vision. People using only their peripheral vision cannot see what is directly in front of them, only that which is up, down, and to the sides. The opposite of peripheral vision is tunnel vision.

Personal emergency response system (PERS). A modified telephone system (and service) purchased through a private company. These telephones provide emergency call buttons, and automatic dialers that contact private operators who take appropriate action based on the emergency. The most noted feature of these systems is one's ability to press a button worn around the neck to contact help in the event of a fall.

"Picking." The inexplicable, sometimes chronic fixation to handle, work at, and remove small items or pieces of something, such as peeling paint, flowers in upholstery, or imaginary lint.

Plateau. To remain in one stage of the disease for a disproportionate or unexpectedly long period of time. Alzheimer's disease has seven stages. People have been known to plateau or remain in one stage for years. Other stages can be entered and left in short periods of time or even skipped.

Privacy lock. A doorknob or lock that is lockable from one side only, often by pushing and turning the inside handle, turning a knob, or pushing a button. Privacy locks are normally found on bathroom doors but have many other uses as well.

Prosthetic. Relating to an assistive device or tool to make up for an inability, disability, or impairment. Examples of prosthetic devices include canes, walkers, glasses, etc.

"Quakes." Rare episodes when the earth suddenly and inexplicably seems to move violently for a person with dementia, causing alarm and possibly a loss of balance.

Quality of life. A term encompassing everything that contributes to one's degree of life satisfaction, pleasure, and comfort. The primary goal for a caregiver is to maintain a high degree of the quality of life for the person she is caring for.

Reality orientation, reality theory, orientation therapy. The practice of correcting someone by helping them realize or understand "what really is" rather than "what they perceive something to be." Examples include correcting your mother when she says she lives in the wrong city or town, that the president of the United States is not Herbert Hoover, or that the man she thinks is her son is really her husband. The opposite of reality theory is validation theory.

Redundant cuing. The use of multiple cues, landmarks, and signals to transmit a single message, improving the possibility that it will be received and understood.

Reminiscence. Reflecting, recalling, and discussing past events and life experiences. It differs from life review in that reminiscence can be either private or shared. Reminiscence is a positive and healthy activity, and much research has resulted in the development and acknowledgment of reminiscence therapy.

Respite. 1) Care and concern for the well-being of the caregiver; 2) temporary care for the person with AD providing rest, relief, and a break for the caregiver.

Reverse funnel effect. The strategy of widening the beginnings and ends of pathways to make them more inviting and recognizable.

Rigidity. A condition sometimes associated with Alzheimer's disease and other age-related disorders whereby legs and/or arms become rigid (sometimes extended) and will not bend. This presents additional problems with space, such as maneuvering in the bathroom, where room might be at a premium, walking, or getting up from the chair or bed.

Rummaging. The inexplicable, sometimes chronic behavior of searching for things. Items sought may demonstrate a theme, such as cardboard boxes, food for the person in the mirror, or preparation for a "trip." At other times they may make no sense at all, just items collected.

Rummaging container. A drawer, trunk, closet, or box specifically intended to be pilfered and searched, containing harmless items of interest to your loved one that if removed will cause no harm or loss.

Seasonal affective disorder (SAD). Consistent agitation or depression that appears to be related to seasonal changes or characteristics, such as overcast skies, shorter days, and less sunlight, cold weather, or being forced to remain indoors for longer periods of time. SAD may be a relative of sundown syndrome or at least have similarities.

Senile dementia, senility. Obsolete terms that poorly and briefly describe what is now recognized as Alzheimer's disease, dementia, and dementia-related disorders. Until quite recently, senility and dementia were falsely considered and accepted as common stages of aging.

"Sense of journey." The cumulative pleasures, discoveries, and occurrences experienced in the course of a journey, whether a trip to the corner drugstore, along the backyard wandering path, or just en route to the dining room. It takes into consideration objects and activities seen, felt, heard, smelled, and otherwise experienced occurring over, under, ahead of, behind, and to the sides of the traveler, as well as unique experiences occurring at different times along the same path.

Shadowing. See Clinging.

Short-term memory. Experiences, learned information, and memories that were acquired recently.

Special place. 1) an area created within a room to ensure safety and provide proximity to family members and family activity, taking into consideration a person's need to share, contribute, and continue to be a part of the family. An example might be a chair in the kitchen from which your family member can supervise meal preparation; 2) a place within the home set up for special purposes and uses. Examples may include a room that only your loved one is allowed to go into, a crafts area in the den, or a bench in the backyard; 3) somewhere that you can take your loved one to calm her, away from sources of agitation (such as mirrors, "strangers," etc.).

Stalling. The inexplicable action of walking and then suddenly stopping. Often the feet stop, but the momentum continues, causing your loved one to fall in a forward direction. It sometimes happens at door openings, upon entering a larger space, or at the end of a stairway.

"Stranger," "intruder." (1) A person in your loved one's life that he no longer recognizes. This can be a family member—a spouse of many years or a son or daughter; (2) an unrecognizable reflection that your loved one sees of himself in a mirror; or (3) an unfamiliar or imaginary person whom your family member blames or accuses for all of the "mysterious" occurences happening in the home ("stolen," missing, misplaced items, etc.).

Sundowning (sundown syndrome). A phenomenon typified by agitation, heightened confusion, or unusual behavior characteristically occurring in the late afternoon or early evening.

Support group. A group of people with common experiences, concerns, and issues that meets to discuss and to support others with similar concerns. We highly recommend support groups for any person involved in caring for someone with Alzheimer's disease. Many support groups encourage you to bring your loved one to the meetings, depending upon his stage or function ability, behavior, acceptance, and understanding of the disease. Contact your local Alzheimer's Association chapter, Area Agency on Aging, or social service organization for information on local support groups. For those who are unable to get out of the house, there are also on-line (computer) support groups that you can contribute to or just listen silently at your computer table.

Tactile impairment. Loss of feeling or difficulties associated with the sense of touch, often occurring in, but not limited to, the hands, feet, arms, or legs. Among the difficulties this imposes are problems walking, temperature sensation, and using the stairs (since one may be unsure when and if his feet have reached firm ground).

Tailgating. Following closely behind someone else, sometimes out the door or into rooms that are intended to be off-limits. This activity often goes unnoticed and can result in elopement if your family member makes it out the door undetected.

Task lighting. Lighting selected and located to focus and assist in specific areas for specific purposes. A special light at your loved one's favorite chair to provide more light for reading and a light at the front door to help you see the lock at night are examples.

Therapeutic environment. Specially prepared surroundings that compensate for unique problems and needs; surroundings that help rather than hinder. A therapeutic environment has good lighting and properly located railings and grab bars. It is forgiving, minimizing the degree of injury from unavoidable accidents and recognizing and removing the causes when possible.

Three-way switch. A wall switch that allows independent control of a single light or electrical outlet from two locations. Three-way switches at the top and bottom of a flight of stairs, for example, would allow you to turn the light on or off from either location.

Threshold. Wooden planks, marble sills, or metal "bridges" installed under doors or changes in flooring material (carpet to vinyl, for example). They can sometimes be unexpected obstacles to unsuspecting travelers with mobility or visual impairments or gait disorders, and for those using wheelchairs or walkers.

Toileting. Normal daily functions requiring the use of the toilet. Toileting includes urinating, moving the bowels, and properly cleaning oneself (or the care receiver) upon completion.

Transfer bench. A product that spans the gap between two locations, assisting a person moving from one location to the other by sitting on it and sliding. Transfer benches may be used to relocate from a wheelchair to the bed, toilet, shower, or chair, or vice versa.

Trigger. Any environmental stimulus that causes a behavioral or cognitive response.

Tripper. A condition, flaw, or object that might cause one to trip or fall. Trippers include worn carpeting, throw rugs, stair runners, thresholds, changes in flooring materials, or a single step. Trippers may be real or perceived. (*See* Visual cliffing.)

Tunnel vision. The tendency or ability to see only that which is in the central part of one's visual field or directly in front of him. Tunnel vision implies the lack or reduction of peripheral vision.

Uniform lighting. General, evenly distributed lighting where there are no contrasting areas of light and dark. In rooms with good uniform lighting, shadows are virtually eliminated because light is coming from and reflected from all directions.

Universal design. The theory of design or environmental modification taking into consideration the needs of persons of all ages, sizes, and conditions.

Validation theory, validation therapy. The concept of buying into a family member's story rather than trying to use logic to correct her. For example, instead of explaining that no one is stealing her clothes (now at the laundry), your response might be, "Oh my, that's terrible. Let's buy a trunk to store them so this doesn't happen again." The confrontation is avoided and you make your family member "right" when probably no other solution is viable. (The opposite of validation therapy is orientation therapy.)

Visual cliffing. The misinterpretation of changes in colors or shades as differences in depth, elevation, or plane. Shadows, for example, may be perceived as steps. The result can be resistance to cross them, stalling, or attempts to jump over the "holes." The perception of a dark strip of flooring as a trench is also an example of visual cliffing. Some caregivers have even taken advantage of this phenomenon and intentionally placed dark mats in front of doorways through which they did not want their loved ones to exit.

Visual impairment. Any difficulty associated with seeing. Visual impairment can be the result of a disease, injury, medication, or an environmental factor. Darkness is a common visual impairment that interferes with the ability to see at night, for example. Some visual impairments can be helped by improving lighting, simplifying pathways, using night lights, taking advantage of contrasting colors, and maximizing reflectivity of walls by the choice of color. If a visual impairment is suspected, the first and most prudent response is to see a doctor.

Wandering. The sometimes incessant tendency to roam, pace back and forth, or repeatedly travel a path in the home or yard; to leave home (*see* Elopement). Wandering can be in search of a specific destination, logical or illogical, or repeating a familiar and comfortable pattern or path, referred to as a wandering path.

Wandering path. An indoor or outdoor trail that either you or your loved one creates for wandering.

"Windows to the world." The views and connections to the outside world for someone who is limited to one location; the portals through which one can see, hear, and experience activity. For someone who might be bedbound, his "windows to the world" might be the door and window.

Suggested Reading

All titles here provide plenty of excellent information on caregiving and related subjects. We highly recommend that you go to your local library or book store and read those that may be of interest.

The Alzheimer's Association. The following books, brochures and pamphlets are written by the Alzheimer's Association and can be ordered by contacting The Alzheimer's Association, 919 North Michigan Avenue, Suite 1000, Chicago, IL 60611-1676; phone (800) 272-3900. The association has a wide variety of excellent publications. When you call, ask for their publications catalogue.

Caregiver's Stress: Signs to Watch Out For . . . Steps to Take. Chicago, Ill.: The Alzheimer's Association, 1995. (Order number PR200Z.)

Family Guide for Alzheimer's Care in Residential Settings. Chicago, Ill.: The Alzheimer's Association, 1992.

Respite Care Guide. Chicago, Ill.: The Alzheimer's Association, 1995. (Order number PF112Z)

Terms & Tips: An Alzheimer's Care Handbook. Chicago, Ill.: The Alzheimer's Association, 1995.

The Alzheimer's Association Materials: Public Catalogue. Chicago, Ill.: The Alzheimer's Association, 1997.

Steps to Planning Activities: Structuring the Day at Home. Chicago, Ill.: Alzheimer's Association, 1996. To order, ask for brochure ED308Z.

The Alzheimer Resource Center of Tallahassee, Inc. *Alzheimer's Disease Resource Book.* Tallahassee, Fla.: The Alzheimer Resource Center of Tallahassee, Inc., 1997.

Andresen, Gayle. *Caring for People with Alzheimer's Disease: A Training Manual for Direct Care Providers.* Baltimore, Md.: Health Professions Press, 1995. Order through Canyonlands Publishing, Inc., 141 South Park Avenue, Tucson, AZ 85719; phone (800) 259-2870.

Aranson, Miriam, ed. *Understanding Alzheimer's Disease.* New York: Scribner, 1988.

Artley, Bob. *Ginny: A Love Remembered.* Iowa: Iowa State University, 1993.

Bayles, Kathryn, and Alfred Kaszniak. *Communicating and Cognition in Normal Aging and Dementia.* Austin, Tex.: Pro-Ed, 1987. Order through Canyonlands Publishing, Inc., 141 South Park Avenue, Tucson, AZ 85719; phone (800) 259-2870.

Brackey, Jolene. *Creating Moments of Joy.* West Lafayette, Ind.: Purdue University Press, 2000. To order, contact the publisher at 1207 South Campus Courts, West Lafayette, IN 47907-1207; phone (800) 933-9637.

Branson, Gary. *Barrier-Free Housing.* White Hall, Va.: Betterway Publications, Inc., 1991.

Brawley, Elizabeth. "Alzheimer's Disease: Designing the Physical Environment." *The American Journal of Alzheimer's Care and Related Disorders & Research* 7 no. 1 (January/February 1992): 3–8.

―――. *Designing for Alzheimer's Disease: Strategies for Creating Better Care Environments.* New York: John Wiley & Sons, 1997.

Bristlow, Lois. *Will I Be Next.* Forest Knolls, Calif.: Elder Books, 1996. To order, contact the publisher at P.O. Box 490, Forest Knolls, CA 94933; phone (800) 909-2673, (415) 488-9002.

Cain, Danny, and Bob Russell. *Blessed Are the Caregivers.* Louisville: Living Word, 1995. To order, call (800) 366-9673.

Cairl, Richard. *Somebody Tell Me Who I Am!* St. Petersburg, Fla.: Caremor Publications, 1995. To order, contact the publisher at 25 Second Street North, Suite 440, St. Petersburg, FL 33701; phone (800) 435-2999, (813) 894-5333.

Calkins, Margaret, and M. Arch. *Design for Dementia: Planning Environments for the Elderly and the Confused.* Owings Mills, Md.: Health Publishing (Division of Williams & Wilkins), 1988.

Caldwell, Marianne. *Gone . . . without a Trace.* Forest Knolls, Calif.: Elder Books, 1995. To order, contact the publisher at P.O. Box 490, Forest Knolls, CA 94933; phone (800) 909-2673, (415) 488-9002.

Cohen, D., and C. Eisdorfer. *Seven Steps to Effective Parent Care: A Planning and Action Guide for Adult Children with Aging Parents.* New York: Putnam, 1994.

Conley, Deborah, and Betty Foster. "Reaching Communities with Alzheimer's Education: Train the Trainer Manual." Omaha, Nebr.: University of Nebraska Medical Center, 1997. To order contact the publisher at 600 South 42nd Street, Omaha, NE 68198-5620; phone (402) 559-7512.

Coughlin, Patricia. *Facing Alzheimer's.* New York: Ballantine Books, 1993.

Cordrey, Cindy. *Hidden Treasures: Music & Memory Activities for People with Alzheimer's.* Washington, D.C.: Center for Books on Aging, Serif Press, Inc., 1994. To order, contact the publisher at 1331 H Street NW, Washington, DC 20005; phone (800) 221-4272, (202) 737-4650.

Deanne, Barbara. *Caring for Your Aging Parents.* Colorado Springs: Nav Press, 1989. To order, contact the publisher at P.O. Box 6000, Colorado Springs, CO 80934; phone (800) 366-7788.

Dykstra, Robert. *She Never Said Good-Bye: One Man's Journey through Loss.* Wheaton, Ill.: H. Shaw Publishers, 1989; Evanston, Ill.: Highland Press, 1990.

Garee, Bettye. *Ideas for Making Your Home Accessible.* Bloomington, Ill.: Accent Special Publications, Cheever Publishing, Inc, 1992.

Gibson, Margaret. "Differentiating Aggressive and Resistive Behaviors in Long-Term Care." *Journal of Gerontological Nursing* 23 no. 4 (April 1997): 21–27.

Glanz, Barbara A. *Care Packages for the Home: Dozens of Ways to Regenerate Spirit Where You Live.* Kansas City, Mo.: Andrews McMeel Pub., 1998.

Gregg, Daphna. "Harvard Health Letter Special Report: Alzheimer's Disease," *Harvard Health Letter* (February 1996).

Grubbs, William McKinley. *In Sickness & in Health: Caring for a Loved One with Alzheimer's Disease.* Forest Knolls, Calif.: Elder Books, 1997. To order, contact the publisher at P.O. Box 490, Forest Knolls, CA 94933; phone (800) 909-2673, (415) 488-9002.

Gruetzner, Howard. *Alzheimer's: A Caregiver's Guide and Sourcebook.* New York: John Wiley & Sons, 1992. To order, contact the publisher at (800) 225-5945.

Guthrie, Donna. *Grandpa Doesn't Know It's Me: A Family Adjusts to Alzheimer's Disease.* New York: Human Sciences Press, 1986.

Haisman, Pam. *Alzheimer's Disease: Caregivers Speak Out.* Ft. Myers, Fla.: Chippendale House Publishers. To order, contact the publisher at P.O. Box 07155, Ft. Myers, FL 33919; phone (800) 247-6553.

Heath, Angela. *Long Distance Caregiving: A Survival Guide for Far Away Caregivers.* Lakewood, Colo.: American Source Books, 1993.

Hewson, Mitchell. *Horticulture as Therapy.* Ontario: HTM, Homewood Health Center, 1994. To order, contact the publisher at 150 Delhi Street, Guelph, Ontario N1E 6K9, Canada; phone (519) 824-1010 ext. 180.

Hodgson, Harriet. *Alzheimer's: Finding the Word: A Communication Guide for Those Who Care.* Minneapolis, Minn.: Chronimed Publishing, 1995. To order, contact the publisher at (800) 848-2793.

Inoue, Yasushi. *Chronicle of My Mother.* Japan: Kodansha International Ltd., 1983.

Kelly, Mary. "Social Interaction among People with Dementia." *Journal of Gerontological Nursing* 23 no. 4 (April 1997): 16–20.

Khachaturian, Zaven, and Teresa Radebaugh. *Alzheimer's Disease: Cause(s), Diagnosis, Treatment, and Care.* Boca Raton, Fla.: CRC Press, 1996.

Mace, Nancy, and Peter Rabins. *The 36-Hour Day.* Baltimore, Md.: The Johns Hopkins University Press, 1991.

Mace, Ronald. *The Accessible Housing Design File: Barrier Free Environments.* New York: Van Nostrand Reinhold, 1991.

Manning, Doug. *When Love Gets Tough: The Nursing Home Decision.* Hereford, Tex.: In-Sight Books, 1993. To order, contact the publisher at Drawer 2058, Hereford, TX 79045; phone (806) 364-7862.

Markin, R. *The Alzheimer's Cope Book: The Complete Care Manual for Patients and Their Families.* New York: Citadel Press, 1992.

McGowin, Diana Friel. *Living in the Labyrinth: A Personal Journey through the Maze of Alzheimer's.* New York: Delacorte Press, 1993.

McLeod, Beth Witrogen. *Caregiving: The Spiritual Journey of Love, Loss, and Renewal.* New York: J. Wiley & Sons, 1999.

McNeil, Caroline. *Alzheimer's Disease: Unraveling the Mystery.* N.p.: [National Institute on Aging], 1995. To order this pamphlet, write for Publication No. 95-3782, National Institute on Aging, Building 31, Room 5C-27, Bethesda, MD 20892, or call (301) 496-1752.

Moskowitz, Francine. *Parenting Your Aging Parents.* Woodland Hills, Calif.: Key Publications, 1991.

Murphy, Beverly Bigtree. *he used to be Somebody: A Journey into Alzheimer's through the Eyes of a Caregiver.* Boulder, Colo.: Gibbs Associates, 1995. To order, contact the publisher at P.O. Box 706, Boulder, CO 80306-0706; phone (800) 792-1592.

NAHB Research Center, Inc., and Barrier Free Environments, Inc. *Residential Remodeling and Universal Design: Making Homes More Comfortable and Accessible.* N.p.: [U.S. Department of Housing and Urban Development, Office of Policy Development and Research], 1996.

Olsen, Richard, Ezra Ehrenkranz, Barbara Hutchings, and M. Arch. *Homes That Help: Advice from Caregivers for Creating a Supportive Home.* Newark, N.J.: New Jersey Institute of Technology, 1993.

Pitzele, Sefra Kobrin. *We Are Not Alone: Learning to Cope with Chronic Illness.* New York: Workman Publishing, 1986.

Powell, Lenore. *Alzheimer's Disease: A Guide for Families.* Reading, Mass.: Addison-Wesley Publishing Co., 1993.

Raschko, Bettyann Boetticher. *Housing Interiors for the Disabled & Elderly.* New York: Van Nostrand Reinhold Company, 1982.

Raymond, Florian. *Surviving Alzheimer's: A Guide for Families.* Forest Knolls, Calif.: Elder Books, 1996. To order, contact the publisher at P.O. Box 490, Forest Knolls, CA 94933; phone (800) 909-2673, (415) 488-9002.

Reisberg, Barry, S. H. Ferris, M. J. de Leon, and T. Crook. "The Global Deterioration Scale for Assessment of Primary Degenerative Dementia." *American Journal of Psychiatry* 139 (1982): 1136-39.

Rob, Caroline. *The Caregiver's Guide.* Boston, Mass.: Houghton Mifflin, 1991.

Roberts, Jeanne. *Taking Care of Caregivers: For Families and Others Who Care for People with Alzheimer's Disease and Other Forms of Dementia.* Palo Alto, Calif.: Bull Publishing Company, 1991. To order, contact the publisher at P.O. Box 208, Palo Alto, CA 94302; phone (415) 322-2855.

Roche, Lyn. *Coping with Caring: Daily Reflections for Alzheimer's Caregivers.* Forest Knolls,

Calif.: Elder Books, 1995. To order, contact the publisher at P.O. Box 490, Forest Knolls, CA 94933; phone (800) 909-2673, (415) 488-9002.

Ronch, Judah. *Alzheimer's Disease: A Practical Guide for Families and Other Caregivers.* New York: The Continuum Publishing Company, 1991.

Rose, Larry. *Show Me the Way to Go Home.* Forest Knolls, Calif.: Elder Books, 1996. To order, contact the publisher at P.O. Box 490, Forest Knolls, CA 94933; phone (800) 909-2673, (415) 488-9002.

Rothert, Gene. *The Enabling Garden: Creating Barrier-Free Gardens.* Dallas, Tex.: Taylor Publishing Co., 1994.

Sheridan, Carmel. *Failure-Free Activities for the Alzheimer's Patient.* Forest Knolls, Calif.: Elder Books, 1987. To order, contact the publisher at P.O. Box 490, Forest Knolls, CA 94933; phone (800) 909-2673, (415) 488-9002.

Sherman, James. *Caregiver's Survival Series.* (4 books) Golden Valley, Minn.: Pathway Books, 1994. To order, contact the publisher at 700 Parkway Terrace, Golden Valley, MN 55416-3439; phone (612) 377-1521.

Schiff, Myra. "Designing Environments for Individuals with Alzheimer's Disease: Some General Principles." *The American Journal of Alzheimer's Care and Related Disorders & Research* 5 no. 3 (May/June 1990): 4–8.

Snyder, Lisa. *Speaking Our Minds: Personal Reflections from Individuals with Alzheimer's.* New York: W.H. Freeman, 1999.

Susik, Helen. *Hiring Home Care Givers.* San Luis Obispo, Calif.: American Source Books, 1995. To order, call (805) 543-5911, (805) 543-4093.

Term, L., and A. Wagner. "Alzheimer's Disease and Depression." *Journal of Consulting and Clinical Psychology* 60 no. 3 (1992): 379–91.

Tideiksaar, Rein. *Falling in Old Age: Its Prevention and Treatment.* New York: Springer Publishing, Co., 1989.

Volicer, Ladislav, and Lisa Bloom-Charette, eds. *Enhancing the Quality of Life in Advanced Dementia.* Philadelphia: Brunner/Mazel, 1999.

Wasch, William K. *Home Planning for Your Later Years: New Designs, Living Options, Smart Decisions, How to Finance It.* [Wilton, Conn.]: Beverly Cracom Publications, 1996. For more information, contact the author at: William K. Wasch Associates, 150 Coleman Road, Middletown, CT; phone (860) 347-2967.

Wenrick, Neta. *So Much More Than Sing-A-Long,* Forest Knolls, Calif.: Elder Books, 1996. To order contact the publisher at P.O. Box 490, Forest Knolls, CA 9493; phone (800) 909-2673, (415) 488-9002.

Wurth, JoEllen. *National Directory of Alzheimer's Specific Residential Care Programs.* Raymore, MO: Foxwood Springs Living Center, Foxwood Springs Institute, 1996. To order contact the publisher at 1500 W. Foxwood Drive, P.O. Box 1172, Raymore, MO 64083; phone (816) 331-3111.

Yale, Robin. *Developing Support Groups for Individuals with Early-Stage Alzheimer's Disease.* Baltimore, Md.: Health Professions Press. Order through Canyonlands Publishing, Inc., 141 South Park Avenue, Tucson, AZ 85719; phone (800) 259-2870.

Yeomans, Kathleen. *The Able Gardener: Overcoming Barriers of Age & Physical Limitations.* Pownal, Vt.: Storey Communications, Inc., 1992.

Index